Radiation Therapy in Hematologic Malignancies

Bouthaina Shbib Dabaja • Andrea K. Ng
Editors

Radiation Therapy in Hematologic Malignancies

An Illustrated Practical Guide

Springer

Editors
Bouthaina Shbib Dabaja
University of Texas
MD Anderson Cancer Center
Houston
Texas
USA

Andrea K. Ng
Dana-Farber Cancer Institute
Harvard University Medical School
Boston
Massachusetts
USA

ISBN 978-3-319-42613-6 ISBN 978-3-319-42615-0 (eBook)
DOI 10.1007/978-3-319-42615-0

Library of Congress Control Number: 2016956483

Printed on acid-free paper

This Springer imprint is published by Springer Nature
The registered company is Springer International Publishing AG
The registered company address is: Gewerbestrasse 11, 6330 Cham, Switzerland

Being compassionate and just constitutes my compass as a physician when serving every patient, and this was instilled in me by my mother Mariam and my father Shbib. Being an orphan at an early age with immense financial hardship, I would have never made it if it were not for my brothers Diaa and Safi who dedicated their lives to provide for me. My husband Mohammad, my eternal source of hope, continuously inspired and brought meaningfulness to my life. James Cox, who saw in me what others did not, along with endless opportunities, shaped my professional career. My mentor and role model, Hagop Kantarjian, who with his continuous help and support, served as a guiding light for all aspects of my professional life. My final dedication is to my children Zaynab and Abbas who honored me with my best achievement in life of being a mother.

Contents

Contributors

Chan Yoon Cheah, MBBS, DMedSc Department of Lymphoma/Myeloma, MD Anderson Cancer Center, Houston, TX, USA

Bouthaina Shbib Dabaja, MD Department of Radiation Oncology, University of Texas MD Anderson Cancer Center, Houston, TX, USA

Andrea Riccardo Filippi, MD Department of Oncology, Board Certification in Radiation Oncology, Torino, Italy

Bradford Hoppe, MD, MPH University of Florida Proton Therapy Institute, Jacksonville, FL, USA

Mario Levis, MD Department of Oncology, University of Torino, Torino, Italy

Yexiong Li, MD Department of Radiation Oncology, Cancer Hospital and Institute, Chinese Academy of Medical Sciences (CAMS) and Peking Union Medical College (PUMC), Beijing, China

N. George Mikhaeel, MD Department of Clinical Oncology and Radiotherapy, Guy's & St Thomas' NHS Foundation Trust and King's Health Partners Academic Health Sciences Centre, London, UK

Sarah A. Milgrom, MD Department of Radiation Oncology, MD Anderson Cancer Center, Houston, TX, USA

Andrea K. Ng, MD, MPH Department of Radiation Oncology, Dana-Farber Cancer Institute, Brigham and Women's Hospital, Harvard Medical School, Boston, MA, USA

Chelsea Pinnix, MD, PhD Department of Radiation Oncology, MD Anderson Cancer Center, Houston, TX, USA

Cristina Piva, MD Department of Oncology, University of Torino, Torino, Italy

John P. Plastaras, MD, PhD University of Pennsylvania, Philadelphia, PA, USA

Umberto Ricardi, MD Department of Oncology, University of Torino, Torino, Italy

Grace L. Smith, MD, PhD, MPH Department of Radiation Oncology, MD Anderson Cancer Center, Houston, TX, USA

Lena Specht, MD, PhD Departments of Oncology and Hematology, Rigshospitalet, University of Copenhagen, Copenhagen, Denmark

Stephanie Terezakis, MD Johns Hopkins School of Medicine, Baltimore, MD, USA

Richard Tsang, MD Department of Radiation Oncology, University of Toronto, Princess Margaret Cancer Centre, Toronto, ON, Canada

Andrew Wirth, MB, BS, MD Department of Radiation Oncology, Peter MacCallum Cancer Centre, East Melbourne, VIC, Australia

Hodgkin Lymphoma

1

Stephanie Terezakis and John P. Plastaras

Abstract
In this chapter, illustrative, early favorable, and unfavorable cases of Hodgkin lymphoma (HL) are presented followed by a detailed discussion of the appropriate evaluation and management, with a focus on the role of radiotherapy.

Clinical Presentation: Combined Modality Therapy for Early-Stage Favorable Patients

A 23-year-old man was in his usual state of health until January 2014 when he first appreciated a non-tender palpable node on the right side of his neck. At that time, he reported mild sweating at night but denied drenching night sweats, fevers, weight loss, chills, or pruritus. He was evaluated for a streptococcal infection and mononucleosis and was treated empirically with amoxicillin for 2 weeks without interval improvement. He ultimately underwent a fine needle aspiration that showed atypical lymphoid infiltrate highly suspicious for Hodgkin lymphoma (HL) with no abnormal population identified on flow cytometry. Excisional biopsy 1 week later confirmed HL, nodular sclerosing type. Laboratory work-ups including complete blood count (CBC), comprehensive metabolic panel (CMP), and erythrocyte sedimentation rate (ESR) were obtained and were all within normal limits. CT of the neck, chest, abdomen, and pelvis with IV contrast was notable for a dominant conglomerate of lymph nodes in the right neck (levels II–III) measuring 5.2 cm in maximal longitudinal dimension. A subsequent PET/CT scan demonstrated multiple hypermetabolic right cervical lymph nodes with maximum SUV of 8.2 (Figs. 1.1 and 1.2). *There were no FDG-avid lesions identified elsewhere.*

S. Terezakis, MD (✉)
Johns Hopkins School of Medicine,
401 N. Broadway, Suite 1440, Baltimore,
MD 21231, USA
e-mail: stereza1@jhmi.edu

J.P. Plastaras, MD, PhD
University of Pennsylvania,
3400 Civic Center Blvd. TRC4W, Philadelphia,
PA 19104, USA
e-mail: Plastaras@uphs.upenn.edu

Pathology

The final pathology demonstrated nodular sclerosis (classic) HL (NSHL). NSHL is composed of Reed-Sternberg (R-S) cells (CD15+) identified in

B.S. Dabaja, A.K. Ng (eds.), *Radiation Therapy in Hematologic Malignancies*,
DOI 10.1007/978-3-319-42615-0_1

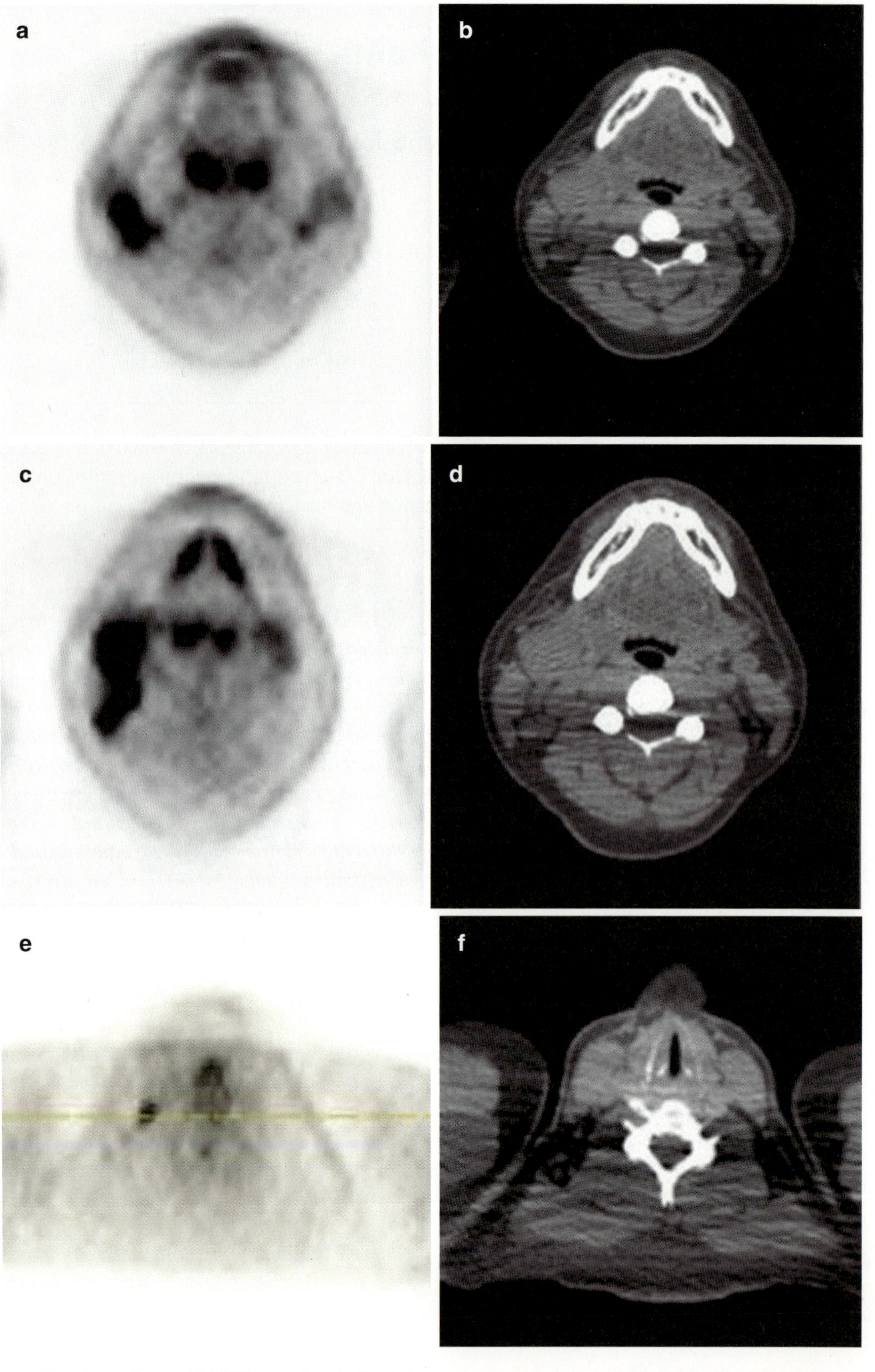

Fig. 1.1 Pre-chemotherapy PET/CT scan (axial slices) demonstrating the extent of disease in the *right* neck

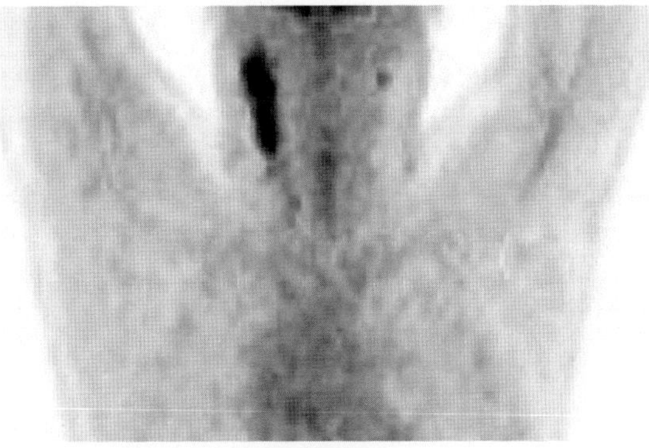

Fig. 1.2 Pre-chemotherapy PET/CT scan (coronal view) demonstrating the extent of disease

a background of predominantly lymphocytes. NSHL is characterized by collagenous bands that divide the lymph node into nodules often containing an R-S cell variant called the lacunar cell. Although NSHL is the most common subtype in all age groups, it is more frequent in adolescents (77 %) and adults (72 %) than in younger children (44 %) [1]. NSHL frequently spreads along contiguous nodal chains as illustrated in this case presentation in which the right neck was involved extending from lymph node levels II–IV.

Staging and Prognostic Factors

After pathology is obtained, patients undergo clinical staging, beginning with a detailed history of systemic symptoms and physical examination. Laboratory studies including CBC and biochemical evaluation with liver function tests (including albumin) should be obtained. Acute-phase reactants, including ESR and C-reactive protein, may be elevated at diagnosis. Patients with "B" symptoms or stage III and IV lymphoma should have a bone marrow biopsy. Given this patient presented with stage IA disease, he did not undergo bone marrow biopsy. Imaging work-up with CT scan of the neck, chest, abdomen, and pelvis with IV contrast is required to define disease involvement and extent [1]. An abdominal and pelvic CT with oral and intravenous contrast can define retroperitoneal and pelvic lymph nodes. HL involving the liver or spleen is suggested by CT findings of definite areas of abnormal density representing lymphomatous deposits. ^{18}F-FDG PET/CT scan is increasingly recognized as the most useful functional staging modality for HL [2]. Areas of abnormal avidity correlate with disease extent, which is essential in staging, and PET scan is critical for assessment of mid-treatment and end-of-treatment response. PET scan, when performed after only two or three cycles of chemotherapy, has prognostic significance in classical HL whether in the initial or relapsed setting [3–5]. A negative mid-treatment PET has been clearly associated with favorable outcomes. While HL patients with a positive mid-treatment PET generally fare worse, the results have been variable given the small number of PET-positive patients seen in these studies. Early metabolic imaging is also being investigated in an effort to reduce chemotherapy toxicity in adequately responding patients while intensifying patients who are slow to respond [6]. Large-scale clinical trials have also used end-of-chemotherapy PET to guide whether and which sites to radiate particularly in the advanced HL setting [7, 8]. There has been a movement to carefully define responses objectively, and ongoing trials and clinical guidelines have used the five-point Deauville criteria based on the mediastinal blood pool and liver as internal benchmarks of uptake [9]. Information gained on the extent of early and end-of-chemotherapy response may help to individually tailor risk-adapted, combined-modality treatment for HL. Currently, and for patients with early favorable HL, HD10 still constitutes the backbone.

In addition to the emerging data on the prognostic significance of response-based imaging, there are several well-established prognostic factors including the stage of disease, presence of bulk, number of involved sites, systemic "B" symptoms, laboratory studies including ESR, and age. Patients presenting with advanced disease (stage III or IV) have a poorer outcome than patients with early-stage disease [10]. "B" symptoms develop as a result of cytokine secretion and are a marker for biologic aggressiveness of disease. ESR, hemoglobin level, and serum albumin have also been reported to predict worse out-

Table 1.1 Definitions of unfavorable risk factors by a specific cooperative group

German Hodgkin Study Group (GHSG)
1. ESR >50 if no B symptoms, ESR >30 if B symptoms
2. Mediastinal mass ratio >0.33
3. >2 nodal sites
4. Any extranodal disease
European Organization for the Research and Treatment of Cancer (EORTC)
1. Age ≥50
2. ESR >50 if no B symptoms, ESR >30 if B symptoms
3. Mediastinal thoracic ratio >0.35
4. >3 nodal sites
National Cancer Institute of Canada (NCIC)
1. Age ≥40
2. Mixed cellularity or lymphocyte depleted histology
3. ESR >50 or any B symptoms
4. Mediastinal mass ratio >0.33 or disease >10 cm
5. >3 nodal sites

comes [11]. HL is typically categorized into "favorable" and "unfavorable" disease based on the constellation of such prognostic factors, and each large cooperative group has defined these categories with specific criteria (See Table 1.1). Therefore, in interpretation of clinical trial data, it is essential to understand the inclusion criteria for "favorable" and "unfavorable" categories to apply the clinical outcomes appropriately.

Our patient presented at a young age, without B symptoms or bulk, with disease confined to one "site" in the right neck, and normal lab values. Therefore, he fell classically into a "favorable" category of disease according to each cooperative group's definition.

Treatment Management

Randomized controlled data have demonstrated the feasibility of lowering the radiation prescription dose particularly in the favorable group of patients. The German Hodgkin Study Group (GHSG) HD10 trial used a 2×2 design to randomize patients to either two or four cycles of ABVD chemotherapy with either 20 Gy- or 30 Gy involved-field radiotherapy (IFRT). There were no significant differences in overall survival and a 5-year freedom-from-treatment failure based on the number of chemotherapy cycles or radiation dose [12]. It is important to note that the GHSG definition of favorable disease differs from both the EORTC and National Cancer Institute of Canada (NCIC) definitions (Table 1.1). In this patient, ABVD was recommended with two cycles followed by 20 Gy of radiation treatment because he met favorable disease criteria per the HD10 trial.

Concerns regarding late radiation toxicity have prompted interest in exploring the feasibility of a chemotherapy-alone approach. A number of trials have compared combined modality therapy with chemotherapy alone, and these studies can be difficult to interpret due to varying inclusion criteria and treatment techniques. Randomized comparisons of combined modality therapy with chemotherapy alone generally show higher rates of relapse with omission of RT. The EORTC-GELA H9-F examined 619 patients with early-stage, favorable disease who had achieved a complete response after six cycles of epirubicin, bleomycin, vinblastine, and prednisone (EBVP) chemotherapy [13]. Following chemotherapy, patients were randomized to observation, 20 Gy of IFRT or 36 Gy of IFRT. There was no difference in a four-year EFS between the two IFRT arms (20 Gy: 84 % vs. 36 Gy: 87 %), and patients in the observation arm experienced a significantly lower four-year EFS of 70 % ($p<0.001$) which resulted in early termination of the observation arm due to prespecified stopping rules. It has been noted that the H9F study employs less intensive chemotherapy than other similarly designed trials, and it has been suggested that this is the reason for a lower EFS in the observation arm [14].

Similarly, in the National Cancer Institute of Canada – Eastern Cooperative Oncology Group (NCIC-ECOG) HD6 trial, 405 patients with early-stage disease were randomized to four to six cycles of ABVD chemotherapy alone versus subtotal nodal irradiation (STNI) with either two cycles of ABVD chemotherapy or no further therapy. Patients in the combined modality arm experienced a trend toward an improved 12-year FFDP compared to patients in the chemotherapy alone arm (92 % vs. 87 %, $p=0.05$), with "unfavorable" patients experiencing a statistically significant difference in FFDP (94 % vs. 86 %, $p=0.01$) [15]. Notably, patients in the combined modality arm experienced worse OS

(87 % vs. 94 %, $p = 0.04$). However, interpretation of the survival results is unclear given an excess of mortality in the combined modality arm from either early toxicity or causes other than lymphoma. Ultimately, the omission of radiation did not adversely affect OS rates in the majority of patients on the HD6 trial. It is critical to be aware that the HD6 trial incorporated more extensive RT with STNI than is delivered with modern radiotherapy. Although the combined modality arm in this study is obsolete, enthusiasts of a chemotherapy-only approach have pointed to the excellent survival results with four to six cycles of ABVD [14]. Therefore, the outcomes of chemotherapy, compared to combined modality therapy delivered with modern techniques, smaller radiation fields, and lower doses, remain to be determined.

A systematic Cochrane review further investigated the omission of RT from combined modality therapy. The analysis included five unconfounded trials and demonstrated that the omission of RT from the combined modality paradigm led to increased risk of relapse [16]. Additionally, two recent analyses using large-scale datasets from the Surveillance, Epidemiology, and End Results (SEER) program and the National Cancer Database have also suggested decreased overall survival in early stage HL patients treated with chemotherapy alone [17, 18].

Excellent survival outcomes and availability of effective salvage therapy do suggest that chemotherapy alone is an option particularly in those patients that are likely to experience morbidity from the late effects of RT. However, there are trade-offs with this approach as it requires more intensive chemotherapy or increased number of chemotherapy cycles, and in the case of relapse, higher doses of RT and/or stem cell transplantation are required resulting in more significant toxicities. To better determine the patients in which to escalate or de-escalate therapy, studies are ongoing to evaluate whether excellent clinical outcomes can be maintained with the omission of RT after a negative interim PET. Although this strategy holds promise, it is not clear yet whether there is predictive power to the interim PET that will guide risk-adapted therapy in the adult population. For example, favorable patients in the H10 trial that had a negative PET after ABVD x 2 cycles received one additional cycle of ABVD without RT. This experimental arm was closed early due to excess treatment failure, and RT was subsequently added to this arm following ABVD completion. There were 16 events of progression in the experimental arm versus 7 in the standard arm at first interim analysis, and the data-monitoring committee concluded that it was unlikely that the experimental arm would have a non-inferior outcome leading to the early closure [19]. The United Kingdom National Cancer Research Institute RAPID trial also explored the role of interim PET in patients with stage I/II disease without B symptoms or mediastinal bulk. Patients with a negative PET scan following three cycles of ABVD were randomized to IFRT versus observation. The trial was designed as a non-inferiority study, and at a median follow-up of 45.7 months, the 3-year PFS was similar between the IFRT and observation arms (IFRT 93.8 vs. observation 90.7 %). However, the 95 % confidence interval for the difference in PFS exceeded the prespecified non-inferiority boundary of 7 %. Additionally, a number of patients randomized to the IFRT arm did not actually receive RT, and therefore, a secondary per-protocol analysis was performed, which showed a significant improvement in PFS with IFRT (3 years PFS with RT: 97.1 % vs. no RT: 90.8 %, $p = 0.02$). The results of this trial are therefore difficult to interpret given the similarity in PFS on the intent-to-treat analysis with a significant difference demonstrated on the per-protocol analysis [20].

Treatment Field and Technique

With the advent of modern chemotherapy, IFRT became the standard radiation technique based on randomized trial data supporting the use of IFRT over an EFRT approach in the context of chemotherapy. Because patients with early-stage HL treated with chemotherapy alone most frequently relapse in the initially involved lymph node(s) [21], efforts have been made to reduce treatment fields to include only the initially involved lymph node(s) and exclude surrounding normal tissues. The EORTC-GELA introduced the concept of INRT [22], which uses all available clinical information, including pre- and post-chemotherapy imaging with CT and FDG-PET scan to define the treatment field. The application of INRT relies on a pre-chemotherapy PET/CT scan to be performed in the treatment position to facilitate fusion with the simulation scan.

However, it is a common scenario that pre-chemotherapy imaging is not available and has not been performed in the treatment position. As a result, the involved site radiation therapy (ISRT) guidelines were developed and similarly target the initially involved lymph nodes, allowing for a

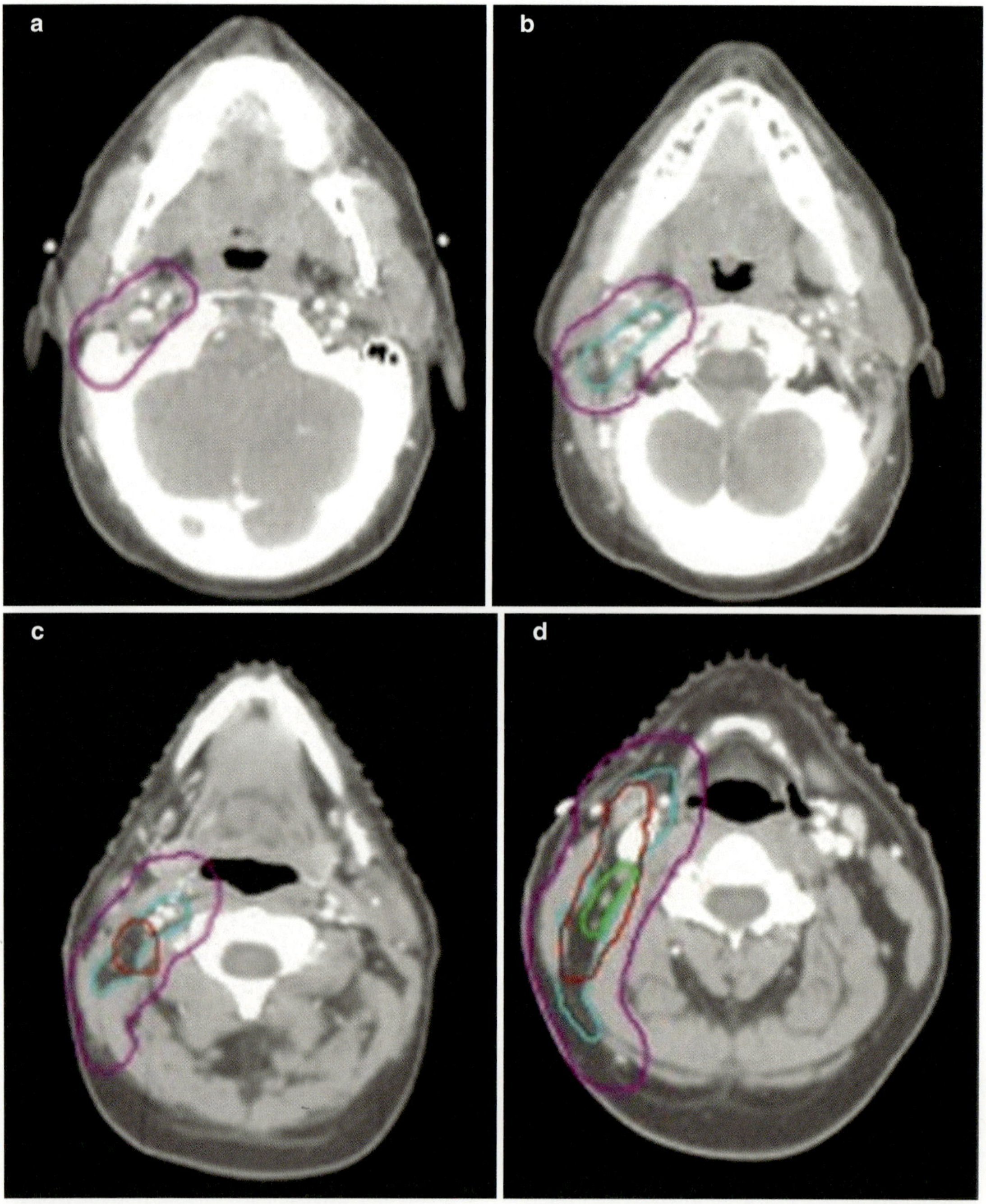

Fig. 1.3 CT simulation scan with contours (axial slices). Pre-chemotherapy GTV (*red*), post-chemotherapy GTV (*green*), CTV (*light blue*), PTV (*pink*)

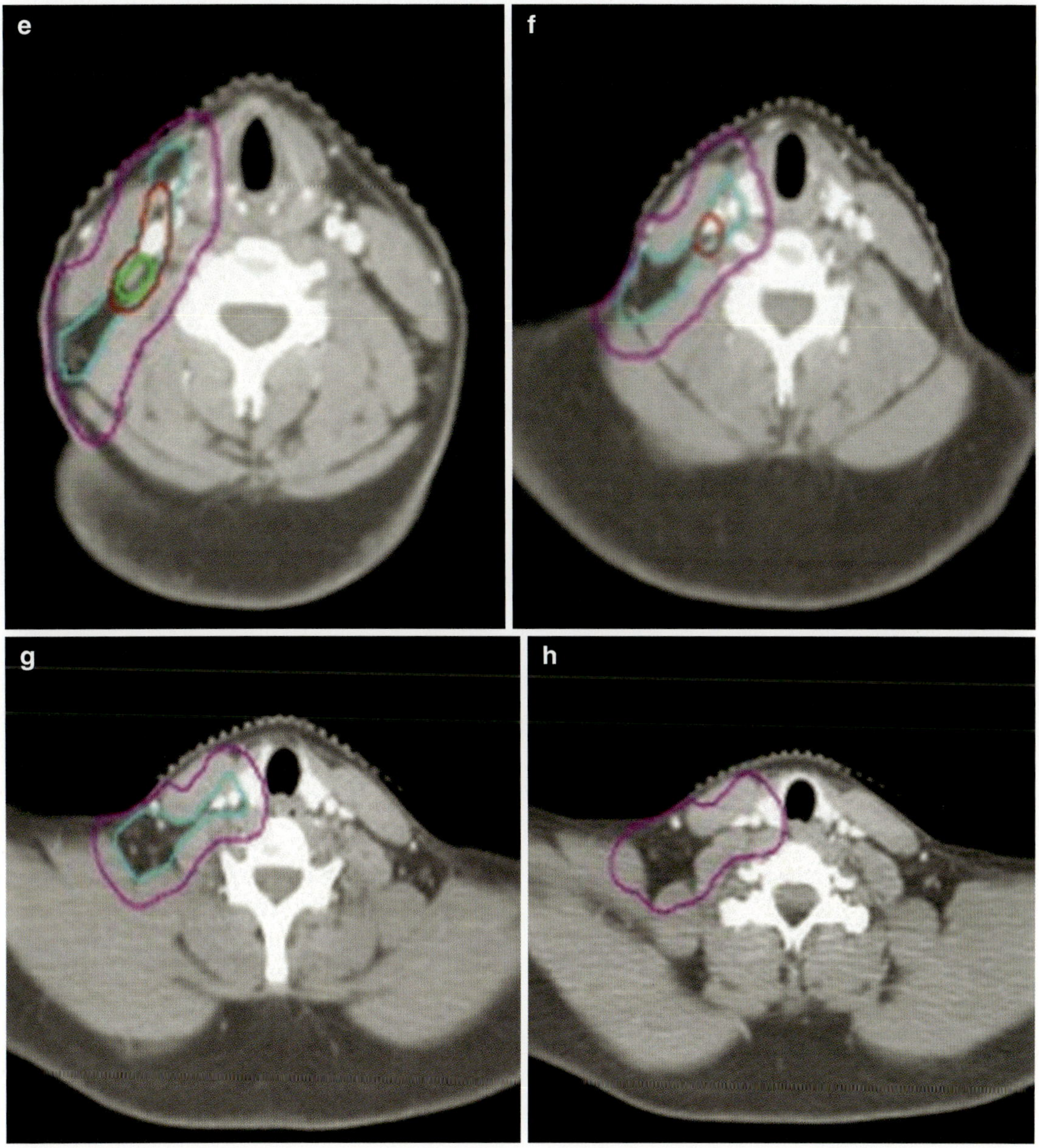

Fig. 1.3 (continued)

potentially larger margin based on the uncertainty introduced by the lack of pre-chemotherapy imaging or inability to fuse such imaging accurately [23]. ISRT fields were developed to take into consideration modern technology with the use of staging PET/CT scans, 3D, and 4D CT-based treatment planning, conformal treatment techniques, and the use of image guidance in an effort to replace the approach of IFRT which was based on 2D treatment planning and bony anatomy.

In this patient, ISRT was utilized to target the initially involved lymph nodes (Fig. 1.3). *A prechemotherapy GTV was constructed to identify the areas of initial involvement. The patient had an excellent response to chemotherapy with no evidence of FDG-avid disease noted on their post-chemotherapy PET/CT scan. Although a PET complete response was achieved, there was evidence of post-chemotherapy residual CT abnormality that was contoured as the post-chemotherapy GTV. The CTV was then designed to encompass both the superior*

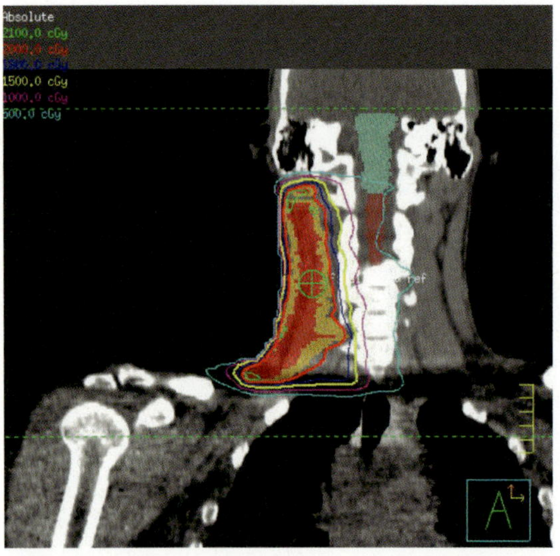

Fig. 1.4 Intensity-modulated radiation therapy plan demonstrating coverage of the CTV (shaded mustard) by the 100 % isodose line (*red*)

and inferior extent but not axial direction of the prechemotherapy GTV (Fig. 1.2). *The CTV was modified to exclude normal anatomy and adjusted to take into account the change in normal anatomic position of the surrounding normal tissues. The CTV was expanded volumetrically to a margin of 5 mm to a final PTV, keeping in mind that this is a neck site with reproducible immobilization, as opposed to a mediastinal location for instance, and therefore does not need as generous of an expansion* (Figs. 1.3 and 1.4).

Low dose radiation delivered to a final dose of 20 Gy in 2 Gy fractions was planned using 3D conformal therapy. Beams were oriented in an AP/PA direction with wedges placed to improve dose homogeneity (Fig. 1.5).

Posttreatment Considerations

Given the evolution of RT field design in the reduction of field size and dose, it is difficult to interpret the current body of literature on RT-related late toxicities, which is heavily derived from patients who were treated with EFRT techniques. The patient described here, reported grade 1 fatigue and grade 1 esophagitis during the course of radiotherapy. At 2 years posttreatment, he has reported no sequelae with resolution of his fatigue as well as esophagitis. Long-term follow-up evaluating thyroid function tests will be important given the location of ISRT.

Long-term follow-up for such patients will be critical to understand how the reduction in field sizes using ISRT and INRT translates in terms of the development of late toxicities [24]. Additionally, initial data on the use of smaller field sizes has suggested that clinical outcomes are not sacrificed with the use of INRT or ISRT. Paumier et al., for example, reported a 92 % 5-year PFS in patients with early-stage HL treated with INRT as per EORTC-GELA guidelines [25]. Similarly, Filippi et al. reported a 3-year relapse-free survival of 99 % in stage IIA patients using an ISRT technique [26]. The current GHSG HD17 trial is open for newly diagnosed intermediate stage Hodgkin lymphoma, delivering two cycles of escalated BEACOPP and two cycles of ABVD followed by assessment of FDG-PET scan. Patients randomized into the standard arm receive IFRT regardless of PET response. Patients randomized into the experimental arm receive no further therapy if their PET is negative and receive INRT in patients if their PET scan is positive.

Clinical Presentation: Combined Modality Therapy for Early-Stage Unfavorable Patients

A 28-year-old man presented with dyspnea on exertion and pleuritic chest pain. Further work-up led to a chest X-ray which revealed mediastinal widening. A chest CT showed an anterior mediastinal mass measuring 9.5 × 5.0 × 4.5 cm, bilateral supraclavicular adenopathy, and presence of pericardial effusion (see Fig. 1.5). *Excisional biopsy of a supraclavicular node showed classical NSHL.*

Staging and Prognostic Factors

The patient's history was notable for a 2-month progressive dyspnea on exertion, but absence of B symptoms or signs of superior vena cava syndrome. His physical examination showed a well-healing biopsy scar in the left supraclavicular area and slight fullness in the right supraclavicular area. He has no other sites adenopathy and no organomegaly. Laboratory studies showed a normal CBC with

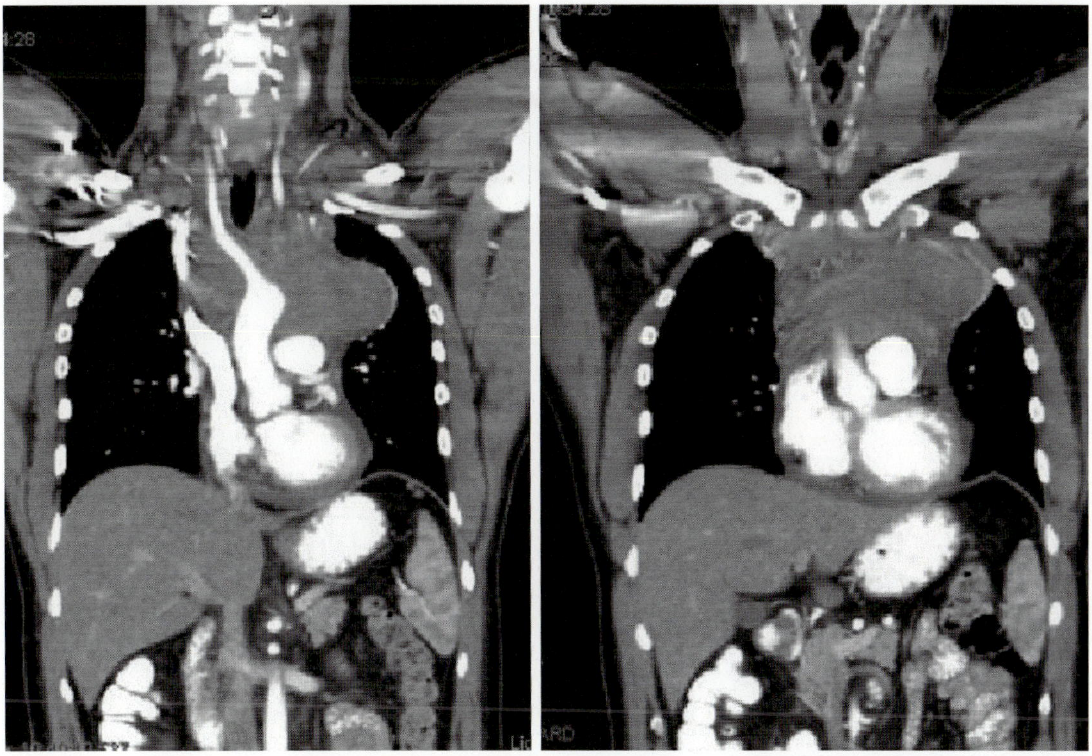

Fig. 1.5 Showing coronal pre-chemotherapy CT images, note the bilateral neck disease, bulky mediastinal mass, and the pericardial effusion

differential, and his ESR was 12 mm/h. PET/CT scan confirmed FDG-avid disease limited to the bilateral supraclavicular fossa and anterior mediastinum (*see* Fig. 1.6). *Although a pericardial effusion was noted, there was no pericardial nodal disease or disease below the diaphragm.*

This patient did not have B symptoms and his laboratory findings are within normal limits. He did not have bulky disease since his mediastinal mass ratio on chest X-ray is <0.33, and his maximal disease dimension is <10 cm. However, he did have three sites of disease (bilateral supraclavicular and mediastinal disease) and is therefore classified as unfavorable according to the GHSG criteria but favorable by the EORTC criteria.

Treatment Management

In the treatment management of early-stage unfavorable-prognosis patients, investigators have explored chemotherapy regimens other than ABVD, the optimal duration of chemotherapy, and optimal radiation dose. Both the EORTC and HD11 studies H9U [27, 28] studies compared 4–6 cycles of ABVD with four cycles of BEACOPP-baseline, followed by involved-field radiation therapy to 20–30 Gy. No significant differences in a 4-year event-free survival (EFS) or overall survival were observed between BEACOPP and ABVD in the EORTC H9U trial. In the GHSG HD11 trial, although there was a significantly higher 5-year freedom-from-treatment failure (FFTF) in the four cycles of baseline BEACOPP arm over the four cycles ABVD arm if followed by 20 Gy of involved-field radiation therapy, no difference was observed, and 30 Gy of involved-field radiation therapy was used. Patients treated with baseline BEACOPP had a higher rate of severe toxicity. The GHSG HD14 trial [29] compared four cycles of ABVD with two cycles of dose-escalated BEACOPP and two cycles of ABVD (2+2 regimen), followed by involved-field irradiation to 30 Gy. Although the 2+2 regimen had a significantly improved 5-year FFTF, it was associated with more acute toxicity,

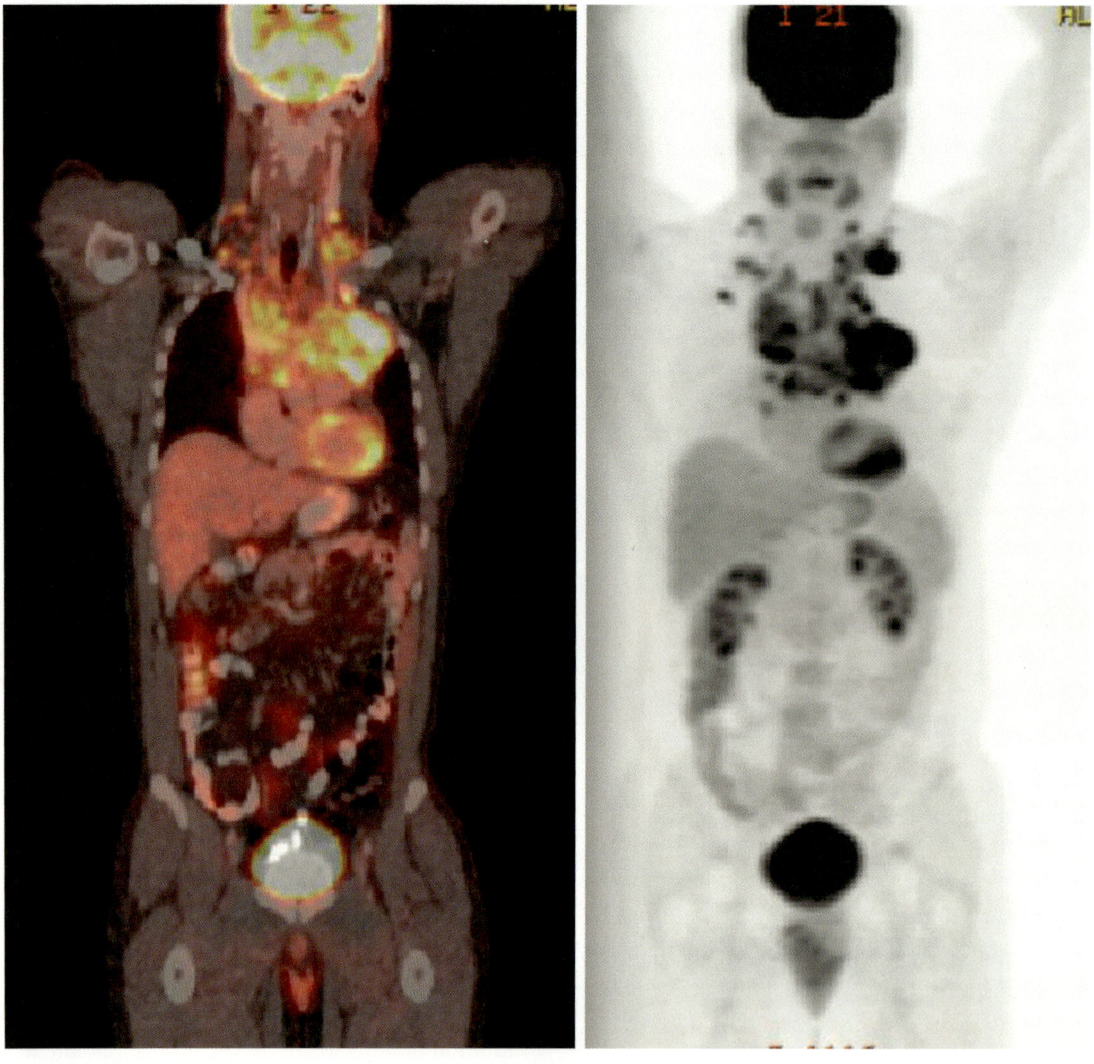

Fig. 1.6 Showing the original disease on the pre-chemotherapy PET/CT

and there was no overall survival advantage. In a subset analysis of E2496 trial of patients with stage I–II bulky disease, there was no significant difference in a 5-year failure-free, and overall survival rates between ABVD and radiotherapy versus Stanford V [30]. Given these data, ABVD remains the most widely accepted chemotherapy regimen for patients with early-stage, unfavorable disease in North America. The question of optimal chemotherapy duration was addressed by the EORTC-H8U and EORTC-H9U trials [27, 31], both showing no difference in EFS between four versus six cycles of chemotherapy, suggesting that in early-stage unfavorable patients, four cycles of ABVD is adequate. However, it should be noted that the GSHG HD11 excluded patients with stage IIB with large mediastinal adenopathy or extranodal disease. Instead, these patients were included in their advanced-stage trials. For patients with early-stage disease with multiple risk factors, a longer course of chemotherapy should therefore be considered.

The question of optimal radiation dose in unfavorable patients was addressed by the previously described GHSG HD11 trial [28] with a 2×2 design comparing 20 Gy versus 30 Gy after four cycles of ABVD or baseline BEACOPP. At a median follow-up of 82 months, the 5-year freedom-from-treatment-failure rates were 81.1 %, 85.3 %, 86.8 %, and 87.0 %, respectively. There was no significant difference in a 5-year FFTF rate between baseline BEACOPP and ABVD when followed by 30 Gy of IFRT; however, inferiority of 20 Gy cannot be excluded after four cycles of ABVD, leading to the authors' conclusion of four cycles of ABVD followed by 30 Gy of radiation therapy as optimal therapy for early-stage, unfavorable HL. Although the GHSG HD11 results do not support radiation dose de-escalation after ABVD in early-stage unfavorable patients, there are single institutional data showing that, especially if there is a complete metabolic response to chemotherapy, doses of 20–25 Gy may be adequate [32, 33].

Our patient has unfavorable disease according to the GHSG criteria, with having three sites of disease as his only risk factor. He received a total of four cycles of ABVD and achieved a complete response (Deauville 2). He then went onto receive ISRT to 30.6 Gy in 17 fractions.

Treatment Field and Technique

ISRT was utilized, targeting the initially involved lymph nodes, including the bilateral supraclavicular and mediastinal nodes, as detailed above. Figure 1.7a, b, *shows the CTV and PTV on the planning CT and superimposed on the pre-chemotherapy CT. The pericardial effusion was not considered part of the CTV, since pericardial effusions in this setting are often reactive in nature, and the suspicion level for any residual microscopic disease is low. Furthermore, its inclusion as part of the target volume would substantially increase doses to the heart.*

The patient was placed in an arms-down position (an arms-down position would be especially important in a young woman to limit the amount of breast tissue in the treatment field). The patient was planned with the deep inspiration breath-hold (DIBH) technique, which has been shown to significantly reduce doses to the lungs, heart, and cardiac substructures. The butterfly IMRT technique of using anterior beams of 300°–30° and posterior beams of 160–210° was used to limit the low-dose bath laterally. Coronal and axial images of the isodose distribution in Fig. 1.8a, b, *show the sparing of the majority of the heart. The DVHs are displayed in* Fig. 1.9. *With the butterfly IMRT technique in DIBH position, a mean heart dose of 5.4 Gy and mean lung dose of 8.8 Gy were achieved. A mean dose to the left coronary artery was 7.1 Gy.*

Posttreatment Considerations

The patient experienced esophagitis and mild fatigue toward the end of the treatment course. At 1-month follow-up, these symptoms largely resolved. As part of follow-up, the patient will undergo annual thyroid function tests. The long-term cardiac risk in this patient is expected to be significantly lower than patients who were treated with full mantle field to higher doses of radiation. Nevertheless, he will benefit from close monitoring of and minimizing traditional cardiac risk factors, including hypertension, hyperlipidemia, and diabetes, and other lifestyle modifications such as healthy diet, regular exercise, and avoiding tobacco use. A baseline cardiology evaluation including resting and stress echocardiogram should be considered approximately 10 years posttreatment. If he were to have had a tobacco history, an annual low-dose chest CT screening for lung cancer should be considered approximately 10 years posttreatment.

Clinical Presentation: Refractory and Relapsed Disease

This patient is a 37-year-old man who was initially diagnosed with upper mediastinal classical HL in 2009. He was treated with ABVD chemotherapy x 6 cycles alone with no further adjuvant therapy. He recurred 6 months later in the mediastinum and received salvage therapy with ICE (e.g., ifosfamide, carboplatin, and etoposide) followed by busulfan/cytoxan preparation regimen with autologous peripheral stem cell transplant shortly thereafter and subsequently attained a CR. Three years later he had a CT scan for follow-up that demonstrated an enlarging mediastinal lesion in the upper mediasti-

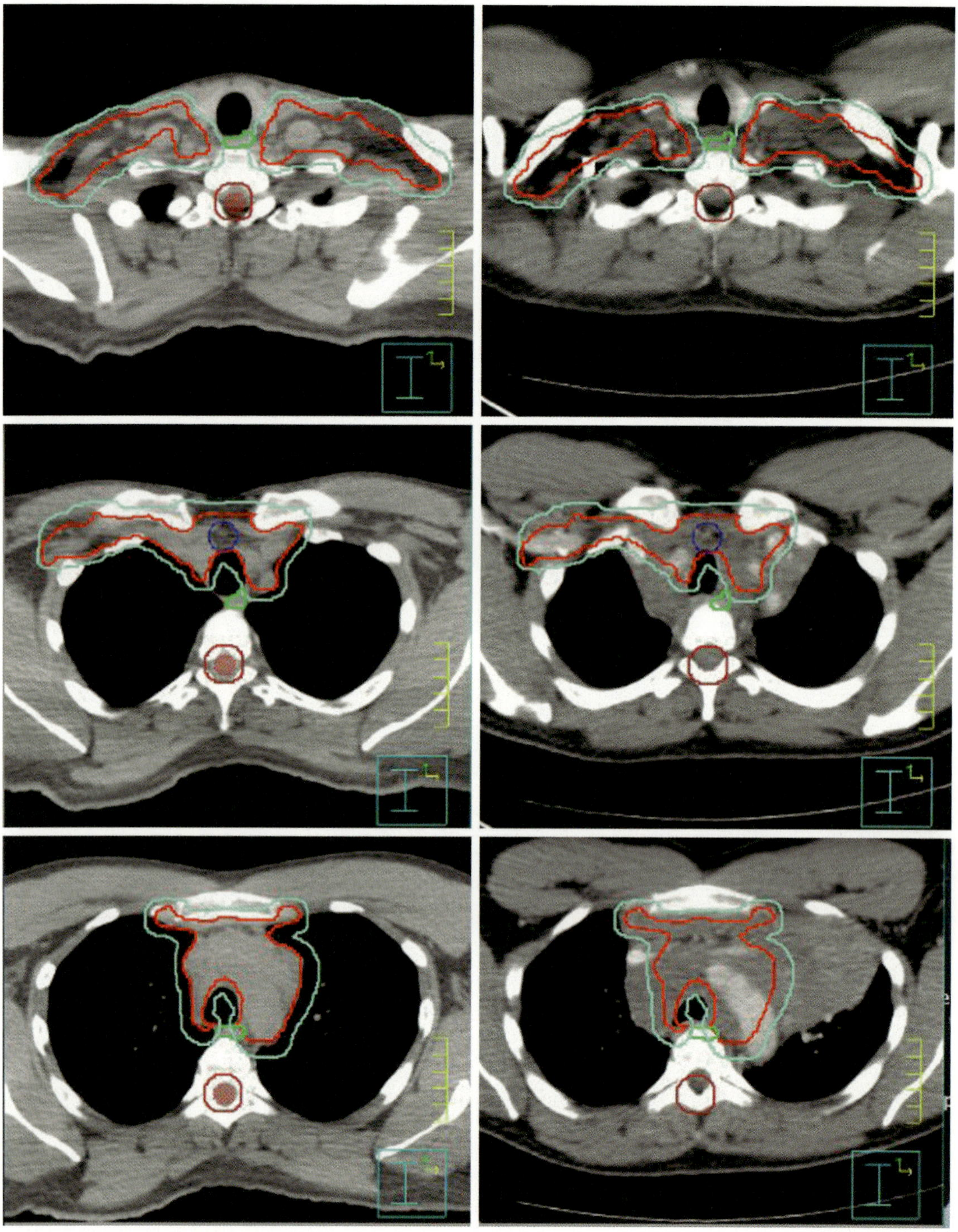

Fig. 1.7 Showing the CTV (*red*) and PTV (*green*). Panel of the left is the CT simulation; panel of the right is the fuse pre-chemotherapy images

num. A PET/CT demonstrated a 3 × 1.9 cm lobulated nodal conglomerate in the superior mediastinum anterior to the upper trachea with an SUV of 11.5 with inferior extension into the retrosternal anterior mediastinum measuring 3.7 × 1.5 cm (Fig. 1.10). *No other disease was identified. The patient underwent core biopsy through an endobronchial approach (EBUS) that confirmed disease recurrence.*

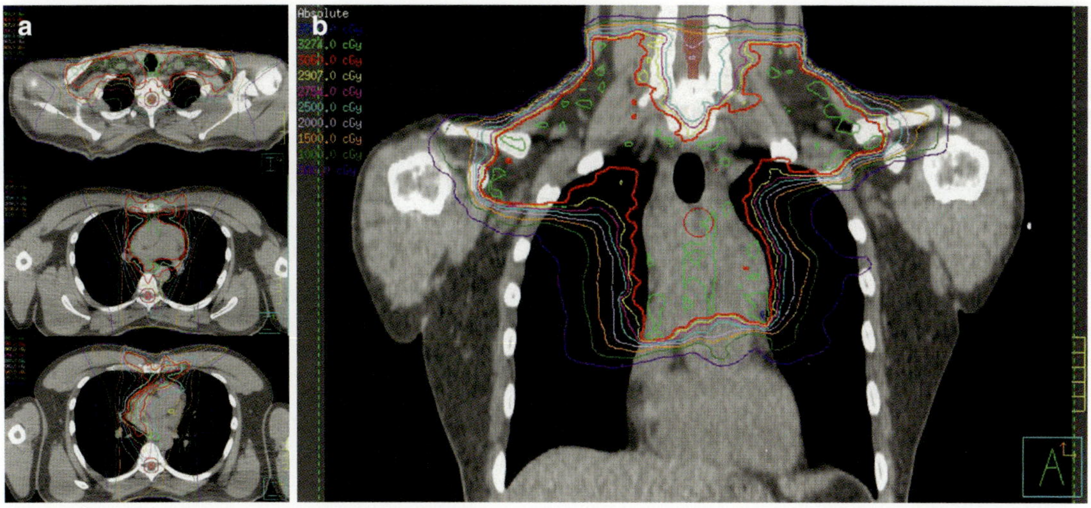

Fig. 1.8 (**a**) Showing the isodose lines, 100 % in red covering PTV and avoiding left ventricle as well as left coronaries. (**b**) Coronal view of the isodose lines, low-dose bath is limited by using butterfly technique. The heart and its structure dose is also limited by using IMRT

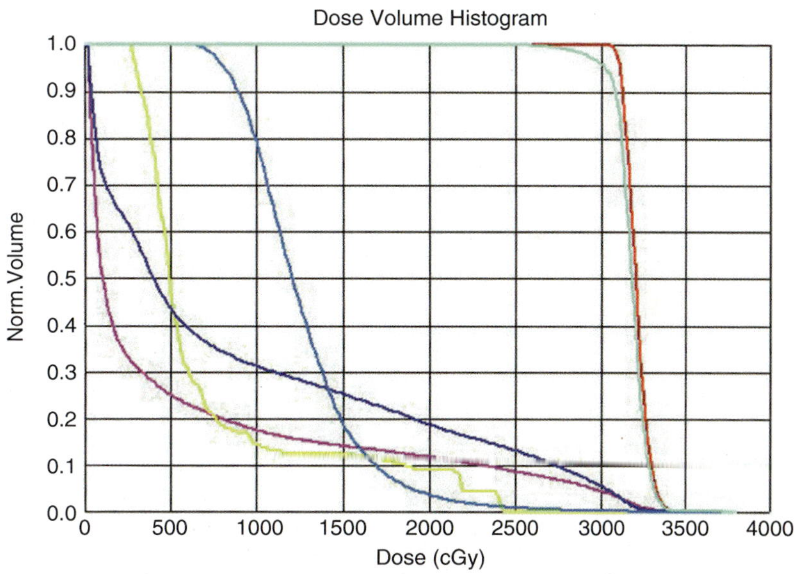

ROI Statistics

Line Type	ROI	Trial or Record	Min.	Max.	Mean	Std. Dev.
	iCTV	Apprvd	2654.1	3734.6	3208.7	67.7
	Heart	Apprvd	17.3	3523.0	542.3	897.6
	LCA	Apprvd	268.0	2430.3	707.4	569.3
	Lungs	Apprvd	13.2	3551.1	877.6	1006.7
	larynx	Apprvd	408.9	3177.2	1259.2	339.4
	pPTV_3060	Apprvd	1756.9	3734.6	3175.3	104.2

Fig. 1.9 Showing dosimetric values of the organs at risk especially the total lung (*blue*) and heart (*pink*)

Pathology, Staging, and Prognostic Factors

Pathology at the time of relapse demonstrated numerous small mature lymphocytes with rare binucleate cells with prominent nucleoli seen. A panel of immunostains demonstrated that the large atypical cells are CD30 and CD15. The background lymphocytes are predominantly CD20-positive B cells. In situ hybridization for EBV (EBER) was negative. The lack of a mixed inflammatory background was unusual, but the morphologic and immunophenotypic findings in the setting of this patient's history were consistent with classical HL. Historically, clinical factors that independently predict for a more favorable outcome in the relapsed setting include nodal relapse site (as opposed to extranodal), early stage at relapse, and response to first-line salvage chemotherapy [1].

Treatment Management

Second and third-line therapies for HL still offer the potential for cure. Relapse occurs most often within 4 years, but late relapse is still possible. There is a spectrum of treatment options including standard chemotherapy (with or without RT), RT alone, or high-dose chemotherapy followed by transplantation with or without RT. High-dose therapy supported by autologous stem cell transplantation (ASCT) has become a standard salvage therapy for

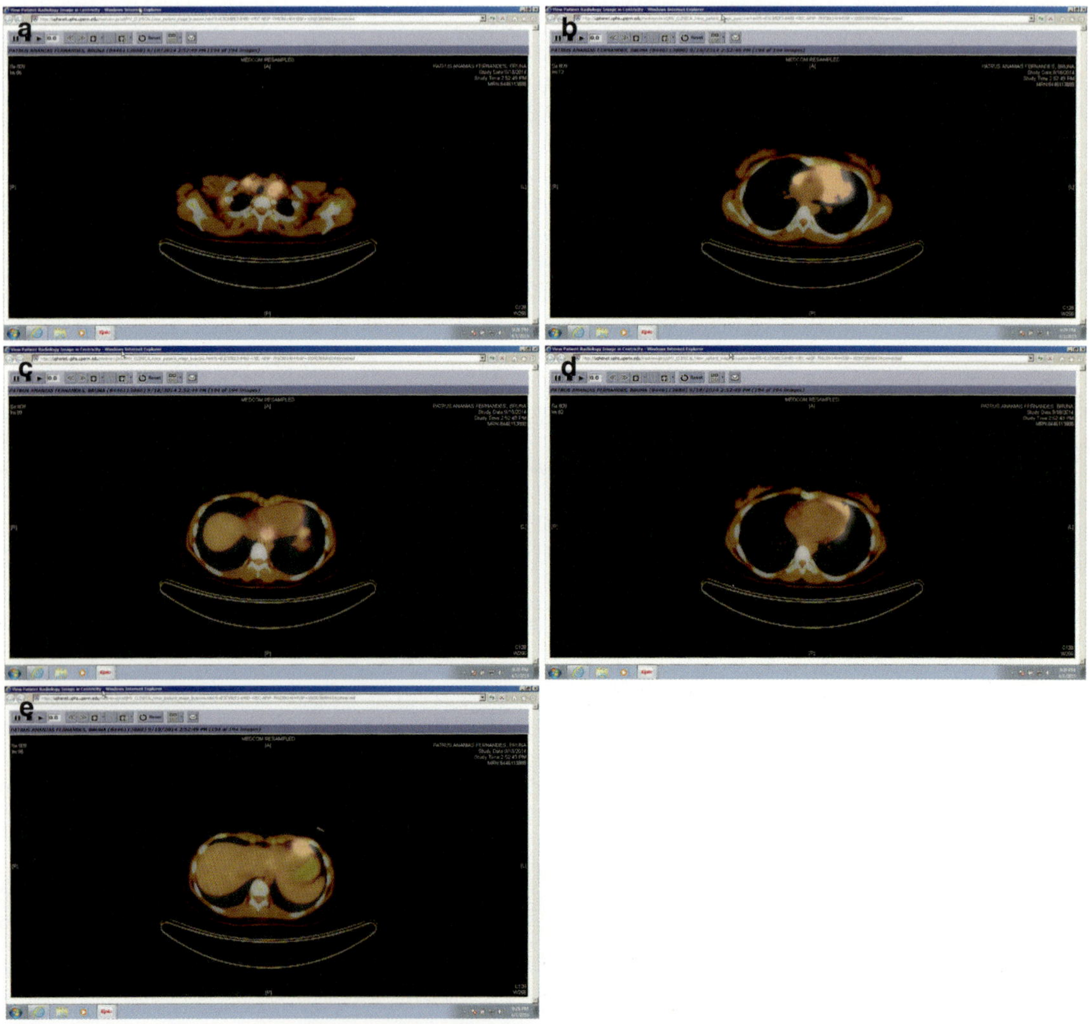

Fig. 1.10 Pre-chemotherapy PET/CT scan (axial slices) demonstrating the extent of disease in the upper mediastinum

patients who relapsed or those with primary refractory disease. Many patients who follow this approach could benefit from integrating RT into the salvage approach. RT, in this context, can be given pre- or post-transplant depending on the clinical scenario. The selection of the most appropriate salvage regimen is based on several factors including the intensity of the primary therapy, whether a complete remission was ever achieved, the durability of the remission, and the extent and location of disease at relapse. In this case, RT alone was recommended given the presence of localized disease and the absence of systemic symptoms with the goal of potentially achieving a prolonged disease-free survival [34]. *Although the patient had failed standard salvage options including ASCT, there is evidence that patients can still achieve a high-response rate to salvage RT in the relapsed/refractory setting.*

Ultimately, systemic failure is the most likely culprit to affect this patient's likelihood for survival. Newer drugs to address systemic failure are promising including targeted therapy with brentuximab vedotin, an antibody-drug conjugate that targets CD30 that has shown excellent results in early clinical trials [35–38]. *A phase-II trial treated 102 patients with relapsed/refractory disease with brentuximab until disease progression or unacceptable toxicity with a goal of maximum of 16 cycles. The median PFS for all patients was 5.6 months, and the median duration of response for those that achieved a CR was 20.5 months. Grade 3 or higher adverse events were recorded in 55 % of the patient cohort with neutropenia (20 %) being the most common* [36] *Brentuximab is currently approved for patients with relapsed HL after ASCT or after at least two prior therapies. It has also been investigated as a bridge to ASCT for patients' refractory to conventional chemotherapy.*

Treatment Field and Technique

Patients with relapsed or primary refractory disease are typically treated with higher doses of RT and thus, may benefit from more advanced treatment techniques such as intensity-modulated radiation therapy (IMRT) or proton therapy to reduce dose to surrounding normal critical structures. In particular, IMRT or proton therapy may be particularly advantageous in treating the thorax to spare dose to the heart, lungs, and developing breast tissue or when treating the abdomen and pelvis to minimize dose to the highly radiosensitive reproductive organs. In addition, higher rates of radiation pneumonitis have been demonstrated in the relapsed/refractory setting, and therefore, strategies to reduce dose to the thorax may be particularly important in this patient population [39, 40, 42]. Recently published data has put forward guidelines that can be used when applying IMRT planning in an effort to respect critical organs while achieving coverage of the target even in relapsed refractory cases. Respecting a lung V5 < 55 % and a mean lung dose of <13.5 Gy was associated with a lower risk of pneumonitis. The use of deep inspiration breath-hold technique was crucial for these plans to be able to meet critical organs restrictions [41]. The risk of pneumonitis with radiation increases in a patient who has been exposed to lung-toxic chemotherapy like bleomycin, brentuximab, or busulfan. Therefore respecting V5 and mean lung dose is essential [41].

The ISRT guidelines were applied in this case to delineate RT volumes localized to the known site of recurrence in the mediastinum incorporating both the PET and CT abnormalities. In certain cases, a larger margin incorporating adjacent nodes may be appropriate in the absence of effective chemotherapy [23]. The GTV was contoured to incorporate the PET/CT abnormalities and then expanded to the CTV with a margin of 1.5 cm respecting normal tissue boundaries including the surrounding lung and bone, which means that 1.5 will be edited accordingly in all cases to end up less than 1.5 cm. A 4D CT scan was obtained to measure respiratory motion. There was minimal motion of the mediastinal mass noted with maximum motion of 3 mm in the lateral direction. The CTV was expanded volumetrically by a margin of 1 cm to the final PTV (Fig. 1.11). An IMRT plan was delivered to a total dose of 45 Gy in 1.8 Gy fractions using image guidance with cone beam CT scan on a daily basis (Fig. 1.12). The CBCT was aligned to the bone and then shifted to the soft tissue mass in the mediastinum.

Posttreatment Considerations

This patient experienced grade 2 esophagitis during the course of therapy as well as grade 1

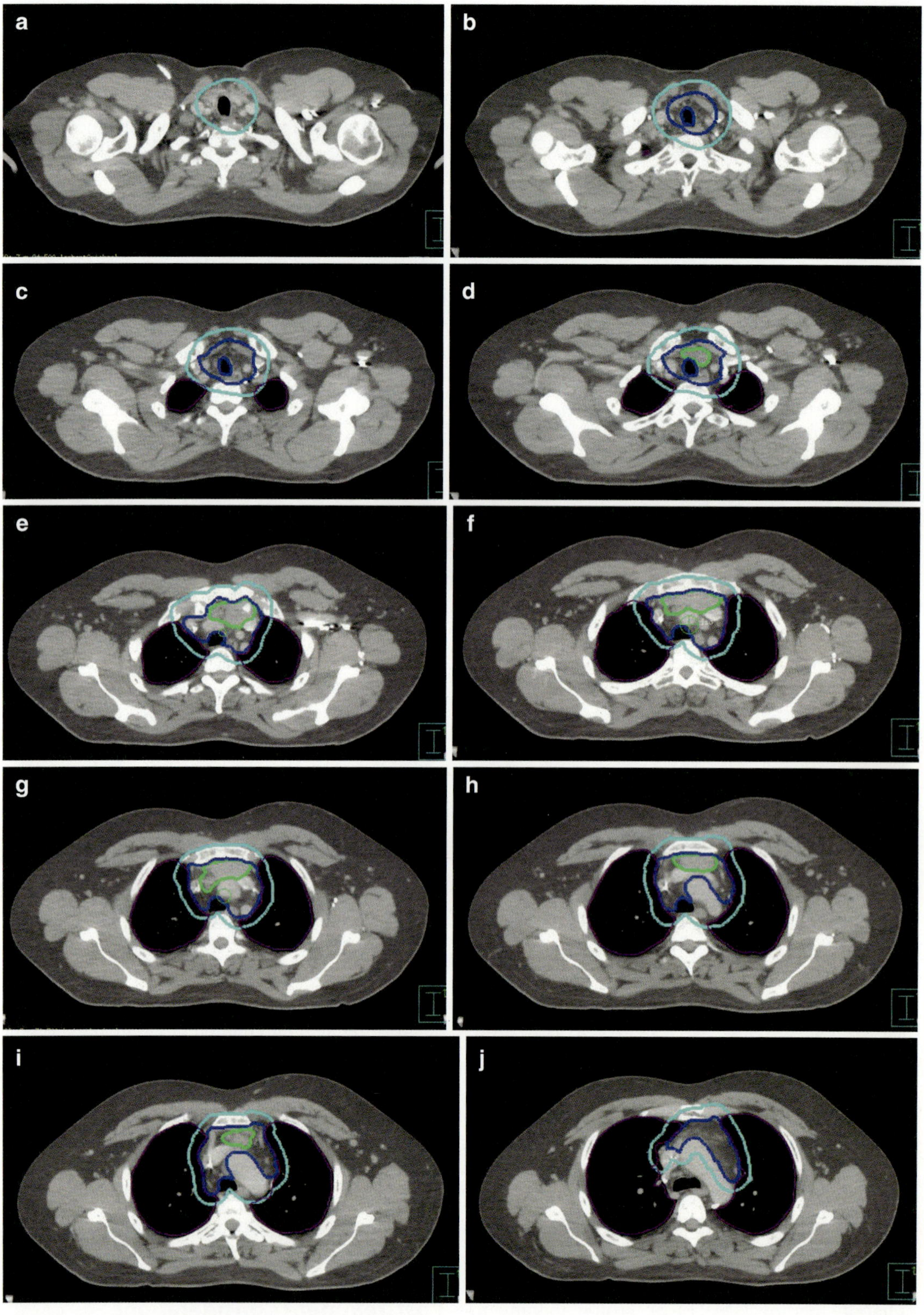

Fig. 1.11 (**a**–l): CT simulation scan with contours (axial slices). GTV (*green*), CTV (*blue*), and PTV (*light blue*)

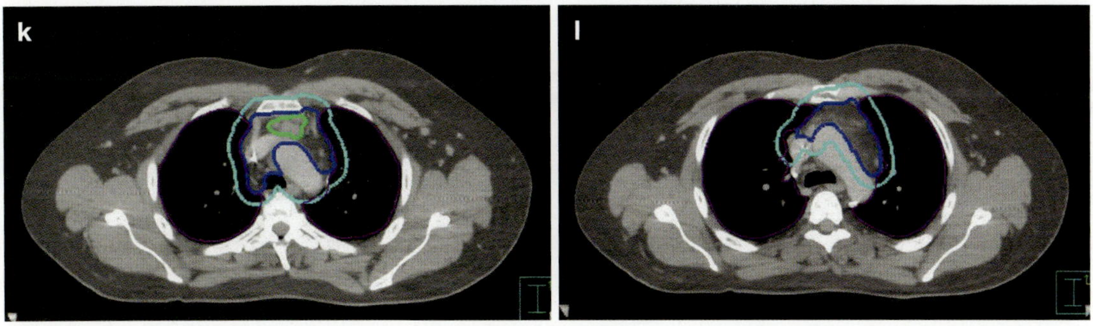

Fig. 1.11 (continued)

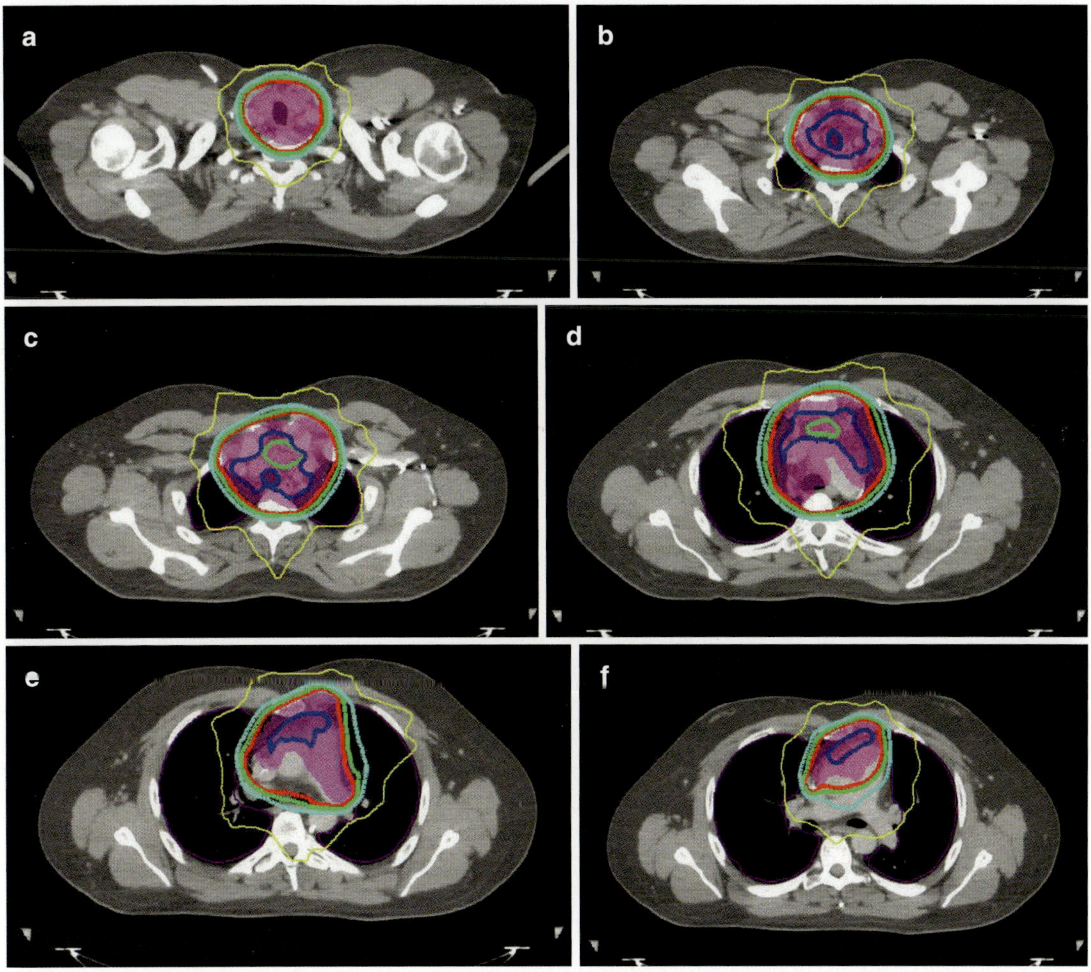

Fig. 1.12 (**a–f**) IMRT plan demonstrating excellent conformal coverage of the PTV (*shaded purple*), CTV (*blue*), and GTV (*green*). (**g**) DVH demonstrating acceptable, low dose delivered to adjacent structures such as the heart and lungs

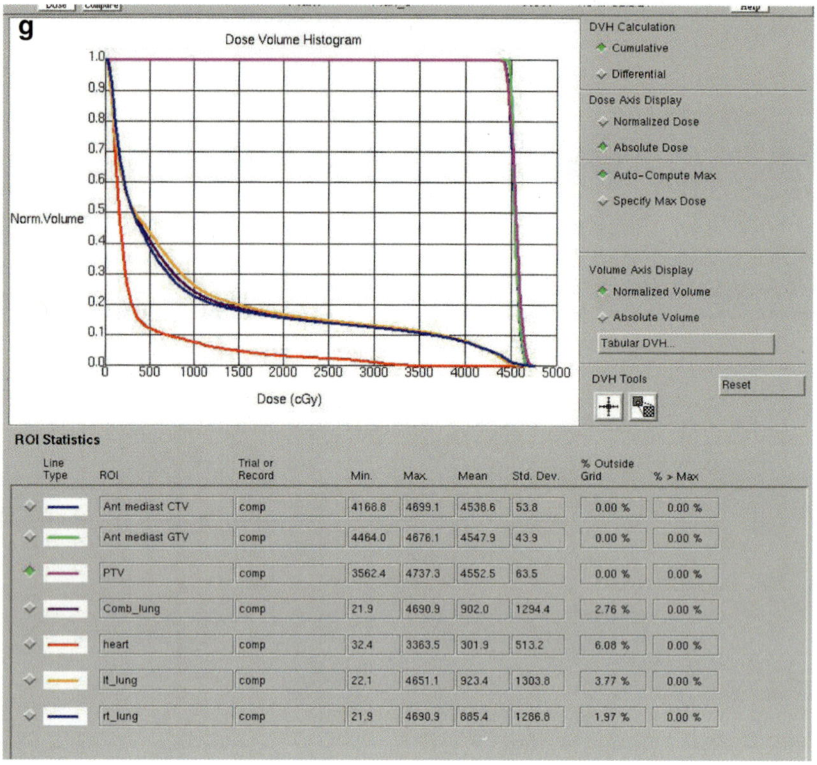

Fig. 1.12 (continued)

fatigue. By 3 months, these acute side effects resolved. The patient will need to be evaluated for long-term cardiopulmonary toxicity given the location of his disease and his prior systemic therapy.

Patients with localized disease can be successfully salvaged with radiation alone. The 5-year freedom from treatment failure after radiation alone was 28 % in a study by the GHSG that examined 4,754 patients from their database, of which 100 patients were treated with RT alone at first treatment failure. Five-year overall survival was 51 %, and significant prognostic factors included B symptoms and stage at relapse. In this study, median RT dose was 40 Gy [34]. Certainly doses of 40 Gy and above are associated with potential long-term cardiopulmonary toxicity, particularly in the context of patients previously treated with adriamycin and bleomycin. However, these concerns must be balanced against the risk of relapse that would be nearly uniformly fatal.

Clinical Presentation: Advanced Stage

A 28-year-old woman developed enlarging, nontender cervical lymphadenopathy, but did not come to medical attention until she developed painful left axillary lymphadenopathy several months later. In the emergency room, she had an upright chest X-ray that showed a widened mediastinum that was greater than 1/3 of the width at the T5/6 level. She had no B symptoms. She was admitted to the hospital and underwent CT of the neck and chest that showed a large mediastinal mass measuring 7.5 × 7.2 cm as well as cervical, supraclavicular, and axillary adenopathy. CT abdomen and pelvis showed enlarged nodes below the diaphragm in the gastrohepatic ligament (3 × 2 cm).

Pathology, Staging, and Prognostic Factors

A biopsy of a cervical lymph node confirmed a diagnosis of nodular sclerosing HL. She had a

PET/CT that demonstrated FDG-avid lymphadenopathy consistent with the CT scan with the mediastinal mass measuring 8 cm and an SUV of 16.6 (Fig. 1.13). *There was also uptake in the region of the gastrohepatic and celiac axis lymph nodes, suspicious for additional sites of lymphomatous involvement.*

In keeping with the aforementioned recommendation for bone marrow biopsy in patients with either stage III/IV disease or B symptoms, this was done but was negative. Thus, she was diagnosed with classic HL, stage IIIAX (X designating bulky disease). Using the advanced-stage international prognostic score (IPS), which is based on seven parameters that predict poor outcome (male sex, age ≥45 years, stage IV, hemoglobin $<10^5$ *g/L, WBC count* $\geq 15 \times 10^9$*/L, lymphocyte count* $<0.6 \times 10^9$*/L or <8 % of differential, albumin <40 g/L), this patient's IPS was 2, based on a low albumin and hemoglobin, putting her into a favorable risk category.* The IPS was developed using 5141 stage III/IV patients treated with multi-agent chemotherapy with or without radiation. The higher the score, the worse the 5 years of progression-free survival ranging from 84 % with a score of 0–42 % for a score of 5 or higher. The IPS still has prognostic value in the era of modern diagnosis and treatment, although the outcomes are generally better, and the range is much narrower than in the original 1998 report [44].

Treatment Management

The cornerstone of treatment for advanced-stage HL is intensive multi-agent chemotherapy, but the choice of regimen is controversial. In the 1970s, 6–8 cycles of ABVD replaced MOPP (mechlorethamine, vincristine, procarbazine, and prednisone) as long-term studies demonstrated improved efficacy with improved toxicity [45, 46]. Through a series of randomized trials (HD9, HD12, HD15), the GHSG has demonstrated that six cycles of dose-escalated BEACOPP have superior freedom from relapse and survival compared to hybrid regimens and other schedules of BEACOPP [7, 47, 48]. However, many practitioners in the United States have been slow to adopt BEACOPP due to its perceived excessive toxic-

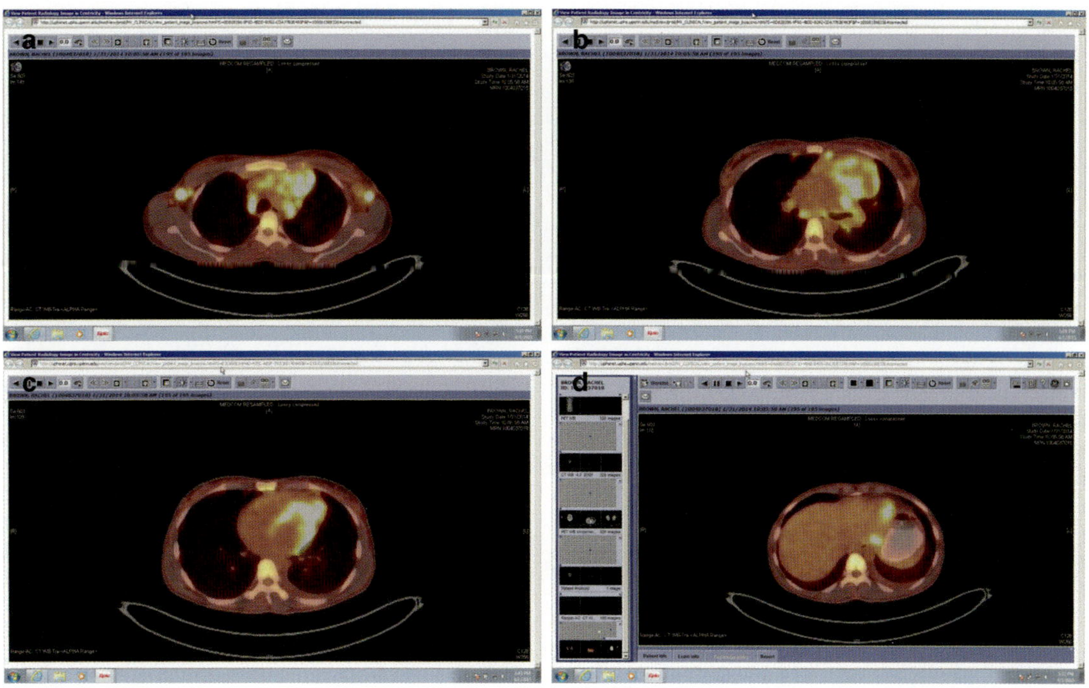

Fig. 1.13 (**a–d**) Stage IIIAX: pre-chemotherapy PET/CT scan (axial slices) demonstrating bulky mediastinal disease, pericardial disease, and gastrohepatic lymphadenopathy

ity, especially related to fertility and second cancers, as well as its requirement for hospital admission. The EORTC 20012 study compared ABVD x 8 vs. BEACOPP (four-escalated/four-standard dose) without radiation in 549 high-risk stage III/IV patients. In their preliminary report at a median follow-up of 3.8 years, they found a progression-free survival difference in favor of BEACOPP (72.8 % vs. 83.4 % at 4 years, HR=0.58, p=0.005) [49]. However, there was not a significant overall survival difference (86.7 % vs. 90.3 % at 4 years, HR=0.71, p=0.208). A Cochrane review evaluated the relative benefits of using an escalated BEACOPP-based regimen compared to an ABVD-based regimen in advanced-stage HL patients. In this analysis of five eligible trials, which did not include EORTC 20012, the authors concluded that advanced-stage HL patients have a progression-free, but no clear, overall survival benefit from escalated BEACOPP compared to ABVD [50]. *This patient opted for treatment with ABVD chemotherapy. After two cycles, she had a PET/CT that showed a very good response overall with resolution of all the disease other than the right supraclavicular region and the mediastinum. The mediastinal mass still measured 6.4×4 cm with an SUV that was 3.6, above the level of the liver (Deauville 3). She went on to get four additional cycles of ABVD, and a final PET/CT showed that the mediastinal mass had shrunk further, now measuring 4.6×1.7 cm. The SUV was 2.6, just above the mean liver SUV (2.2). The patient was referred for consideration of radiotherapy after a multidisciplinary review.*

The decision to add radiotherapy after effective chemotherapy in advanced-stage patients is difficult but depends on what chemotherapy was given as well as the anatomic response (CT-based) and metabolic response (PET-based). When using an intensive regimen such as escalated BEACOPP, the role of radiation is quite selective. In the HD12 trial done in the pre-PET era, patients with initially large disease (>5 cm) and those with residual disease after BEACOPP-based chemotherapy were randomly assigned to radiotherapy with 30 Gy or no RT. They found that radiation improved disease control, especially in those patients with CT-detected residual disease [48]. In the GHSG HD15 trial, which compared various schedules/cycles of BEACOPP, radiotherapy was reserved for subjects with PET-positive residual masses that measured at least 2.5 cm [7]. In these patients treated with BEACOPP, PET-negative patients had an impressive 4-year PFS of 91.5 %; however PET-positive patients who were irradiated had a 4-year PFS of 86.1 %. Interestingly, those PET-positive patients that had poor shrinkage by CT (less than 40 %) had an even greater risk of relapse [51]. When less intensive chemotherapy regimens are used, the role of radiation becomes less clear, but indicators such as initial bulk, residual disease on CT, and FDG-avidity are commonly used to argue for the addition of RT to patients in apparent remission after chemotherapy. The EORTC randomized stage III/IV patients in complete remission after treatment with MOPP/AVD chemotherapy to IFRT (30 Gy) or observation. There was no difference with the addition of radiation in patients in a CR [52]. The patients who only achieved a partial response were all radiated with IFRT, and their PFS and OS were similar to those patients in a CR [53]. The authors argued that this equivalence with complete responders argues in favor of radiating sites of residual disease. In this patient, she not only had a residual mass after six cycles of ABVD that was minimally FDG-avid, but her interim PET/CT after two cycles showed only a partial response. Interim PET responses after two cycles of ABVD are actually more predictive than the IPS in advanced-stage patients [54]. The predictive value of PET response after two cycles was confirmed using the Deauville scale, with 1–3 scored as negative and 4–5 as positive. The 3-year PFS was 28 % for those with positive interim scans and 95 % for patients with negative interim scans [55]. The precise way to use interim PET/CTs is still being studied, but her negative interim scan suggests that she will have a good prognosis provided that her residual masses are controlled.

Treatment Field and Technique

Radiotherapy of patients with stage III/IV requires a realistic understanding of how radiation fits into the picture. Patients are generally referred for anatomic residual in a few limited sites in a patient that has achieved a CR everywhere else. The concept of ISRT in the advanced-stage patient abandons the goal of trying to radiate every previously PET-avid site of disease. Rather, RT is focused on the anatomic residual GTV, plus CTV expansions to account for errors in fusion of the pre-chemotherapy scans [23]. Doses have ranged from 20 to 30 Gy in the trials where radiotherapy has been tested in advanced-stage patients in CR. In the modern era, where radiation oncologists are asked to treat residual masses that may or not be PET-avid, 30 Gy is a reasonable choice based on the EORTC and HD15 studies [7, 53]. *In this patient, the CTV encompassed the residual mass as well as the adjacent regions involved initially by PET-avid disease. In order to minimize pulmonary toxicity, the axillae were excluded, especially since they responded completely.* Cardiac toxicity is a difficult problem when there is contiguous extension of the residual disease along (or directly anterior to) the heart. Conformal treatments like IMRT or proton therapy may be considered in order to maximally spare the heart, lung, and breast tissue. In advanced-stage patients who have generally received multiple cycles of multi-agent chemotherapy and who have a slimmer margin of benefit from radiation, careful attention should be paid to organs at risk. Figure 1.14 *shows representative axial images of the CT simulation scan showing CTV (red) and PTV (blue) to the area of mediastinal residual disease but also including the original mediastinal FDG avid sites. The sites omitted were bilateral axillae, pre-cardiac disease, bilateral neck, and abdominal disease.* To support this treatment approach, MD Anderson Cancer Center published a retrospective study on 104 patients with stage III Hodgkin lymphoma and showed an improvement in local control and disease-free survival and overall survival when treating the initially bulky disease sites. This was true mainly for mediastinal locations although benefits were also seen for both bulky axillary and neck locations. Since the

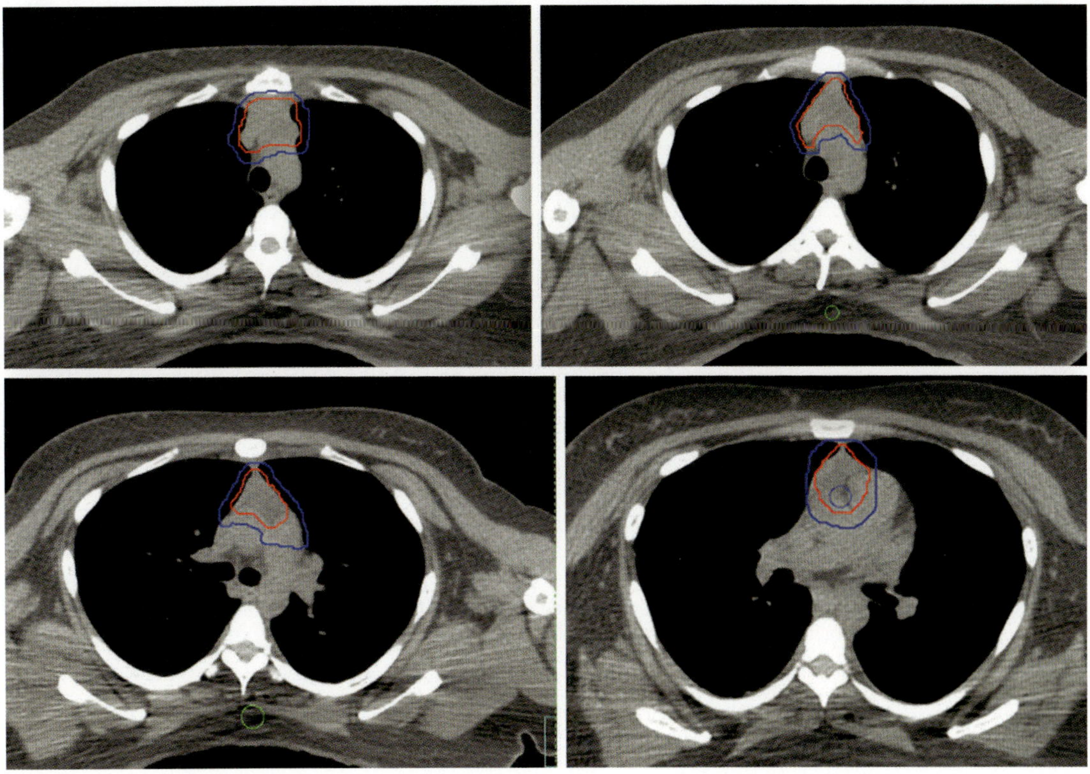

Fig. 1.14 Showing the axial images of the CT simulation, CTV (*red*), and PTV (*blue*)

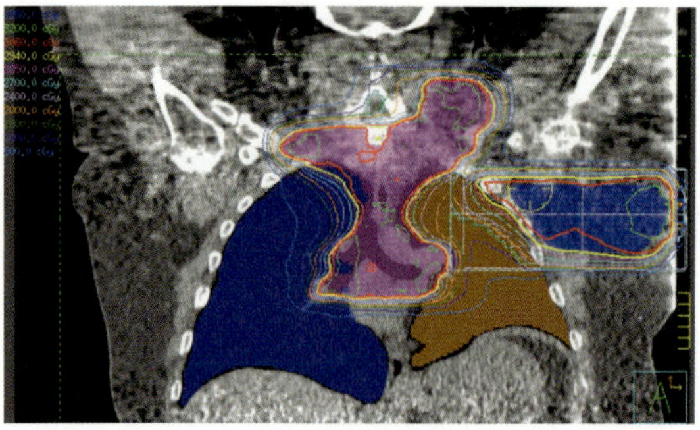

Fig. 1.15 Increased lung dose in patients when attempting to include both mediastinal and axillary diseases

abdominal disease relapse was very low, the authors recommended not to include originally involved abdominal disease [64].

Additionally, adding either the axilla or the pre-cardiac disease will increase the toxicity to the lung and heart and will outweigh the benefit in this case. Figure 1.15 shows how the lung dose will increase substantially when trying to include both mediastinum and axilla, especially when breath hold is not feasible.

Clinical Presentation: Large Volume Disease and Toxicity Limitations, When to Omit Radiation

An 18-year-old woman noticed bilateral cervical adenopathy that did not resolve with antibiotics. An excisional biopsy revealed nodular sclerosing Hodgkin lymphoma, and subsequent PET/CT demonstrated hypermetabolic nodes in the bilateral necks, mediastinum, periesophageal, and left diaphragmatic regions (Fig. 1.16). *An upright CXR confirmed that she had bulky mediastinal disease. She had no B symptoms, her ESR was 2, and her other laboratory studies were unremarkable. Thus, she had stage IIAX classic HL, an unfavorable disease due to the number of sites of disease and bulk. She was put on prednisone while she underwent egg banking, and her cervical adenopathy partially resolved. An echocardiogram revealed normal ejection fraction and no valvular abnormalities. Her pulmonary function tests were unremarkable.*

Her interim PET/CT after three cycles of ABVD showed a complete metabolic response (Deauville 2), but there was still a residual mass in the mediastinum and along the left side of the heart. The left-sided pericardiophrenic disease shrank to 1 × 1 cm. She developed a cough, and pulmonary function tests showed a decrement in her DLCO, so her fourth cycle of ABVD was given without bleomycin, and she was started on prednisone for bleomycin pneumonitis. She was referred for consideration of radiotherapy. In this case, the decision to use combined modality therapy is not so clear.

Cardiac and Pulmonary Toxicity

Figure 1.17 *shows a photon plan using an anterior-posterior/posterior-anterior field arrangement prescribed to 30 Gy. The mean lung dose is 11.6 Gy, and the lung V20 is 30 %. The mean heart dose is 29 Gy*. The risks and benefits of a combined modality approach in this case may favor using chemotherapy alone, especially with regard to acute pulmonary and late cardiovascular risks. The risk of radiation pneumonitis in lymphoma patients is generally lower than the risk in lung cancer patients, who often have significant smoking history and comorbid chronic obstructive pulmonary disease. The risk of pneumonitis in patients treated initially with chemotherapy and consolidative radiation ranges from 3 to 13 % [41, 43]. Koh et al. recommended keeping mean lung doses below 14 Gy and V20 less than 36 % [43]. Fox et al. noted that mean lung doses above 13.5 Gy and V20 over 33.5 % predicted for radiation pneumonitis [40]. Cella et al. found that symptomatic radiation pneumonitis occurred more frequently with a left-lung V30 cutoff of 32 % [56]. *In this patient, the mean lung dose (11.6 Gy) and V20 (30 %) predict a relatively low risk of clinically significant radiation pneumonitis, but one must keep in mind that she had developed symptomatic bleomycin-induced pneumonitis that required a course of steroids. Although bleomycin exposure in particular has not been shown to increase the risk of radiation*

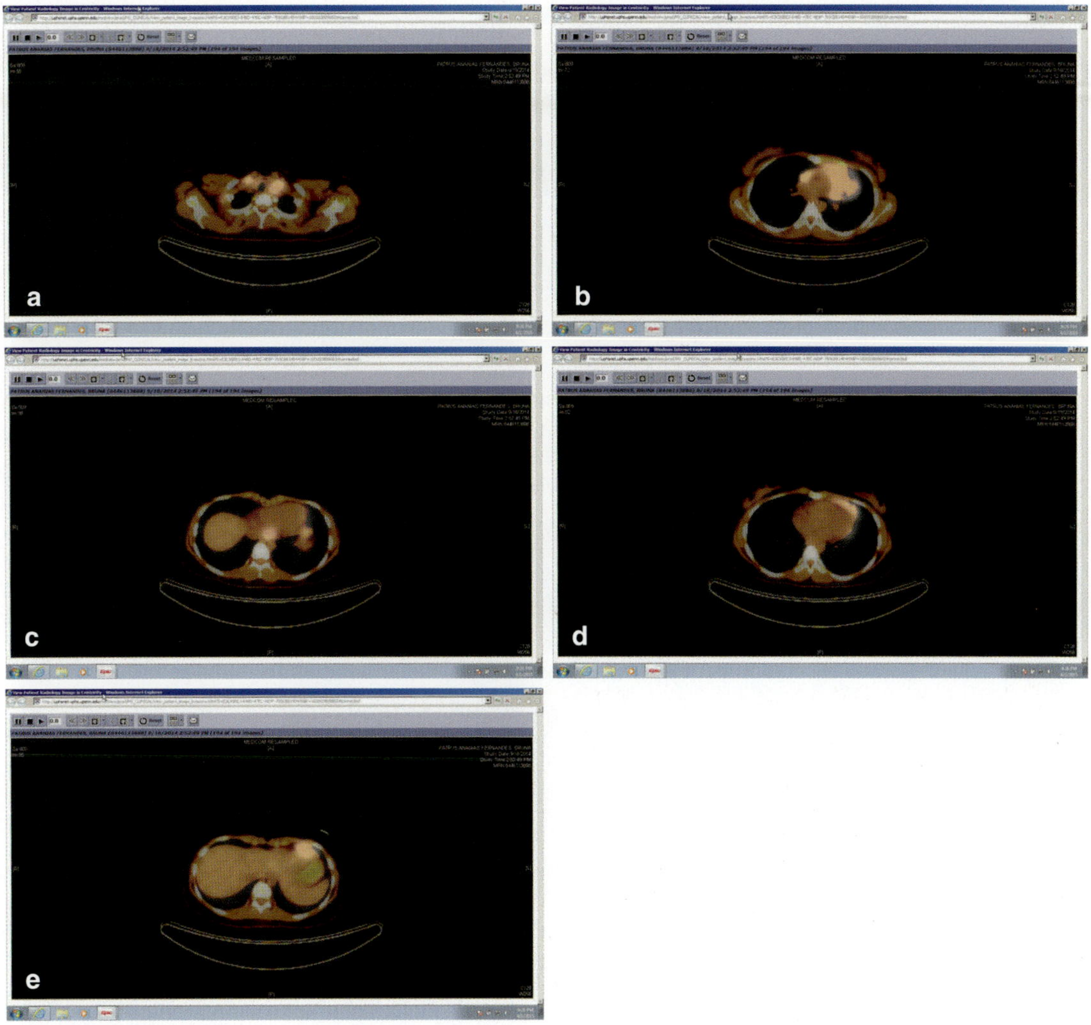

Fig. 1.16 Stage IIAX: pre-chemotherapy PET/CT scan (axial slices) demonstrating bulky mediastinal disease, pericardial disease, and gastrohepatic lymphadenopathy

pneumonitis, it is generally advisable to obtain pulmonary function testing and delay radiotherapy until patients have fully recovered from bleomycin-induced pneumonitis if possible.

In the kilovoltage era, many thought that the heart was radioresistant, but with the advent of megavoltage linear accelerators, it became clear that the heart should be protected when possible. Exactly how much radiation dose the heart can tolerate depends in part on how long patients are followed [57]. In a study of 1,279 Hodgkin patients treated between 1969 and 1998, the rates of clinically significant cardiac events accumulated over time: 2.2 % at 5 years, 4.5 % at 10 years, 9.6 % at 15 years, and 16 % at 20 years [58]. Late cardiac complications include both ischemic and valvular problems. In a study of 1,474 HL survivors treated between 1965 and 1995, the 30-year cumulative incidence of cardiovascular disease was 34.5 % (12.9 % myocardial infarction and 19.7 % valvular problems) [59]. The risk of cardiac complications also depends on how closely you look. Wethal and colleagues reported on a longitudinal study of Hodgkin lymphoma survivors treated with ~40 Gy without cardiac shielding using serial echocardiography at a

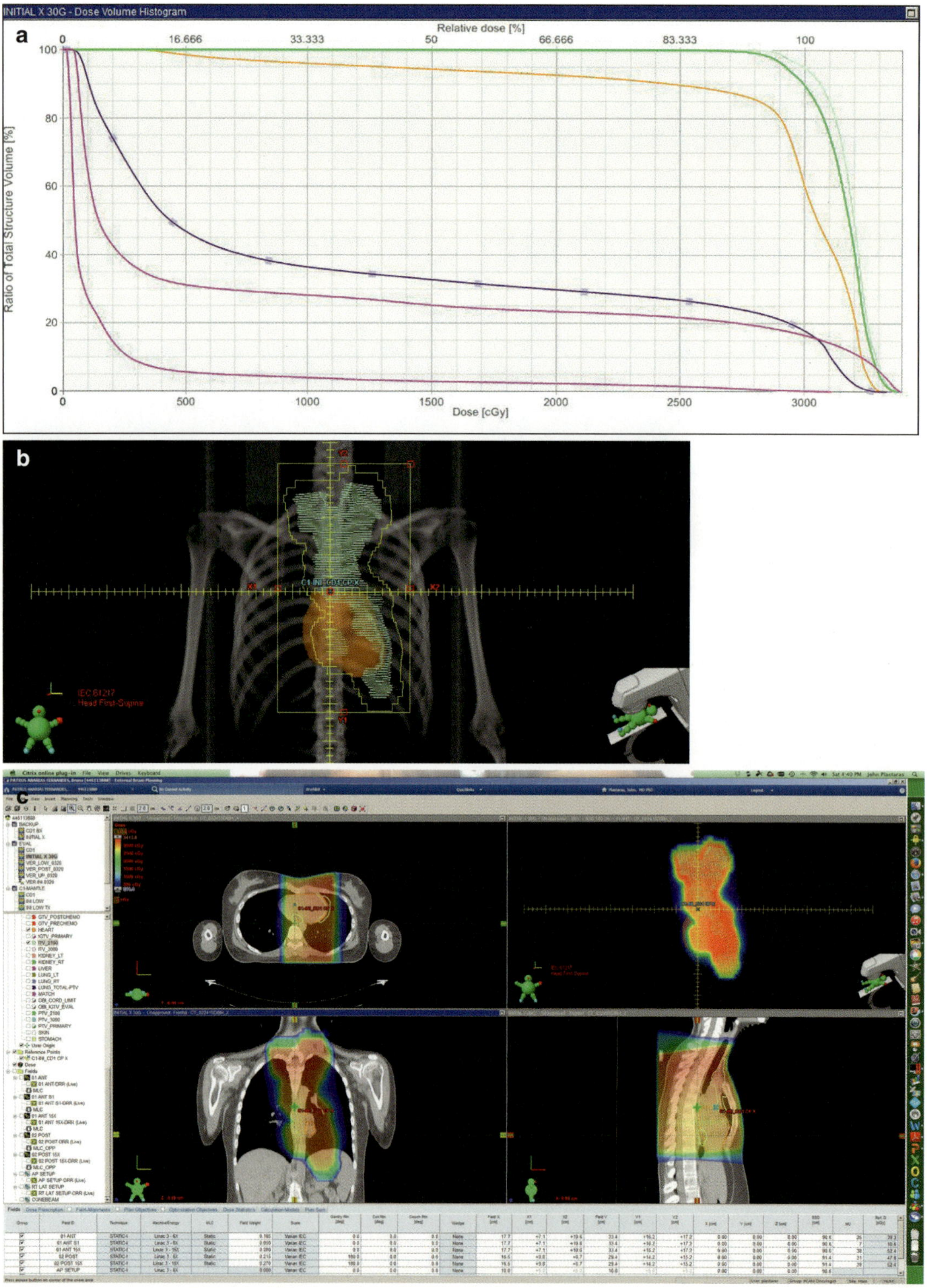

Fig. 1.17 Large volume stage IIAX. Unacceptable AP-PA plan prescribed to 30 Gy: (**a**) DVH demonstrating a high dose to the heart (*orange*, mean heart dose 29 Gy) and borderline acceptable dose to the lungs (*dark purple*) and breast (*pink*). (**b**) AP field beam's eye view showing the CTV (*green*) and heart (*orange*). (**c**) Dose-color wash of AP-PA plan showing axial (*top*) and coronal (*bottom*) views

median of 22 years after treatment. They found that 39 % of survivors had developed late mild to severe aortic stenosis [60]. Some attempts have been made to model the risk of cardiac disease based on dosimetric parameters. The risk of severe valvular problems appears to be correlated with dose, increasing from a factor of 1.4-fold at 30 Gy up to 11.8-fold over 40 Gy [61]. There is a paucity of data that predict toxicity related to partial volumetric parameters in lymphoma survivors; however, mean heart dose has been hypothesized to be a determinant of radiation-related cardiac disease in breast cancer with a relative risk of 7.4 %/Gy [62]. Although this estimate may be flawed based on the methods used to reconstruct implied dose volume histograms on phantoms, there are other data that corroborate the risk of late cardiac toxicity with low-moderate radiation doses. A meta-analysis has linked low to moderate doses of radiation to cardiovascular disease at an estimated excess risk of 2.5 %/Sv [63]. *In this patient, is a mean heart dose of 29 Gy safe? We would argue that such a plan is unacceptable. In an 18-year-old with a highly curable disease, 30-year toxicity is very important. Rather than expose her to excess risk from late radiation complication with the plan shown in* Fig. 1.17, *alternative strategies should be used.*

Although it may be tempting to stop after four cycles given her complete metabolic response after three cycles, the H10 trial suggests that this approach is fraught with risk of a high relapse rate [19]. *This patient was treated with two additional cycles of modified chemotherapy (AVD) without bleomycin due to her pulmonary reaction. The chemotherapy-only arm of the HD6 trial did have good long-term survival, and six cycles of A(B) VD for this young woman with unfavorable risk stage IIA HL are a reasonable alternative to combined-modality therapy.*

Posttreatment Considerations

This patient tolerated the rest of her chemotherapy without complications. She resumed normal menstrual cycles 4 months after finishing therapy. Given the exposure to Adriamycin, it was recommended that she follow a regular exercise routine aimed at cardiovascular health. She did not smoke and was advised not to start as she headed off to college as she followed the recommended survivorship follow-up plan [24].

Conclusions

The management of patients with HL should be customized based on a variety of factors including pathologic, radiologic, and response criteria. Radiation fields and doses have substantially reduced over time as we have learned how to better incorporate radiation with optimized combined modality management. In addition, patient factors including comorbidities, family history, and reliability for follow-up affect management and influence the decision regarding the radiation approach utilized. Unanswered questions remain to further tailor radiotherapy fields and approaches in an effort to define the optimum therapeutic ratio for each patient.

References

1. Terezakis S, Hudson MM, Constine LS. Hodgkin's disease. In: Halperin EC, Constine LS, Tarbell NJ, Kun LE, editors. Pediatric radiation oncology. 5th ed. Philadelphia: Lippincott Williams and Wilkins; 2011. p. 137–65.
2. Jerusalem G, Warland V, Najjar F, et al. Whole-body 18F-FDG PET for the evaluation of patients with Hodgkin's disease and non-Hodgkin's lymphoma. Nucl Med Commun. 1999;20(1):13–20.
3. Gallamini A, Rigacci L, Merli F, et al. The predictive value of positron emission tomography scanning performed after two courses of standard therapy on treatment outcome in advanced stage Hodgkin's disease. Haematologica. 2006;91(4):475–81.
4. Hutchings M, Loft A, Hansen M, et al. FDG-PET after two cycles of chemotherapy predicts treatment failure and progression-free survival in Hodgkin lymphoma. Blood. 2006;107(1):52–9.
5. Moskowitz AJ, Yahalom J, Kewalramani T, et al. Pretransplantation functional imaging predicts outcome following autologous stem cell transplantation for relapsed and refractory Hodgkin lymphoma. Blood. 2010;116(23):4934–7.

6. Friedman DL, Chen L, Wolden S, et al. Dose-intensive response-based chemotherapy and radiation therapy for children and adolescents with newly diagnosed intermediate-risk hodgkin lymphoma: a report from the Children's Oncology Group Study AHOD0031. J Clin Oncol. 2014;32(32):3651–8.
7. Engert A, Haverkamp H, Kobe C, et al. Reduced-intensity chemotherapy and PET-guided radiotherapy in patients with advanced stage Hodgkin's lymphoma (HD15 trial): a randomised, open-label, phase 3 non-inferiority trial. Lancet. 2012;379(9828):1791–9.
8. Kobe C, Dietlein M, Franklin J, et al. Positron emission tomography has a high negative predictive value for progression or early relapse for patients with residual disease after first-line chemotherapy in advanced-stage Hodgkin lymphoma. Blood. 2008;112(10):3989–94.
9. Barrington SF, Qian W, Somer EJ, et al. Concordance between four European centres of PET reporting criteria designed for use in multicentre trials in Hodgkin lymphoma. Eur J Nucl Med Mol Imaging. 2010;37(10):1824–33.
10. Smith RS, Chen Q, Hudson MM, et al. Prognostic factors for children with Hodgkin's disease treated with combined-modality therapy. J Clin Oncol. 2003;21(10):2026–33.
11. Specht L. Prognostic factors in Hodgkin's disease. Semin Radiat Oncol. 1996;6(3):146–61.
12. Engert A, Plütschow A, Eich HT, et al. Reduced treatment intensity in patients with early-stage Hodgkin's lymphoma. N Engl J Med. 2010;363(7):640–52.
13. Eghbali H, Brice P, Creemers G, et al. Comparison of three radiation dose levels after EBVP regimen in favorable supradiaphragmatic clinical stages I-II Hodgkin's lymphoma: preliminary results of the EORTC-GELA H9-F trial. Blood. 2005;106(11).
14. Straus DJ. Radiotherapy should be omitted in most patients. Clin Adv Hematol Oncol. 2014;12(4): 247–9.
15. Meyer RM, Gospodarowicz MK, Connors JM, et al. ABVD alone versus radiation-based therapy in limited-stage Hodgkin's lymphoma. N Engl J Med. 2012;366(5):399–408.
16. Herbst C, Rehan FA, Skoetz N, et al. Chemotherapy alone versus chemotherapy plus radiotherapy for early stage hodgkin lymphoma. Cochrane Database Syst Rev. 2011;(2).
17. Koshy M, Rich SE, Mahmood U, Kwok Y. Declining use of radiotherapy in stage I and II Hodgkin's disease and its effect on survival and secondary malignancies. Int J Radiat Oncol Biol Phys. 2012;82(2):619–25.
18. Parikh R, Yahalom J, Talcott J, et al. Early-stage Hodgkin disease: the utilization of radiation therapy and its impact on overall survival. Int J Radiat Oncol Biol Phys. 2014;90(1):S5.
19. Raemaekers JM, Andre MP, Federico M, et al. Omitting radiotherapy in early positron emission tomography-negative stage I/II hodgkin lymphoma is associated with an increased risk of early relapse: clinical results of the preplanned interim analysis of the randomized EORTC/LYSA/FIL H10 trial. J Clin Oncol. 2014;32(12):1188–94.
20. Radford J, Illidge T, Counsell N, Hancock B, Pettengell R, Johnson P, et al. Results of a trial of PET-directed therapy for early-stage Hodgkin's lymphoma. N Engl J Med. 2015;372(17):1598–607.
21. Shahidi M, Kamangari N, Ashley S, Cunningham D, Horwich A. Site of relapse after chemotherapy alone for stage I and II Hodgkin's disease. Radiother Oncol. 2006;78(1):1–5.
22. Girinsky T, van der Maazen R, Specht L, Aleman B, Poortmans P, Lievens Y, et al. Involved node radiotherapy (INRT) in patients with early Hodgkin lymphoma: concepts and guidelines. Radiother Oncol. 2006;79(3):270–7.
23. Specht L, Yahalom J, Illidge T, Berthelsen AK, Constine LS, Eich HT, et al. Modern radiation therapy for Hodgkin lymphoma: field and dose guidelines from the international lymphoma radiation oncology group (ILROG). Int J Radiat Oncol Biol Phys. 2014;89(4):854–62.
24. Ha CS, Hodgson DC, Advani R, et al. ACR appropriateness criteria follow-up of Hodgkin lymphoma. J Am Coll Radiol. 2014;11(11):1026–33.
25. Paumier A, Ghalibafian M, Beaudre A, Ferreira I, Pichenot C, Messai T, et al. Involved-node radiotherapy and modern radiation treatment techniques in patients with Hodgkin lymphoma. Int J Radiat Oncol Biol Phys. 2011;80(1):199–205.
26. Filippi AR, Ciammella P, Piva C, Ragona R, Botto B, Gavarotti P, et al. Involved-site image guided intensity modulated versus 3D conformal radiation therapy in early stage supradiaphragmatic Hodgkin lymphoma. Int J Radiat Oncol Biol Phys. 2014;89(2):370–5.
27. Thomas J, Fermé C, Noordijk EM, Eghbali H, Henry-Amar M. The EORTC-GELA treatment strategy in clinical stages I-II HL: results of the H9-F and H9-U trials. International Symposium on Hodgkin Lymphoma; Cologne, Presentation. 2007.
28. Eich HT, Diehl V, Görgen H, Pabst T, Markova J, Debus J, et al. Intensified chemotherapy and dose-reduced involved-field radiotherapy in patients with early unfavorable Hodgkin's lymphoma: final analysis of the German Hodgkin Study Group HD11 trial. J Clin Oncol. 2010;28(27):4199–206.
29. von Tresckow B, Plütschow A, Fuchs M, Klimm B, Markova J, Lohri A, et al. Dose-intensification in early unfavorable Hodgkin's lymphoma: final analysis of the German Hodgkin Study Group HD14 trial. J Clin Oncol. 2012;30(9):907–13.
30. Advani RH, Hong F, Fisher RI, Bartlett NL, Robinson KS, Gascoyne RD, et al. Randomized phase III trial comparing ABVD plus radiotherapy with the Stanford V regimen in patients with stages I or II locally extensive, bulky mediastinal Hodgkin lymphoma: a subset analysis of the North American Intergroup E2496 Trial. J Clin Oncol. 2015;33(17):1936–42.
31. Ferme C, Eghbali H, Meerwaldt JH, Rieux C, Bosq J, Berger F, et al. Chemotherapy plus involved-field radiation in early-stage Hodgkin's disease. EORTC-

GELA H8 Trial. N Engl J Med. 2007;357(19): 1916–27.
32. Laskar S, Kumar DP, Khanna N, Menon H, Sengar M, Arora B, et al. Radiation therapy for early stage unfavorable Hodgkin lymphoma: is dose reduction feasible? Leuk Lymphoma. 2014;55(10):2356–61.
33. Torok JA, Wu Y, Prosnitz LR, Kim GJ, Beaven AW, Diehl LF, et al. Low-dose consolidation radiation therapy for early stage unfavorable Hodgkin lymphoma. Int J Radiat Oncol Biol Phys. 2015;92(1): 54–9.
34. Josting A, Nogová L, Franklin J, et al. Salvage radiotherapy in patients with relapsed and refractory Hodgkin's lymphoma: a retrospective analysis from the German Hodgkin Lymphoma Study Group. J Clin Oncol. 2005;23(7):1522–9.
35. Gopal AK, Chen R, Smith SE, et al. Durable remissions in a pivotal phase 2 study of brentuximab vedotin in relapsed or refractory Hodgkin lymphoma. Blood. 2015;125(8):1236–43.
36. Younes A, Gopal AK, Smith SE, et al. Results of a pivotal phase II study of brentuximab vedotin for patients with relapsed or refractory Hodgkin's lymphoma. J Clin Oncol. 2012;30(18):2183–9.
37. Younes A, Bartlett NL, Leonard JP, et al. Brentuximab vedotin (SGN-35) for relapsed CD30-positive lymphomas. N Engl J Med. 2010;363(19):1812–21.
38. Gopal AK, Bartlett NL, Forero-Torres A, et al. Brentuximab vedotin in patients aged 60 years or older with relapsed or refractory CD30-positive lymphomas: a retrospective evaluation of safety and efficacy. Leuk Lymphoma. 2014;55(10):2328–34.
39. Plastaras JP, Mesina A, Grover S, et al. Factors for radiation pneumonitis in patients with lymphoma treated with chemotherapy and photon or proton radiation therapy. http://dx.doi.org/10.1016/j.ijrobp.2014.05.2005.
40. Fox AM, Dosoretz AP, Mauch PM, et al. Predictive factors for radiation pneumonitis in Hodgkin lymphoma patients receiving combined-modality therapy. Int J Radiat Oncol Biol Phys. 2012;83(1):277–83.
41. Pinnix CC, Smith GL, Milgrom S, Osborne EM, Reddy JP, Akhtari M, et al. Predictors of radiation pneumonitis in patients receiving intensity modulated radiation therapy for Hodgkin and non-Hodgkin lymphoma. Int J Radiat Oncol Biol Phys. 2015;92(1):175–82.
42. Girinsky T, Pichenot C, Beaudre A, et al. Is intensity-modulated radiotherapy better than conventional radiation treatment and three-dimensional conformal radiotherapy for mediastinal masses in patients with Hodgkin's disease, and is there a role for beam orientation optimization and dose constraints assigned to virtual volumes? Int J Radiat Oncol Biol Phys. 2006;64(1):218–26.
43. Koh ES, Sun A, Tran TH, et al. Clinical dose-volume histogram analysis in predicting radiation pneumonitis in Hodgkin's lymphoma. Int J Radiat Oncol Biol Phys. 2006;66(1):223–8.
44. Moccia AA, Donaldson J, Chhanabhai M, et al. International prognostic score in advanced-stage Hodgkin's lymphoma: altered utility in the modern era. J Clin Oncol. 2012;30(27):3383–8.
45. Santoro A, Bonadonna G, Valagussa P, et al. Long-term results of combined chemotherapy-radiotherapy approach in Hodgkin's disease: superiority of ABVD plus radiotherapy versus MOPP plus radiotherapy. J Clin Oncol. 1987;5(1):27–37.
46. Canellos GP, Anderson JR, Propert KJ, et al. Chemotherapy of advanced Hodgkin's disease with MOPP, ABVD, or MOPP alternating with ABVD. N Engl J Med. 1992;327(21):1478–84.
47. Diehl V, Franklin J, Pfreundschuh M, et al. Standard and increased-dose BEACOPP chemotherapy compared with COPP-ABVD for advanced Hodgkin's disease. N Engl J Med. 2003;348(24):2386–95.
48. Borchmann P, Haverkamp H, Diehl V, et al. Eight cycles of escalated-dose BEACOPP compared with four cycles of escalated-dose BEACOPP followed by four cycles of baseline-dose BEACOPP with or without radiotherapy in patients with advanced-stage Hodgkin's lymphoma: final analysis of the HD12 trial of the German Hodgkin Study Group. J Clin Oncol. 2011;29(32):4234–42.
49. Carde P, Karrasch M, Fortpied C, et al. ABVD (8 cycles) versus BEACOPP (4 escalated cycles ≥ 4 baseline) in stage III-IV high-risk Hodgkin lymphoma (HL): first results of EORTC 20012 Intergroup randomized phase III clinical trial. J Clin Oncol. 2012;30(Suppl):510s, abstr 8002.
50. Bauer K, Skoetz N, Monsef I, et al. Comparison of chemotherapy including escalated BEACOPP versus chemotherapy including ABVD for patients with early unfavourable or advanced stage Hodgkin lymphoma. Cochrane Database Syst Rev. 2011;8:CD007941.
51. Kobe C, Kuhnert G, Kahraman D, et al. Assessment of tumor size reduction improves outcome prediction of positron emission tomography/computed tomography after chemotherapy in advanced-stage Hodgkin lymphoma. J Clin Oncol. 2014;32(17):1776–81.
52. Aleman BM, Raemaekers JM, Tirelli U, et al. Involved-field radiotherapy for advanced Hodgkin's lymphoma. N Engl J Med. 2003;348(24):2396–406.
53. Aleman BM, Raemaekers JM, Tomiŝiĉ R, et al. Involved-field radiotherapy for patients in partial remission after chemotherapy for advanced Hodgkin's lymphoma. Int J Radiat Oncol Biol Phys. 2007;67(1):19–30.
54. Gallamini A, Hutchings M, Rigacci L, et al. Early interim 2-[18F]fluoro-2-deoxy-D-glucose positron emission tomography is prognostically superior to international prognostic score in advanced-stage Hodgkin's lymphoma: a report from a joint Italian-Danish study. J Clin Oncol. 2007;25(24):3746–52.
55. Gallamini A, Barrington SF, Biggi A, et al. The predictive role of interim positron emission tomography for Hodgkin lymphoma treatment outcome is confirmed using the interpretation criteria of the Deauville five-point scale. Haematologica. 2014;99(6):1107–13.

56. Cella L, Liuzzi R, D'Avino V, et al. Pulmonary damage in Hodgkin's lymphoma patients treated with sequential chemo-radiotherapy: predictors of radiation-induced lung injury. Acta Oncol. 2014;53(5):613–9.
57. Hodgson DC. Late effects in the era of modern therapy for Hodgkin lymphoma. Hematology Am Soc Hematol Educ Program. 2011;2011:323–9.
58. Galper SL, Yu JB, Mauch PM, et al. Clinically significant cardiac disease in patients with Hodgkin lymphoma treated with mediastinal irradiation. Blood. 2011;117(2):412–8.
59. Aleman BM, van den Belt-Dusebout AW, De Bruin ML, et al. Late cardiotoxicity after treatment for Hodgkin lymphoma. Blood. 2007;109(5):1878–86.
60. Wethal T, Lund MB, Edvardsen T, et al. Valvular dysfunction and left ventricular changes in Hodgkin's lymphoma survivors. A longitudinal study. Br J Cancer. 2009;101(4):575–81.
61. Cutter DJ, Schaapveld M, Darby SC, et al. Risk of valvular heart disease after treatment for Hodgkin lymphoma. J Natl Cancer Inst. 2015;107(4):djv 008.
62. Darby SC, Ewertz M, McGale P, et al. Risk of ischemic heart disease in women after radiotherapy for breast cancer. N Engl J Med. 2013;368(11):987–98.
63. Little MP, Azizova TV, Bazyka D, et al. Systematic review and meta-analysis of circulatory disease from exposure to low-level ionizing radiation and estimates of potential population mortality risks. Environ Health Perspect. 2012;120(11):1503–11.
64. Phan J, Mazloom A, Abboud M, Salehpour M, Reed V, Zreik T, Shihadeh F, Fisher C, Wogan C, Dabaja BS. Consolidative radiation therapy for stage III Hodgkin lymphoma in patients who achieve complete response after ABVD chemotherapy. Am J Clin Oncol. 2011;34(5):499–505. doi:10.1097/COC.0b013e3181f477a8.

Diffuse Large B-Cell Lymphoma

2

N. George Mikhaeel and Lena Specht

Abstract

In this chapter, illustrative cases of diffuse large B-cell lymphoma (DLBCL) are presented, followed by a discussion of the appropriate evaluation and management, with a focus on the role of radiotherapy.

Clinical Presentation: Combined Modality Therapy for Early-Stage Diffuse Large B-Cell Lymphoma

A 34-year-old man with no prior morbidities or admissions to a hospital noticed a swelling in the right side of the neck in the beginning of January 2012. He was referred to an ENT surgeon in March 2012. On clinical examination the patient had a 5×3×2 cm lymph node in the right submandibular region. No other abnormalities. No B symptoms. Performance status 0.

N.G. Mikhaeel, MD (✉)
Department of Clinical Oncology and Radiotherapy, Guy's & St Thomas' NHS Foundation Trust and King's Health Partners Academic Health Sciences Centre, Westminster Bridge Road, London SE1 7EH, UK
e-mail: George.Mikhaeel@gstt.nhs.uk

L. Specht, MD, PhD
Department of Oncology and Hematology, Rigshospitalet, University of Copenhagen, Blegdamsvej 9, Copenhagen 2100, Denmark
e-mail: lena.specht@regionh.dk

Pathology

An enlarged lymph node was removed for microscopic examination. It showed a lymph node with totally effaced architecture, dominated by diffuse proliferation of large centroblastic cells with vesicular nuclei, sometimes with membrane-bound nucleoli. Scattered mitoses and apoptotic cells. Scattered reactive lymphocytes. The tumor cells were positive for CD20, CD79a, CD10, BCL2, CD38, and in focal areas for CD30. They were negative for CD3, CD5, CD15, CD23, CD43, and Cyclin D1. Ki-67 was 70 %. A diagnosis of diffuse large B-cell lymphoma (DLBCL), centroblastic variant, and germinal center B-cell-like (GCB) type was made.

There are three common morphologic variants of DLBCL, centroblastic, immunoblastic, and anaplastic [1]. The centroblastic variant is the most common one. Gene expression profiling has identified two subgroups of DLBCL, germinal center B-cell-like (GCB), and activated peripheral B-cell-like (ABC) [2–4]. The GCB-subgroup has a better prognosis than the ABC-subgroup also with modern rituximab-containing chemotherapy

B.S. Dabaja, A.K. Ng (eds.), *Radiation Therapy in Hematologic Malignancies*,
DOI 10.1007/978-3-319-42615-0_2

[5]. Gene profiling studies of the tumor microenvironment have also shown prognostic influence of the nonmalignant cell populations [5]. Immunophenotypical subdivision into GCB and non-GCB has been proposed by several groups [6–10]. CD10 positivity is invariably associated with the GCB type. However, the immunophenotypical subdivisions have not consistently been shown to be prognostic, and they have not gained wide use in the clinical management of patients [11]. CD20 is virtually always positive, and it is the basis for the effect of anti-CD20 antibodies. BCL2 occurs in 20–30 % of cases and may indicate transformation from a follicular lymphoma, but it does not seem to have prognostic importance, at least in the GCB-subgroup [8]. The proliferation fraction as detected by Ki67 staining is usually high (well over 40 %) and may be greater than 90 %. However, in most studies it did not show prognostic importance [7, 12, 13]. Recent research has demonstrated a particularly poor prognosis if there is *both* MYC translocation *and* BCL2 or BCL6 expression, so-called double hit [14–16]. MYC and BCL6 were not performed in the present patient.

Staging and Prognostic Factors

The patient was referred to a hematological department and was staged with clinical examination, blood tests, whole-body PET/CT, and bone marrow biopsy. An enlarged PET+ lymph node measuring 3 cm in largest diameter was found in the right side of the neck close to the site where the diagnostic lymph node was removed (see Fig. 2.1). *The largest diameter of the combined conglomerate of the involved lymph nodes was less than 7.5 cm. No other pathological lesions were found. LDH was normal. The bone marrow biopsy was negative. The patient was therefore in stage IA according to the Ann Arbor classification* [17] *with involvement solely in the right upper neck.*

Prognostic indices have been developed for aggressive lymphomas. This patient had no risk factors according to the International Prognostic Index (IPI) (risk factors: Ann Arbor stage III–IV, >1 extranodal site, high LDH, age >60 years, performance status ≥2 (ECOG)) [18], *according to the age-adjusted IPI (risk factors: Ann Arbor stage III–IV, high LDH, performance status ≥2 (ECOG))* [18], *and according to the modified IPI for early-stage disease (risk factors: age >60 years, stage II disease, high LDH, performance status ≥2 (ECOG))* [19]. *Bulky disease is usually defined as 7.5 cm. Therefore, this patient had localized non-bulky disease, stage IA, with no risk factors.*

Treatment Management

The patient was treated with three cycles of R-CHOP (rituximab, cyclophosphamide, adriamycin, vincristine, prednisone) given every 3 weeks. After this, the patient was treated with radiation therapy (RT) to the initially involved lymphoma volume (involved site radiotherapy (ISRT) [20]*) to a dose of 30 Gy given in 15 fractions with five fractions per week. Apart from some pain on swallowing, which was treated with paracetamol, he had no acute side effects. PET/CT scanning performed 2 months after the end of RT showed complete metabolic response. On CT a small residual node measuring 1.2 × 0.7 cm could be seen in the right upper neck. The patient has since been seen for regular follow-up. There has been no sign of recurrence for 2½ years.*

Brief systemic treatment with immunochemotherapy plus ISRT is an excellent treatment for patients with low-risk, non-bulky, early-stage DLBCL with a 2-year progression-free and overall survival over 90 % [21]. Randomized trials testing the value of RT are only available from the pre-rituximab era [19, 22–24]. They have been criticized for many reasons [25], and they are of limited interest after the introduction of rituximab.

The NCCN Guidelines mention as an alternative six cycles of R-CHOP with or without subsequent ISRT [26]. Full chemotherapy is probably advisable in patients with risk factors, such as bulky disease or an elevated LDH, although no randomized trials exist to support this. However, full chemotherapy comes at the price of an

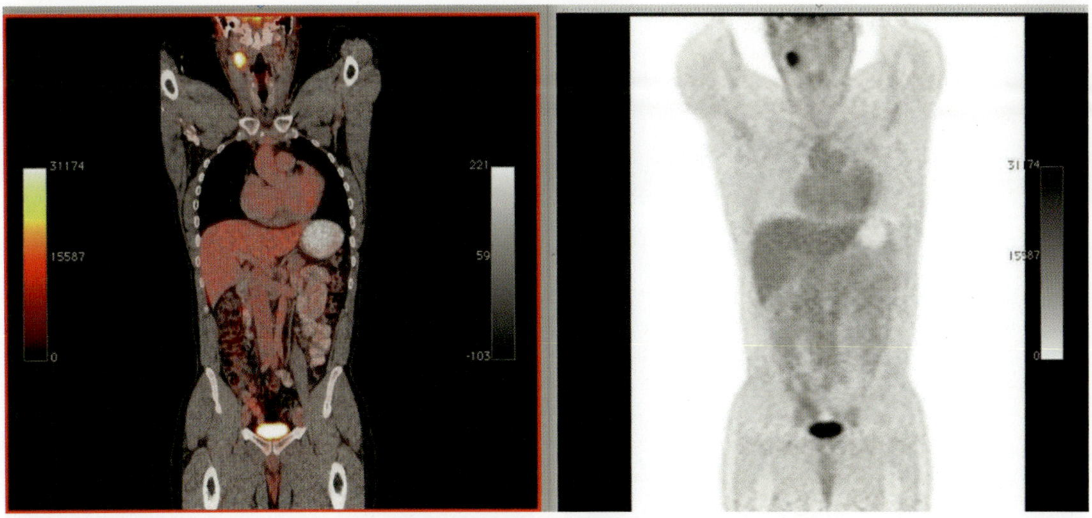

Fig. 2.1 Pre-chemotherapy-staging PET/CT scan of patient with early-stage diffuse large B-cell lymphoma

increased risk of cardiac failure from anthracyclines [27]. Even with full chemotherapy, omission of RT will lead to a decrease in the chance of durable local control [28].

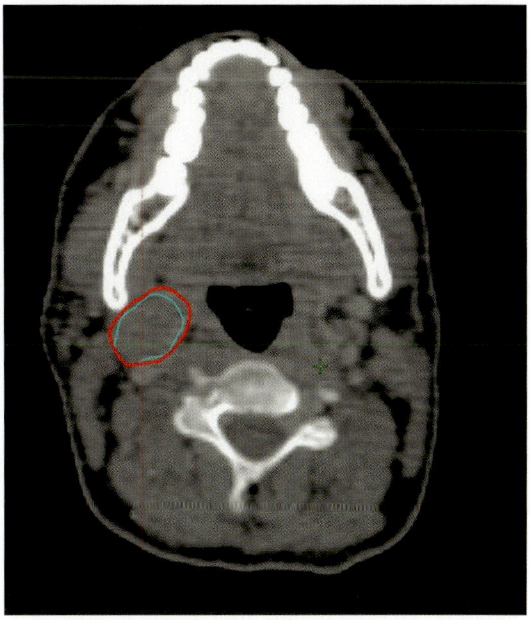

Fig. 2.2 Pre-chemotherapy PET/CT scan. PET+ volume: *light blue*. GTV: *red*

Treatment Volume and Technique

In the combined modality setting, modern immunochemotherapy is relied upon to eradicate microscopic disease. RT is delivered as consolidation therapy after the systemic chemotherapy. The detailed guidelines on modern RT for nodal non-Hodgkin lymphoma have been recently published by the International Lymphoma Radiation Oncology Group (ILROG) [20].

The clinical target volume (CTV) that should be irradiated to the prescribed dose should encompass the initial macroscopically involved lymphoma volume (GTV) before any intervention. The pre-chemotherapy-staging PET/CT scan of the patient is seen in Fig. 2.1. The GTV was contoured on this scan, the PET positive volume was contoured in light blue, and the whole GTV as seen on CT was contoured in red (see Fig. 2.2).

The patient's planning CT scan after the end of the immunochemotherapy was performed with the patient in roughly the same position as the pre-chemotherapy-staging PET/CT scan. This allowed fusion of the pre- and post-chemotherapy images, and the GTV was imported to the planning CT image (*see* Fig. 2.3).

The CTV was then contoured on the post-chemotherapy, planning CT scan using information from the pre-chemotherapy PET/CT scan, but

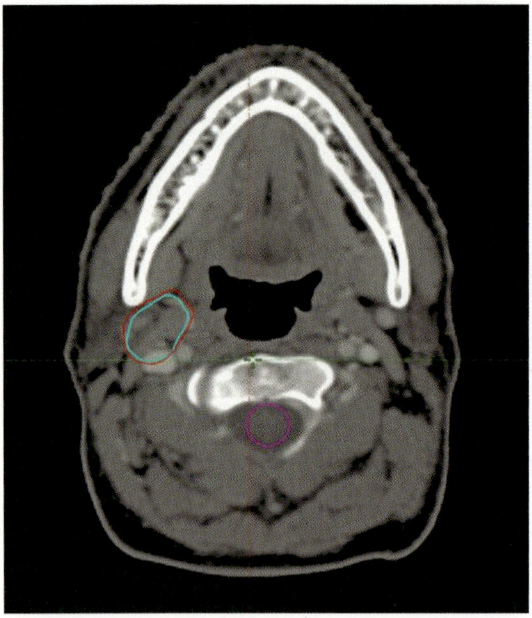

Fig. 2.3 Post-chemotherapy-planning CT scan: Pre-chemo GTV: *red*. Pre-chemo PET+ GTV: *light blue*. (Pre- and post-chemotherapy images were fused with some adjustment for slightly different positions in the two images)

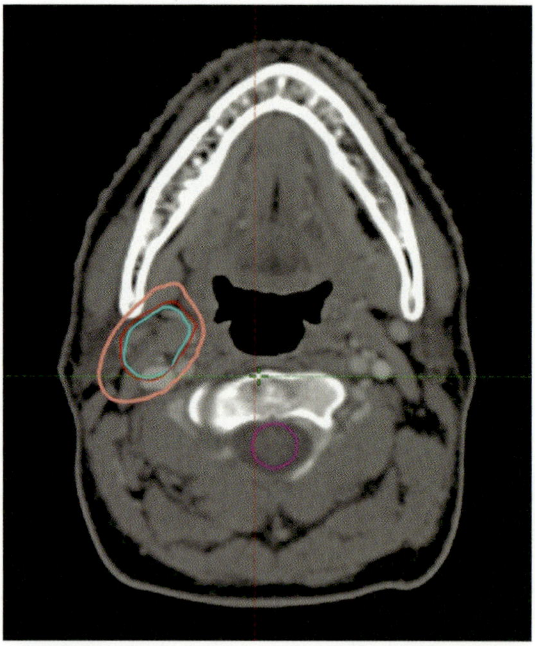

Fig. 2.4 Post-chemotherapy-planning CT scan. CTV: *pink*. Pre-chemotherapy GTV: *red*. Pre-chemotherapy PET + volume: *light blue*

taking into account tumor shrinkage and other anatomic changes. The CTV encompasses the GTV and the tissue volume which contained the lymph node, which was removed for diagnosis. The CTV was modified to account for anatomical changes during chemotherapy, excluding normal structures such as muscles that were clearly never involved. The CTV was also modified and sometimes enlarged to account for uncertainties in the image fusion and the position of the patient. The CTV in this patient is shown in pink in Fig. 2.4.

As there is very little movement in the neck, no internal target volume (ITV) was contoured. A planning target volume was created adding a margin of 5 mm to the CTV to account for setup uncertainties in patient positioning and alignment of the beams during treatment planning and through all treatment sessions, see Fig. 2.5.

Treatment planning was then performed, using volumetric arc treatment, and the prescribed dose volume conforms excellently to the PTV (*see* Fig. 2.6*a–c*).

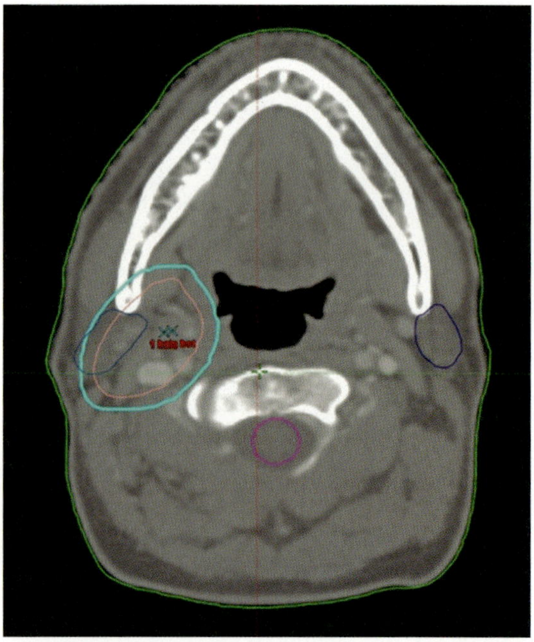

Fig. 2.5 Post-chemotherapy-planning CT scan. CTV: *pink*. PTV: *Light blue*

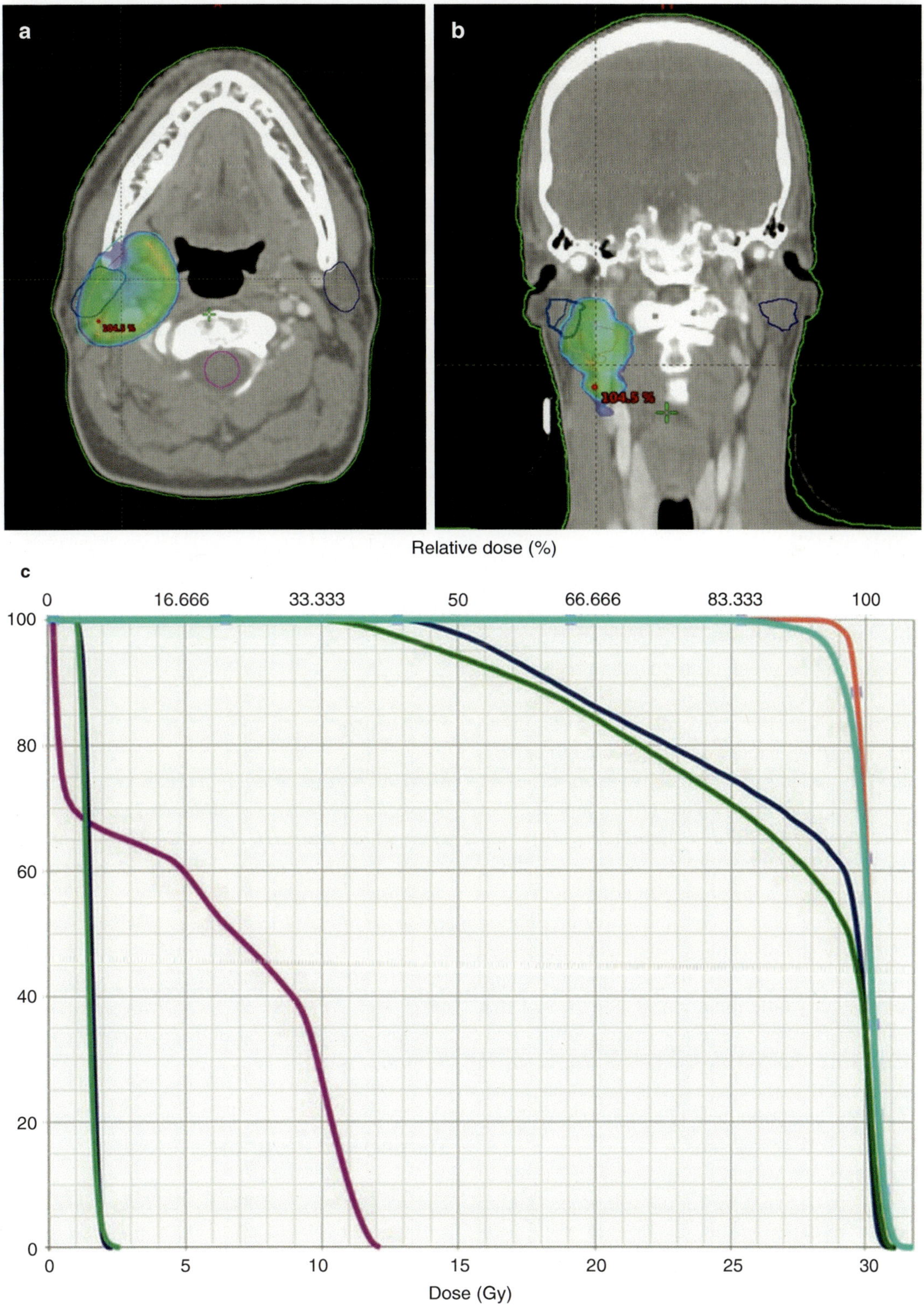

Fig. 2.6 (**a**) Treatment plan, showing doses above 95 % of prescribed dose. (**b**) Treatment plan in coronal view. (**c**) Dose/volume histogram. CTV: *pink*. PTV: *light blue*. Spinal cord: *purple*. *Right and left* parotids: *dark blue*. *Right and left* submandibular gland: *green*

The prescribed radiation dose was 30 Gy in 15 fractions with five fractions per week. The choice of dose was based on the large prospective, randomized trial from the United Kingdom, showing no difference between doses of 30 Gy and 40 Gy in high-grade lymphomas [29].

Posttreatment Considerations

As can be seen from the treatment plan, some of the right side of the pharynx will receive close to the prescribed dose. This means that, when the patient is about 1 week into the treatment, some pain and discomfort may be elicited from this area, in particular when the patient eats. This condition should be treated with analgesics. It is an acute side effect, and it is expected to resolve about 2 weeks after the end of therapy.

The lymphoma was originally located very close to the right parotid and submandibular glands; hence, particular attention was given to spare these glands as much as possible.

About 50 % of the right submandibular gland receives the prescribed dose of 30 Gy. Fortunately, the submandibular gland tolerates doses up to 36 Gy, and the patient is not expected to experience any reduction in the saliva from the right submandibular gland. The left submandibular gland receives very little radiation.

About 80 % of the right parotid receives 26 Gy or more, which is the constraint normally used in head and neck cancer, and the saliva production from these glands will be somewhat decreased after RT. However, as the left parotid gland receives very little radiation, it is expected that there will be very little xerostomia after treatment. Still, the patient should be instructed in good oral hygiene and regular dental examinations. The radiation dose is so low that osteoradionecrosis is not an issue.

Most patients like this one, who are treated to small volumes with conformal techniques and to modest radiation doses, experience very little long term side effects from the treatment. As mentioned above, a patient like this one, with stage IA DLBCL, GCB type, no risk factors and no bulky disease, has a very good chance (over 90 %) of being permanently cured with brief immunochemotherapy followed by ISRT to 30 Gy [21, 28, 30].

Clinical Presentation: Diffuse Large B-Cell Lymphoma, Bulky Abdominal Mass, and Primary Refractory Disease

A 58-year-old female with no previous medical history presented with abdominal pain and nausea. On examination, there was an ill-defined mass in the right upper quadrant. An infection work-up including virology was negative. A CT scan of the abdomen revealed a large abdominal mass 14.3 × 10.3 cm in the axial dimension and 13 cm in the craniocaudal dimension with medial displacement of the right kidney. There was external compression of the inferior vena cava without complete obstruction. A CT-guided percutaneous biopsy showed diffuse large B-cell lymphoma (DLBCL).

Pathology

Microscopic examination of the mediastinal mass biopsy showed sheets of malignant large lymphocytes which were CD79a+, CD20+ confirming B-cell origin. Further immunohistochemistry confirmed activated B-cell subtype of DLBCL, which is MUM1+, BCL2+, BCL6+, p53+, CD30+/−, CD10+/− with proliferation fraction (Ki67) > 90 %. In situ hybridization showed no MYC, IgH, BCL2, or BCL6 rearrangements. The subclassification of DLBCL is discussed under the previous case.

Staging and Prognostic Factors

The patient was referred to the lymphoma team and was staged with clinical examination, blood tests (including CBC, serum biochemistry, LDH), whole-body FDG-PET/CT, and bone marrow biopsy (BMB). PET/CT revealed stage II disease with large abdominal mass spanning over the

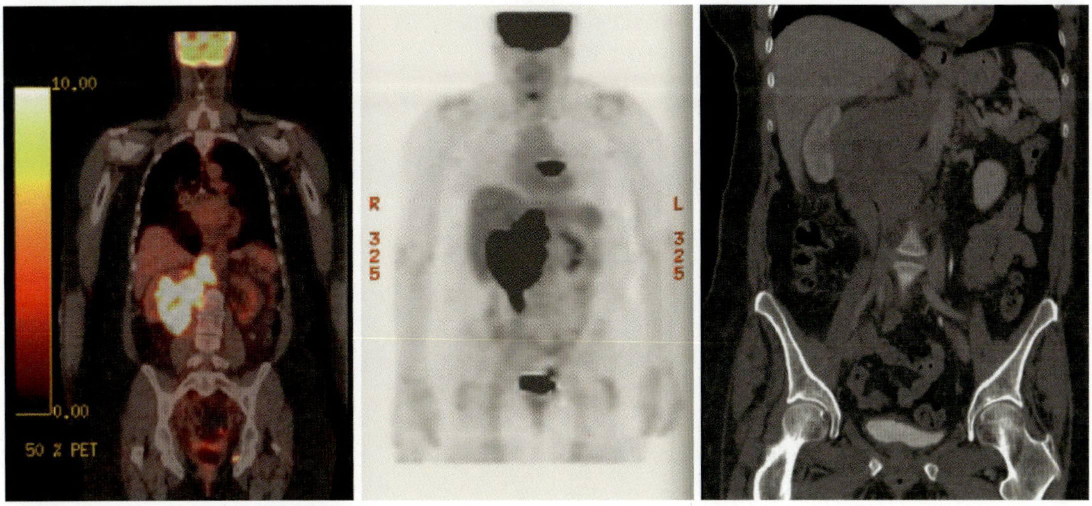

Fig. 2.7 Initial PET/CT and CT abdomen showing right bulky abdominal mass

upper and lower mesenteric area with increased FDG uptake (SUVmax 18.5). There was no evidence of involvement above the diaphragm (see Fig. 2.7*). Prognostic indices are discussed under the previous case.*

Treatment Management

The case was discussed in the lymphoma multidisciplinary meeting (MDM), and the histological diagnosis and the stage of disease (IIA bulky) were confirmed. The International Prognostic Index (IPI) was 1 (elevated LDH), i.e., low-risk group, and the age-adjusted IPI was also 1. A treatment plan was recommended to administer R-CHOP-21 immunochemotherapy given every 3 weeks for six cycles followed by consolidation radiotherapy (RT) to the bulky disease site.

The treatment of choice for advanced DLBCL (stage III+IV or early stage with bulky disease) is immunochemotherapy with R-CHOP-21 (rituximab, cyclophosphamide, doxorubicin, vincristine, prednisone given on day 1 every 21 days) for six cycles. R-CHOP has been shown to be superior to CHOP alone in phase 3 randomized trials [31–33]. Although CHOP given every 14 days (CHOP-14) is superior to CHOP-21, the same does not hold true when rituximab is added. A large phase 3 randomized study showed that there was no difference between R-CHOP-21 and R-CHOP-14 [34]. Eight cycles of chemotherapy have not been found to be better than six cycles [35].

This patient had bulky disease which is a recognized risk factor, although it is not included in the IPI which classifies her as "low risk" (IPI 0–1) [18]. A significant proportion of recurrences occur in previous sites of involvement, particularly the bulky sites. RT to sites of bulky disease has been traditionally used as a consolidation after chemotherapy. Single institution series report significantly better PFS and OS in patients who receive RT to initial bulky sites with local control usually in the region of 90–100 % [28, 36, 37]. However, with improvements in chemotherapy outcome with the addition of rituximab, the value of consolidation RT has been questioned. The MInT study, which tested CHOP-like chemotherapy with or without rituximab in young patients (<60) with good prognosis and showed a definite benefit from adding rituximab in these low-risk patients, was analyzed with respect to the presence of bulky disease. The analysis included 823 patients and revealed that rituximab reduced but did not eliminate the poor prognostic effect of bulky disease [38]. An updated analysis with 6 years follow-up showed that RT seemed to eliminate the adverse effect of bulky disease [39]. More recent evidence from the German RICOVER-60 study suggests that consolidation RT to sites of bulky disease (≥7.5 cm) or extranodal sites improves PFS (3-y PFS 88 v 62 %, $p<0.001$) and OS (3-y OS 90 v 65 %, $p=001$) in R-CHOP-treated patients over 60 years of age [40]. Another German study (UNFOLDER study, DSHNHL 2004–3; ClinicalTrials.gov identifier NCT00278408) evaluated the role of consolidation RT in patients aged 18–60 with an age-adjusted IPI score of 1 or score 0 with bulky tumor (≥7.5 cm). Patients were randomized into 14-day versus 21-day cycles of R-CHOP and consolidative RT versus observation after chemotherapy. The no-RT arms were closed when interim analysis revealed significantly worse EFS with the omission of RT (3-year EFS 65 % vs. 81 % with combined modality therapy) [12th international conference on malignant lymphoma, Lugano, Switzerland, 2013]. The final results of this study are eagerly awaited, but the current evidence supports a role for consolidation RT to sites of bulky (≥7.5 cm) disease. Therefore a recommendation to give consolidation RT for the site of bulky disease was made by the multidisciplinary team.

An alternative approach would be to decide on consolidation RT on the basis of response to full course of chemotherapy as assessed by PET/CT with RT only added if there is evidence of residual FDG activity. This approach has not been tested in clinical trials and there is evidence suggesting that the presence of a residual mass (>2 cm) in the context of complete metabolic response confers an increased risk of relapse compared to patients with no residual mass [41].

The patient received three cycles of R-CHOP at full dose, and a repeat PET/CT scan showed reduction in the size of the mass (10 × 7.5 cm). There was also partial metabolic response with reduction in the FDG uptake (SUVmax 11.7) and the residual uptake was scored as Deauville score 5 (*see* Fig. 2.8). *She received further three cycles and a repeat PET/CT scan after a total of six cycles showed further reduction of the uptake (SUVmax 8, Deauville score 4) and the size of the mass* (*see* Fig. 2.9).

Interim imaging is usually done during a course of chemotherapy to monitor response to treatment. PET/CT is better than CT in showing early response during a course of chemotherapy [42]. Patients with early complete metabolic response tend to have a better outcome than patients with residual activity. However, the difference between the two groups is variable in various studies in DLBCL [43–48]. Treatment modification (response-adapted therapy) based on interim PET (iPET) scanning is currently being tested in several randomized studies in Hodgkin lymphoma and aggressive non-Hodgkin lymphoma. To date there has been no evidence that an early change of treatment improves outcome in DLBCL, and there is no established alternative therapy, so the information of iPET is only of prognostic value and should not be used to change treatment unless it shows no response or progressive disease. Therefore treatment with the most effective regime (R-CHOP) was continued despite the presence of residual activity on iPET.

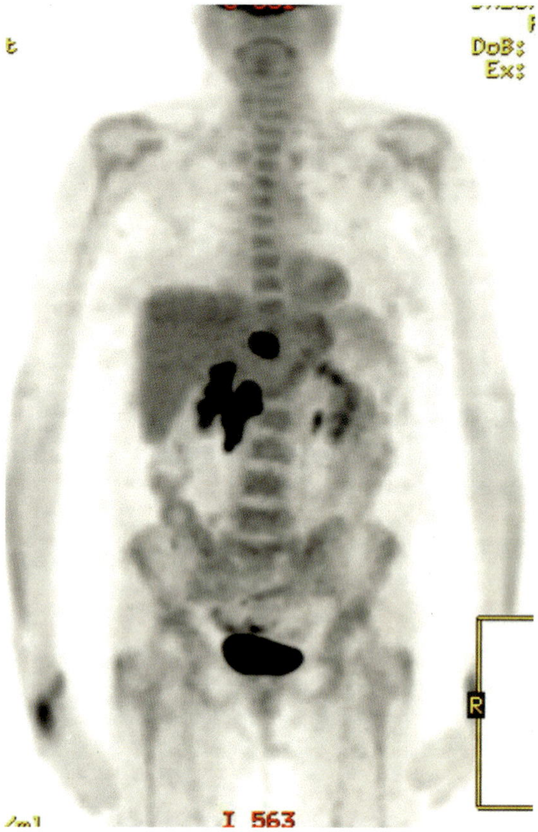

Fig. 2.8 Large residual mass with Deauville 5 after three cycles of R-CHOP

The case was discussed again in the lymphoma MDM, and a plan for salvage treatment was made. Primary refractory DLBCL is usually defined as disease progression or failure to

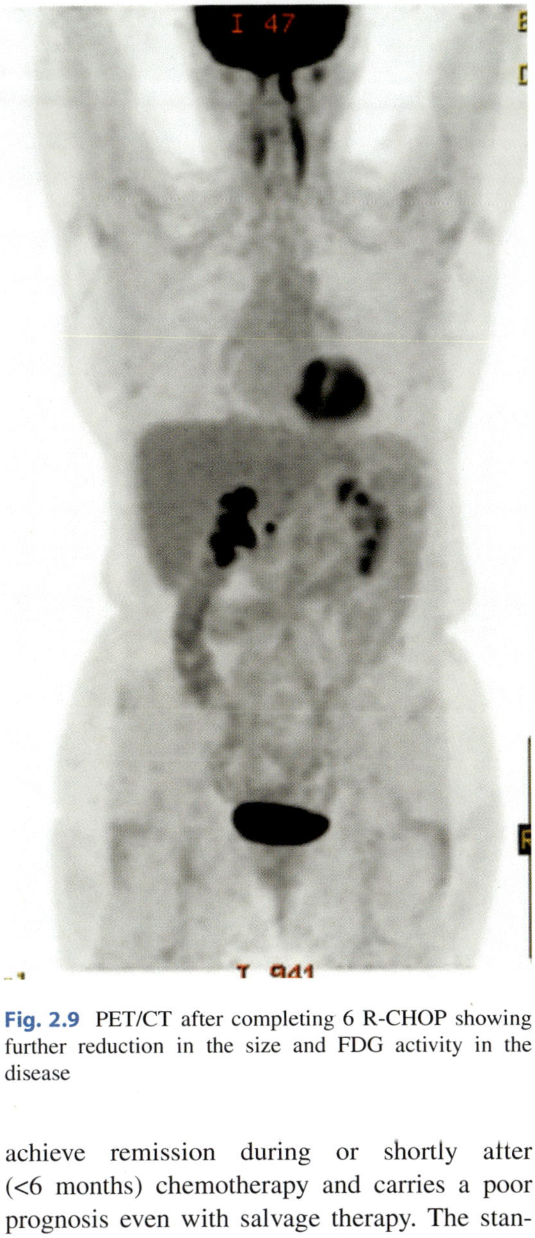

Fig. 2.9 PET/CT after completing 6 R-CHOP showing further reduction in the size and FDG activity in the disease

achieve remission during or shortly after (<6 months) chemotherapy and carries a poor prognosis even with salvage therapy. The standard salvage therapy after failure of R-CHOP involves inducing a remission with a salvage chemotherapy regime followed by high-dose chemotherapy and autologous hematopoietic stem cell transplant (SCT) for fit patients. However, the CORAL study showed that the effectiveness of salvage chemotherapy after R-CHOP is worse than after CHOP as it appears that R-CHOP-failures define a worse prognostic group (response rate was 51 % v 83 % in rituximab-treated and rituximab-naive patients) which translated into a worse outcome (3y EFS of 21 vs. 47 %, respectively) [49]. In addition, patients who relapsed within <1 year and received rituximab in first-line therapy had a particularly poor outcome. None of the commonly used salvage regimes (e.g., DHAP, ESHAP, ICE, GPD, IGEV) has proven to be better than the rest, and there is a need to improve the effectiveness of salvage chemotherapy in rituximab-treated patients.

One approach to improve the outcome of salvage treatment in this poor-prognosis group is to add RT when feasible. This is based on the findings from patterns of failure analysis suggesting that 50–75 % of failures after SCT occur in sites of previous involvement [50]. However, the timing and exact impact of peri-transplant RT are not established. Many clinicians choose to add RT after transplant to ensure control of systemic disease and avoid risk of overlapping toxicity, particularly pneumonitis with mediastinal irradiation. In some situations where response to salvage chemotherapy is suboptimal, RT can be given prior to SCT to induce a remission and improve the chance of successful outcome.

There is no prospective evidence of improved outcome with peri-transplant RT. However, retrospective studies suggest that RT improves local control, PFS, and in at least one recent study OS. A retrospective study from the University of Rochester on 176 patients showed that RT improved disease-specific survival and OS and that the benefit was greater for R-CHOP-treated patients than CHOP-treated patients, presumably because of the more resistant disease in patients for whom R-CHOP failed [51].

The patient received two cycles of R-ICE, a repeat PET/CT scan showed maximal reduction of the size to 6 × 5 cm and an FDG avidity of 5.7 (Deauville 4) (see Fig. 2.10). The patient went on to receive high-dose stem cell transplant. At the completion of transplant and on day 30, a repeated PET scan finally showed a residual soft tissue mass of 4 × 5 cm with an FDG avidity of 3.7 and a Deauville of 3, and patient was declared in remission. At that time the patient was referred to receive consolidation radiotherapy to the abdominal mass (see Fig. 2.11). The patient received 46 Gy to the residual non-FDG-avid mass integrated with 36 Gy to the original disease site. She remains in remission 16 months after completing her radiation with no side effects especially in reference to both kidneys and the liver.

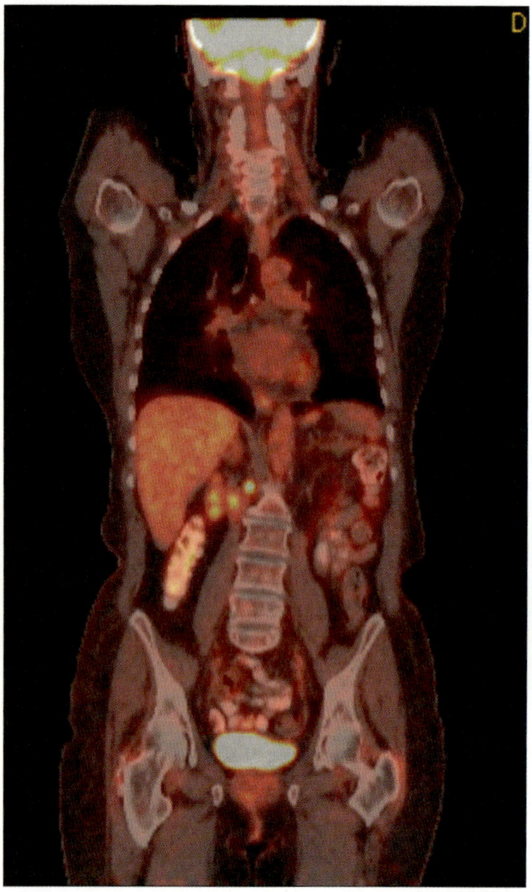

Fig. 2.10 PET/CT after two cycles of RICE showing a mass of 6×5 cm with Deauville of 4

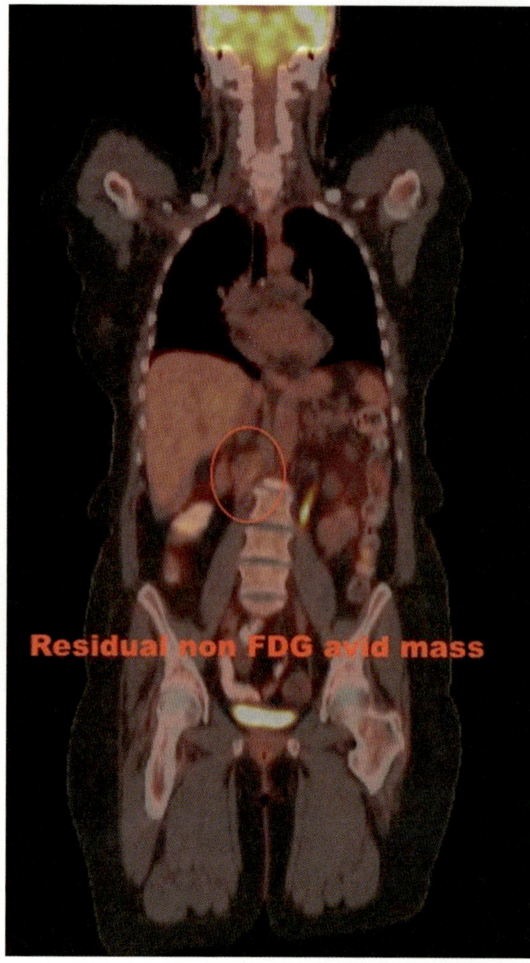

Fig. 2.11 PET/CT showing non-FDG-avid residual mass

Treatment Volume and Technique

Before starting the simulation a renal scan (differential kidney function scan) was performed, in anticipation of inclusion of at least part of the right kidney in the radiation field. This showed the left kidney contributes 60 % of the total renal function versus 40 % in the right kidney. The patient was simulated in a supine position with the arms by the side, using deep inspiration breath-hold technique. The patient was instructed to be NPO (nothing per os) 6 h prior to presenting for her simulation. A CT simulation was obtained from above the diaphragm to the iliac crest. A planning CT scan was acquired and was used to define the radiation volume together with information from the initial staging PET/CT and the post-transplant PET/CT. The aim was to treat the current extent of disease using the concept of involved site radiotherapy (ISRT) as defined by the recently published ILROG guidelines [20]. The CTV was outlined covering the extent of the original mass from the initial imaging while taking into consideration the reduction in volume of the mass returning the kidney back into its normal location. An isotropic margin of 8 mm was added to create the PTV. A small margin to PTV was allowed in this case, owing to the fact we used deep inspiration breath hold that accounted for the internal motion. A plan was created using anteroposterior beam arrangement with an intensity modulated radiation therapy to achieve the best conformity (see Figs. 2.12 and 2.13). A dose of 46 Gy in 20 fractions to the refractory residual mass seen on CT, while the initial site of disease that responded to R-CHOP received 36 Gy in 20 fractions, treated 5 days a week for a total of 4 weeks. The plan allowed ade-

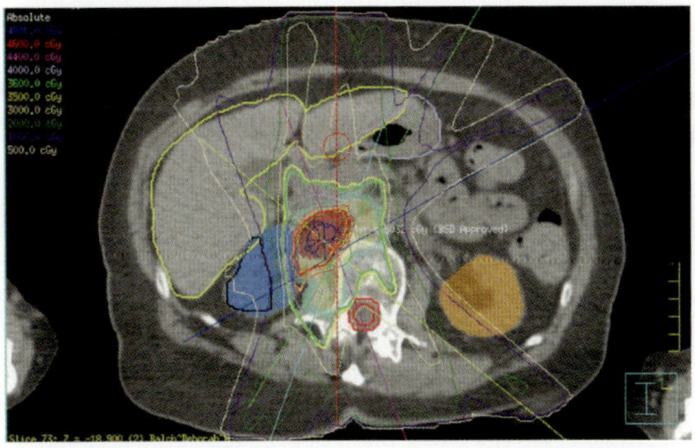

Fig. 2.12 Showing axial images of the IMRT plan

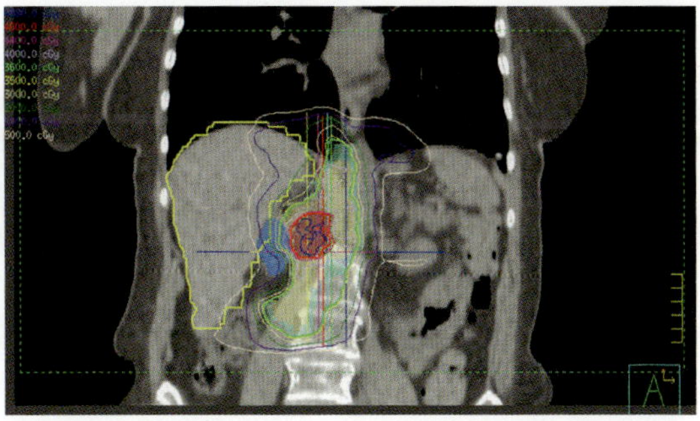

Fig. 2.13 Showing coronal view of the IMRT plan

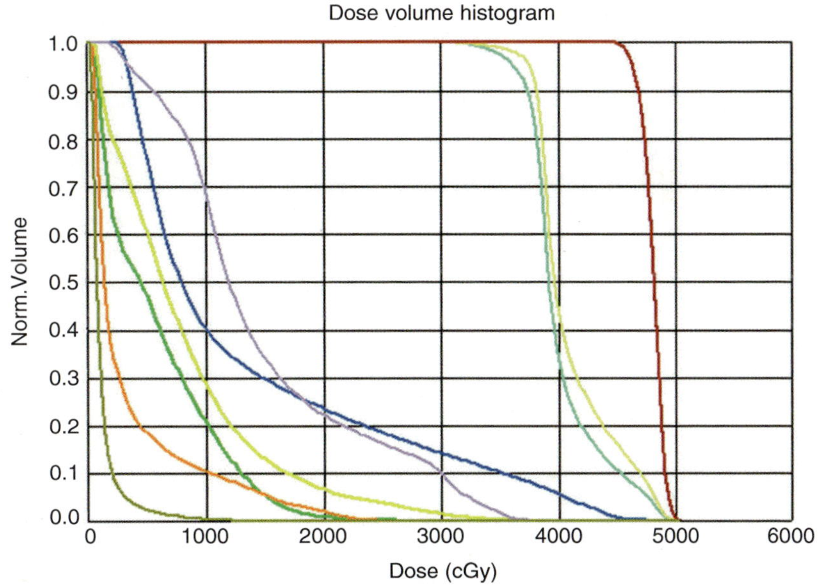

ROI Statistics

Line Type	ROI	Trial or Record	Min.	Max.	Mean	Std. Dev.
	PTV_	BSD Approved	2441.5	5009.0	3999.2	318.4
	CTV 36	BSD Approved	2482.5	5009.0	4084.1	337.2
	integrated boost to 46	BSD Approved	4361.5	5009.0	4798.3	90.8
	Esophagus	BSD Approved	62.5	2610.4	579.7	481.8
	Kidney_R	BSD Approved	225.7	4737.0	1348.5	1178.5
	Kidney_L	BSD Approved	55.7	2462.8	347.6	464.0
	Liver	BSD Approved	50.0	3657.3	797.7	663.4

Fig. 2.14 Dose-volume histogram

quate coverage of PTV (V95: 98.9 %) while minimizing the dose to organs at risk. The right kidney V10 and V20 were 40 % and 22 %, respectively; the left kidney V10 and V20 were 10 % and 2 %, respectively; the liver V20 of 7 % and mean liver dose of 7.9 Gy (see Fig. 2.14).

Although the standard dose for consolidation radiotherapy is usually 30 Gy [29], refractory disease usually requires higher dose to overcome the resistance.

Posttreatment Considerations

Treatment was delivered as planned without interruption. The patient experienced moderate fatigue, which was cumulative and increased as treatment progressed. She also experienced moderate abdominal distension and nausea, which started at the end of the second week, manifesting as discomfort after meals, and was treated with dietary modification and antiemetics.

Acknowledgment I would likwwo express my gratitude to Dr. Anne Kiil Berthelsen from the PET Centre and the Oncology Department and Ms. Deborah Schut from the Section of Radiation Oncology at Rigshospitalet for their help with the PET and radiotherapy figures, respectively.

References

1. Swerdlow SH, Campo E, Harris NL, Jaffe ES, Pileri SA, Stein H, Thiele J, Vardiman JW, editors. WHO Classification of tumours of haematopoietic and lymphoid tissues. Lyon: IARC; 2008.
2. Alizadeh AA, Eisen MB, Davis RE, Ma C, Lossos IS, Rosenwald A, Boldrick JC, Sabet H, Tran T, Yu X, Powell JI, Yang L, Marti GE, Moore T, Hudson Jr J, Lu L, Lewis DB, Tibshirani R, Sherlock G, Chan WC, Greiner TC, Weisenburger DD, Armitage JO, Warnke R, Staudt LM. Distinct types of diffuse large B-cell lymphoma identified by gene expression profiling. Nature. 2000;403:503–11.
3. Rosenwald A, Wright G, Chan WC, Connors JM, Campo E, Fisher RI, Gascoyne RD, Muller-Hermelink HK, Smeland EB, Giltnane JM, Hurt EM, Zhao H, Averett L, Yang L, Wilson WH, Jaffe ES, Simon R, Klausner RD, Powell J, Duffey PL, Longo DL, Greiner TC, Weisenburger DD, Sanger WG, Dave BJ, Lynch JC, Vose J, Armitage JO, Montserrat E, Lopez-Guillermo A, Grogan TM, Miller TP, LeBlanc M, Ott G, Kvaloy S, Delabie J, Holte H, Krajci P, Stokke T, Staudt LM. The use of molecular profiling to predict survival after chemotherapy for diffuse large-B-cell lymphoma. N Engl J Med. 2002;346:1937–47.
4. Shipp MA, Ross KN, Tamayo P, Weng AP, Kutok JL, Aguiar RC, Gaasenbeek M, Angelo M, Reich M, Pinkus GS, Ray TS, Koval MA, Last KW, Norton A, Lister TA, Mesirov J, Neuberg DS, Lander ES, Aster JC, Golub TR. Diffuse large B-cell lymphoma outcome prediction by gene-expression profiling and supervised machine learning. Nat Med. 2002;8:68–74.
5. Lenz G, Wright G, Dave SS, Xiao W, Powell J, Zhao H, Xu W, Tan B, Goldschmidt N, Iqbal J, Vose J, Bast M, Fu K, Weisenburger DD, Greiner TC, Armitage JO, Kyle A, May L, Gascoyne RD, Connors JM, Troen G, Holte H, Kvaloy S, Dierickx D, Verhoef G, Delabie J, Smeland EB, Jares P, Martinez A, Lopez-Guillermo A, Montserrat E, Campo E, Braziel RM, Miller TP, Rimsza LM, Cook JR, Pohlman B, Sweetenham J, Tubbs RR, Fisher RI, Hartmann E, Rosenwald A, Ott G, Muller-Hermelink HK, Wrench D, Lister TA, Jaffe ES, Wilson WH, Chan WC, Staudt LM. Stromal gene signatures in large-B-cell lymphomas. N Engl J Med. 2008;359:2313–23.
6. Choi NC, Timothy AR, Kaufman SD, Carey RW, Aisenberg AC. Low dose fractionated whole body irradiation in the treatment of advanced non-Hodgkin's lymphoma. Cancer. 1979;43:1636–42.
7. Colomo L, Lopez-Guillermo A, Perales M, Rives S, Martinez A, Bosch F, Colomer D, Falini B, Montserrat E, Campo E. Clinical impact of the differentiation profile assessed by immunophenotyping in patients with diffuse large B-cell lymphoma. Blood. 2003;101:78–84.
8. Hans CP, Weisenburger DD, Greiner TC, Gascoyne RD, Delabie J, Ott G, Muller-Hermelink HK, Campo E, Braziel RM, Jaffe ES, Pan Z, Farinha P, Smith LM, Falini B, Banham AH, Rosenwald A, Staudt LM, Connors JM, Armitage JO, Chan WC. Confirmation of the molecular classification of diffuse large B-cell lymphoma by immunohistochemistry using a tissue microarray. Blood. 2004;103:275–82.
9. Meyer PN, Fu K, Greiner TC, Smith LM, Delabie J, Gascoyne RD, Ott G, Rosenwald A, Braziel RM, Campo E, Vose JM, Lenz G, Staudt LM, Chan WC, Weisenburger DD. Immunohistochemical methods for predicting cell of origin and survival in patients with diffuse large B-cell lymphoma treated with rituximab. J Clin Oncol. 2011;29:200–7.
10. Muris JJ, Meijer CJ, Vos W, Van Krieken JH, Jiwa NM, Ossenkoppele GJ, Oudejans JJ. Immunohistochemical profiling based on Bcl-2, CD10 and MUM1 expression improves risk stratification in patients with primary nodal diffuse large B cell lymphoma. J Pathol. 2006;208:714–23.
11. Gutierrez-Garcia G, Cardesa-Salzmann T, Climent F, Gonzalez-Barca E, Mercadal S, Mate JL, Sancho JM, Arenillas L, Serrano S, Escoda L, Martinez S, Valera A, Martinez A, Jares P, Pinyol M, Garcia-Herrera A, Martinez-Trillos A, Gine E, Villamor N, Campo E, Colomo L, Lopez-Guillermo A. Gene-expression profiling and not immunophenotypic algorithms predicts prognosis in patients with diffuse large B-cell lymphoma treated with immunochemotherapy. Blood. 2011;117:4836–43.
12. Saez AI, Saez AJ, Artiga MJ, Perez-Rosado A, Camacho FI, Diez A, Garcia JF, Fraga M, Bosch R, Rodriguez-Pinilla SM, Mollejo M, Romero C, Sanchez-Verde L, Pollan M, Piris MA. Building an outcome predictor model for diffuse large B-cell lymphoma. Am J Pathol. 2004;164:613–22.

13. Winter JN, Weller EA, Horning SJ, Krajewska M, Variakojis D, Habermann TM, Fisher RI, Kurtin PJ, Macon WR, Chhanabhai M, Felgar RE, Hsi ED, Medeiros LJ, Weick JK, Reed JC, Gascoyne RD. Prognostic significance of Bcl-6 protein expression in DLBCL treated with CHOP or R-CHOP: a prospective correlative study. Blood. 2006;107:4207–13.
14. Green TM, Young KH, Visco C, Xu-Monette ZY, Orazi A, Go RS, Nielsen O, Gadeberg OV, Mourits-Andersen T, Frederiksen M, Pedersen LM, Moller MB. Immunohistochemical double-hit score is a strong predictor of outcome in patients with diffuse large B-cell lymphoma treated with rituximab plus cyclophosphamide, doxorubicin, vincristine, and prednisone. J Clin Oncol. 2012;30:3460–7.
15. Horn H, Ziepert M, Becher C, Barth TF, Bernd HW, Feller AC, Klapper W, Hummel M, Stein H, Hansmann ML, Schmelter C, Moller P, Cogliatti S, Pfreundschuh M, Schmitz N, Trumper L, Siebert R, Loeffler M, Rosenwald A, Ott G. MYC status in concert with BCL2 and BCL6 expression predicts outcome in diffuse large B-cell lymphoma. Blood. 2013;121:2253–63.
16. Johnson NA, Slack GW, Savage KJ, Connors JM, Ben-Neriah S, Rogic S, Scott DW, Tan KL, Steidl C, Sehn LH, Chan WC, Iqbal J, Meyer PN, Lenz G, Wright G, Rimsza LM, Valentino C, Brunhoeber P, Grogan TM, Braziel RM, Cook JR, Tubbs RR, Weisenburger DD, Campo E, Rosenwald A, Ott G, Delabie J, Holcroft C, Jaffe ES, Staudt LM, Gascoyne RD. Concurrent expression of MYC and BCL2 in diffuse large B-cell lymphoma treated with rituximab plus cyclophosphamide, doxorubicin, vincristine, and prednisone. J Clin Oncol. 2012;30:3452–9.
17. Carbone PP, Kaplan HS, Musshoff K, Smithers DW, Tubiana M. Report of the committee on Hodgkin's disease staging classification. Cancer Res. 1971;31:1860–1.
18. The International Non-Hodgkin's Lymphoma Prognostic Factors Project. A predictive model for aggressive non-Hodgkin's lymphoma. N Engl J Med. 1993;329:987–94.
19. Miller TP, Dahlberg S, Cassady JR, Adelstein DJ, Spier CM, Grogan TM, LeBlanc M, Carlin S, Chase E, Fisher RI. Chemotherapy alone compared with chemotherapy plus radiotherapy for localized intermediate- and high-grade non-Hodgkin's lymphoma. N Engl J Med. 1998;339:21–6.
20. Illidge T, Specht L, Yahalom J, Aleman B, Berthelsen AK, Constine L, Dabaja BS, Dharmarajan K, Ng A, Ricardi U, Wirth A. Modern radiation therapy for nodal non Hodgkin lymphoma – target definition and dose guidelines from the International Lymphoma Radiation Oncology Group (ILROG). Int J Radiat Oncol Biol Phys. 2014;89:49–58.
21. Persky DO, Unger JM, Spier CM, Stea B, LeBlanc M, McCarty MJ, Rimsza LM, Fisher RI, Miller TP. Phase II study of rituximab plus three cycles of CHOP and involved-field radiotherapy for patients with limited-stage aggressive B-cell lymphoma: Southwest Oncology Group study 0014. J Clin Oncol. 2008;26:2258–63.
22. Bonnet C, Fillet G, Mounier N, Ganem G, Molina TJ, Thieblemont C, Ferme C, Quesnel B, Martin C, Gisselbrecht C, Tilly H, Reyes F. CHOP alone compared with CHOP plus radiotherapy for localized aggressive lymphoma in elderly patients: a study by the Groupe d'Etude des Lymphomes de l'Adulte. J Clin Oncol. 2007;25:787–92.
23. Horning SJ, Weller E, Kim K, Earle JD, O'Connell MJ, Habermann TM, Glick JH. Chemotherapy with or without radiotherapy in limited-stage diffuse aggressive non-Hodgkin's lymphoma: Eastern Cooperative Oncology Group study 1484. J Clin Oncol. 2004;22:3032–8.
24. Reyes F, Lepage E, Ganem G, Molina TJ, Brice P, Coiffier B, Morel P, Ferme C, Bosly A, Lederlin P, Laurent G, Tilly H. ACVBP versus CHOP plus radiotherapy for localized aggressive lymphoma. N Engl J Med. 2005;352:1197–205.
25. Wirth A. The rationale and role of radiation therapy in the treatment of patients with diffuse large B-cell lymphoma in the Rituximab era. Leuk Lymphoma. 2007;48:2121–36.
26. NCCN Clinical practice guidelines in oncology, non-hodgkin's lymphomas version 2.2015. 2015. www.nccn.org
27. Moser EC, Noordijk EM, van Leeuwen FE, le Cessie S, Baars JW, Thomas J, Carde P, Meerwaldt JH, van Glabbeke M, Kluin-Nelemans HC. Long-term risk of cardiovascular disease after treatment for aggressive non-Hodgkin lymphoma. Blood. 2006;107:2912–9.
28. Phan J, Mazloom A, Medeiros LJ, Zreik TG, Wogan C, Shihadeh F, Rodriguez MA, Fayad L, Fowler N, Reed V, Horace P, Dabaja BS. Benefit of consolidative radiation therapy in patients with diffuse large B-cell lymphoma treated with R-CHOP chemotherapy. J Clin Oncol. 2010;28:4170–6.
29. Lowry L, Smith P, Qian W, Falk S, Benstead K, Illidge T, Linch D, Robinson M, Jack A, Hoskin P. Reduced dose radiotherapy for local control in non-Hodgkin lymphoma: a randomised phase III trial. Radiother Oncol. 2011;100:86–92.
30. Aanaes K, Kristensen E, Ralfkiaer EM, von Buchwald C, Specht L. Improved prognosis for localized malignant lymphomas of the head and neck. Acta Otolaryngol. 2010;130:626–31.
31. Coiffier B, Lepage E, Briere J, Herbrecht R, Tilly H, Bouabdallah R, Morel P, Van Den NE, Salles G, Gaulard P, Reyes F, Lederlin P, Gisselbrecht C. CHOP chemotherapy plus rituximab compared with CHOP alone in elderly patients with diffuse large-B-cell lymphoma. N Engl J Med. 2002;346:235–42.
32. Pfreundschuh M, Trumper L, Osterborg A, Pettengell R, Trneny M, Imrie K, Ma D, Gill D, Walewski J, Zinzani PL, Stahel R, Kvaloy S, Shpilberg O, Jaeger U, Hansen M, Lehtinen T, Lopez-Guillermo A, Corrado C, Scheliga A, Milpied N, Mendila M, Rashford M, Kuhnt E, Loeffler M. CHOP-like chemo-

therapy plus rituximab versus CHOP-like chemotherapy alone in young patients with good-prognosis diffuse large-B-cell lymphoma: a randomised controlled trial by the MabThera International Trial (MInT) Group. Lancet Oncol. 2006;7:379–91.
33. Sehn LH, Donaldson J, Chhanabhai M, Fitzgerald C, Gill K, Klasa R, MacPherson N, O'Reilly S, Spinelli JJ, Sutherland J, Wilson KS, Gascoyne RD, Connors JM. Introduction of combined CHOP plus rituximab therapy dramatically improved outcome of diffuse large B-cell lymphoma in British Columbia. J Clin Oncol. 2005;23:5027–33.
34. Cunningham D, Hawkes EA, Jack A, Qian W, Smith P, Mouncey P, Pocock C, Ardeshna KM, Radford JA, McMillan A, Davies J, Turner D, Kruger A, Johnson P, Gambell J, Linch D. Rituximab plus cyclophosphamide, doxorubicin, vincristine, and prednisolone in patients with newly diagnosed diffuse large B-cell non-Hodgkin lymphoma: a phase 3 comparison of dose intensification with 14-day versus 21-day cycles. Lancet. 2013;381:1817–26.
35. Pfreundschuh M, Schubert J, Ziepert M, Schmits R, Mohren M, Lengfelder E, Reiser M, Nickenig C, Clemens M, Peter N, Bokemeyer C, Eimermacher H, Ho A, Hoffmann M, Mertelsmann R, Trumper L, Balleisen L, Liersch R, Metzner B, Hartmann F, Glass B, Poeschel V, Schmitz N, Ruebe C, Feller AC, Loeffler M. Six versus eight cycles of bi-weekly CHOP-14 with or without rituximab in elderly patients with aggressive CD20+ B-cell lymphomas: a randomised controlled trial (RICOVER-60). Lancet Oncol. 2008;9:105–16.
36. Dorth JA, Prosnitz LR, Broadwater G, Diehl LF, Beaven AW, Coleman RE, Kelsey CR. Impact of consolidation radiation therapy in stage III-IV diffuse large B-cell lymphoma with negative post-chemotherapy radiologic imaging. Int J Radiat Oncol Biol Phys. 2012;84:762–7.
37. Shi Z, Das S, Okwan-Duodu D, Esiashvili N, Flowers C, Chen Z, Wang X, Jiang K, Nastoupil LJ, Khan MK. Patterns of failure in advanced stage diffuse large B-cell lymphoma patients after complete response to R-CHOP immunochemotherapy and the emerging role of consolidative radiation therapy. Int J Radiat Oncol Biol Phys. 2013;86:569–77.
38. Pfreundschuh M, Ho AD, Cavallin-Stahl E, Wolf M, Pettengell R, Vasova I, Belch A, Walewski J, Zinzani PL, Mingrone W, Kvaloy S, Shpilberg O, Jaeger U, Hansen M, Corrado C, Scheliga A, Loeffler M, Kuhnt E. Prognostic significance of maximum tumour (bulk) diameter in young patients with good-prognosis diffuse large-B-cell lymphoma treated with CHOP-like chemotherapy with or without rituximab: an exploratory analysis of the MabThera International Trial Group (MInT) study. Lancet Oncol. 2008;9:435–44.
39. Pfreundschuh M, Kuhnt E, Trumper L, Osterborg A, Trneny M, Shepherd L, Gill DS, Walewski J, Pettengell R, Jaeger U, Zinzani PL, Shpilberg O, Kvaloy S, de Nully BP, Stahel R, Milpied N, Lopez-Guillermo A, Poeschel V, Grass S, Loeffler M, Murawski N. CHOP-like chemotherapy with or without rituximab in young patients with good-prognosis diffuse large-B-cell lymphoma: 6-year results of an open-label randomised study of the MabThera International Trial (MInT) Group. Lancet Oncol. 2011;12:1013–22.
40. Held G, Murawski N, Ziepert M, Fleckenstein J, Poschel V, Zwick C, Bittenbring J, Hanel M, Wilhelm S, Schubert J, Schmitz N, Loffler M, Rube C, Pfreundschuh M. Role of radiotherapy to bulky disease in elderly patients with aggressive B-cell lymphoma. J Clin Oncol. 2014;32:1112–8.
41. Dabaja BS, Phan J, Mawlawi O, Medeiros LJ, Etzel C, Liang FW, Podoloff D, Oki Y, Hagemeister FB, Chuang H, Fayad LE, Westin JR, Shihadeh F, Allen PK, Wogan CF, Rodriguez MA. Clinical implications of positron emission tomography-negative residual computed tomography masses after chemotherapy for diffuse large B-cell lymphoma. Leuk Lymphoma. 2013;54:2631–8.
42. Barrington SF, Mikhaeel NG, Kostakoglu L, Meignan M, Hutchings M, Mueller SP, Schwartz LH, Zucca E, Fisher RI, Trotman J, Hoekstra OS, Hicks RJ, O'Doherty MJ, Hustinx R, Biggi A, Cheson BD. Role of imaging in the staging and response assessment of lymphoma: consensus of the International Conference on Malignant Lymphomas Imaging Working Group. J Clin Oncol. 2014;32:3048–58.
43. Casasnovas RO, Meignan M, Berriolo-Riedinger A, Bardet S, Julian A, Thieblemont C, Vera P, Bologna S, Briere J, Jais JP, Haioun C, Coiffier B, Morschhauser F. SUVmax reduction improves early prognosis value of interim positron emission tomography scans in diffuse large B-cell lymphoma. Blood. 2011;118:37–43.
44. Haioun C, Itti E, Rahmouni A, Brice P, Rain JD, Belhadj K, Gaulard P, Garderet L, Lepage E, Reyes F, Meignan M. [18F]fluoro-2-deoxy-D-glucose positron emission tomography (FDG-PET) in aggressive lymphoma: an early prognostic tool for predicting patient outcome. Blood. 2005;106:1376–81.
45. Itti E, Meignan M, Berriolo-Riedinger A, Biggi A, Cashen AF, Vera P, Tilly H, Siegel BA, Gallamini A, Casasnovas RO, Haioun C. An international confirmatory study of the prognostic value of early PET/CT in diffuse large B-cell lymphoma: comparison between Deauville criteria and DeltaSUVmax. Eur J Nucl Med Mol Imaging. 2013;40:1312–20.
46. Mikhaeel NG, Hutchings M, Fields PA, O'Doherty MJ, Timothy AR. FDG-PET after two to three cycles of chemotherapy predicts progression-free and overall survival in high-grade non-Hodgkin lymphoma. Ann Oncol. 2005;16:1514–23.
47. Pregno P, Chiappella A, Bello M, Botto B, Ferrero S, Franceschetti S, Giunta F, Ladetto M, Limerutti G, Menga M, Nicolosi M, Priolo G, Puccini B, Rigacci L, Salvi F, Vaggelli L, Passera R, Bisi G, Vitolo U. Interim 18-FDG-PET/CT failed to predict the outcome in diffuse large B-cell lymphoma patients treated at the diagnosis with rituximab-CHOP. Blood. 2012;119:2066–73.

48. Safar V, Dupuis J, Itti E, Jardin F, Fruchart C, Bardet S, Vera P, Copie-Bergman C, Rahmouni A, Tilly H, Meignan M, Haioun C. Interim [18F]fluorodeoxyglucose positron emission tomography scan in diffuse large B-cell lymphoma treated with anthracycline-based chemotherapy plus rituximab. J Clin Oncol. 2012;30:184–90.
49. Gisselbrecht C, Glass B, Mounier N, Singh GD, Linch DC, Trneny M, Bosly A, Ketterer N, Shpilberg O, Hagberg H, Ma D, Briere J, Moskowitz CH, Schmitz N. Salvage regimens with autologous transplantation for relapsed large B-cell lymphoma in the rituximab era. J Clin Oncol. 2010;28:4184–90.
50. Mundt AJ, Williams SF, Hallahan D. High dose chemotherapy and stem cell rescue for aggressive non-Hodgkin's lymphoma: pattern of failure and implications for involved-field radiotherapy. Int J Radiat Oncol Biol Phys. 1997;39:617–25.
51. Biswas T, Dhakal S, Chen R, Hyrien O, Bernstein S, Friedberg JW, Fisher RI, Liesveld J, Phillips G, Constine LS. Involved field radiation after autologous stem cell transplant for diffuse large B-cell lymphoma in the rituximab era. Int J Radiat Oncol Biol Phys. 2010;77:79–85.

Follicular Lymphoma: Treatment for Early-Stage, Grades 1 and 2, and Advanced-Stage Disease

3

Bradford Hoppe

Abstract
Follicular lymphoma is the second most common non-Hodgkin lymphoma histology diagnosed and the most common of the indolent histologies. Radiotherapy remains an important treatment modality for patients with follicular lymphoma. Among patients with early-stage disease, definitive treatment with radiotherapy remains the standard of care to doses of 24–30 Gy using involved-site radiotherapy. For patients with advanced disease, low-dose radiotherapy (2 Gy/fraction × two fractions) remains an excellent palliative treatment with durable control for approximately 18 months. Utilizing two different clinical scenarios, this chapter discusses epidemiology, staging, and treatment options and provides an in-depth overview of the radiotherapy treatment field design and plan evaluation for follicular lymphoma.

Clinical Presentation

Case 1

A 68-year-old male was seen by his primary care physician for new onset swelling in his right groin. The patient denied any B symptoms, recent trauma, or recent infectious history, and a 4-cm non-painful mass was palpated in the right groin area, movable and not painful.

Case 2

An 82-year-old female with multiply relapsed stage IV follicular lymphoma (FL) following immunotherapy and chemotherapy presented with a large bulky abdominal mass.

In 2014, approximately 70,000 cases of non-Hodgkin lymphoma (NHL) were diagnosed in the United States [1]. NHL is made up of about 60 different subtypes, and FL is the second most common (~20 % of all NHL diagnoses); FL is the most common of all indolent histologies.

FL generally affects older patients with a median age of 60 years, and it rarely affects children or adolescents [2, 3]. The most common presenting symptom is painless peripheral adenopathy that waxes and wanes in size over time, and B symptoms are found in about 20 % of

B. Hoppe, MD, MPH
University of Florida Proton Therapy Institute, 2015 North Jefferson St., Jacksonville, FL 32206, USA
e-mail: bhoppe@floridaproton.org

B.S. Dabaja, A.K. Ng (eds.), *Radiation Therapy in Hematologic Malignancies*,
DOI 10.1007/978-3-319-42615-0_3

patients. About 80 % of patients are diagnosed with stage III or IV disease [2, 3].

Pathology and Comment on What Is Typical and What Is the Meaning of Markers and Their Implications

Case (1). The right groin lymph node demonstrated grade 1 FL with diffuse areas. Immunohistochemical stains revealed CD10-positive, BCL6-positive, and BCL2-positive disease.

Case (2). Although a repeat biopsy to confirm that the FL had not developed into a higher-grade lymphoma was considered, the patient was not a candidate for additional chemotherapy; furthermore, the biopsy would have been highly invasive for the patient.

When NHL is being considered in the differential diagnosis, excisional biopsy of the lymph node is preferred to a core needle biopsy to better evaluate pattern and grade.

FL is a B-cell lymphoma that is derived from germinal center cells of a lymph node. The World Health Organization (WHO) describes specific growth patterns and grading of FL [4]. The growth pattern of FL within the lymph node can be described as follicular, focally follicular, follicular and diffuse, or diffuse. The following grading system is based on the number of centroblasts in the follicles: grade 1, 5 or fewer centroblasts per high-power field (hpf); grade 2, 6–15 per hpf; grade 3A, more than 15 per hpf with centrocytes intermingled with the centroblasts; and grade 3B, more than 15 per hpf with pure sheets of centroblasts.

Normal follicle center cells express CD10 and BCL6 markers and are negative for BCL2, while the follicular dendritic cells express CD21. FL cells, on the other hand, are usually positive for BCL2 (~85 %) and, in higher-grade FL, might be negative for CD10 [5]. Additionally, FL can have a characteristic t(14;18) translocation which moves BCL2 adjacent to a promoter gene that leads to overexpression of BCL2 antiapoptotic protein that can be detected by polymerase chain reaction (PCR) or by fluorescence in situ hybridization (FISH). Higher-grade tumors can have a BCL6 rearrangement.

Staging and Prognostic Factors and What Is It Based on

Case (1). The patient underwent a positron emission tomography (PET)-computed tomography (CT) scan and CT of the neck, chest, abdomen, and pelvis. The scans demonstrated right groin adenopathy with a maximum standardized uptake value (SUV max) of 8.4 (Fig. 3.1a, b). *The patient's blood work was normal, and his bone marrow was negative. His FL International Prognostic Index (FLIPI) and FLIPI2 scores were both 1, consistent with a low risk for FLIPI1 and an intermediate risk for FLIPI2.*

Case (2). The patient had a PET-CT scan ordered for a 10 × 7-cm mesenteric lymph node mass within the right side of the mid abdomen with an SUV max of 18.2 and several enlarged hypermetabolic mesenteric and para-aortic lymph nodes surrounding it. Additionally, the patient had bilateral pelvic, inguinal, axillary, and cervical lymph nodes present (Fig. 3.2a, b). *Considering the patient had known extensive relapsed disease, a PET-CT scan was not necessary, and a CT of the chest/abdomen/pelvis would suffice in this scenario.*

Staging of FL follows that of other NHLs using the Ann Arbor system. Work-up should include a patient medical history and physical examination (focused on the lymphatic region) for evaluation of B symptoms, extent of disease, and performance status. Blood work should include a complete blood count, a lactate dehydrogenase test (LDH), a beta-2 (B2) microglobulin test, a comprehensive metabolic panel test, hepatitis B testing, and a pregnancy test for women of child-bearing age. Bone marrow biopsy should be performed in all cases. Imaging should include a diagnostic CT scan of the chest/abdomen/pelvis with consideration of a CT of the neck and/or a PET-CT scan. PET-CT scans are important if considering definitive treatment with radiation for early-stage FL. Wirth et al. demonstrated that a PET-CT scan upstaged patients who were thought to have early-stage (I/II) FL by conventional assessment to stage III/IV in 31 % of the cases [6]. Additionally, PET-CT scan showed more extensive stage I/II disease

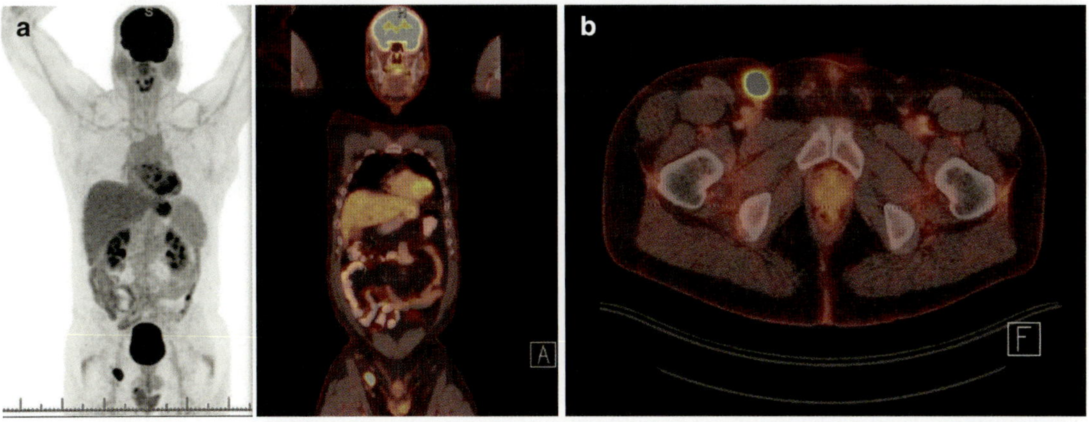

Fig. 3.1 (**a**) Coronal PET image showing the right groin mass. (**b**) Axial PET imaging showing the right groin mass

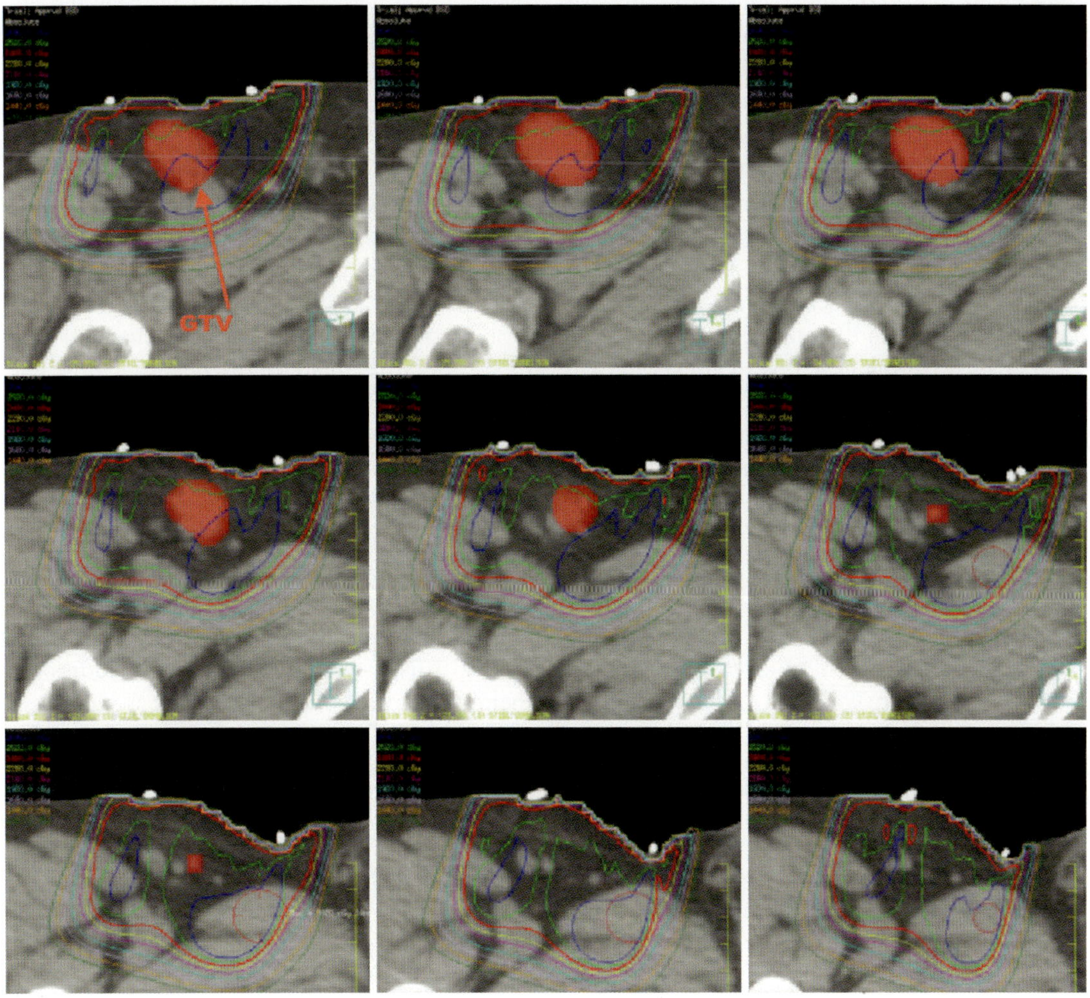

Fig. 3.2 Showing the coverage of the groin mass

than previously thought, which would increase the radiation field in 14 % of the cases.

In a large pooled analysis that led to the development of the FLIPI, several important clinical features were observed, including an even distribution of disease between the sexes (male, 51 %, female, 49 %), 63 % of patients under 60 years old, 22 % with stage I/II disease, 19 % with B symptoms, 35 % with five or more nodal sites, 38 % with extranodal involvement (other than bone marrow), 48 % with bone marrow involvement, 22 % with splenic involvement, 41 % with elevated serum B2 microglobulin, 21 % with elevated LDH, 18 % with hemoglobin below 120 g/L, and 10 % with albumin <35 g/L [2]. The factors that were found to be most prognostic for outcomes were age ≥60 years, stage III/IV disease, hemoglobin <120 g/L, elevated LDH, and >4 involved nodal sites. Based on these factors, the following risk groups were created: low risk, 0–1 factor; intermediate risk, 2 factors; and high risk, 3 or more factors. The 5-year and 10-year overall survival rates are 91 %, and 71 % for low-risk disease were 78 and 51 % for intermediate-risk disease and 53 and 36 % for high-risk disease.

In a follow-up project that involved a more modern patient cohort treated in the era of rituximab, a FLIPI2 was developed [7]. The factors found to have the strongest prognosis were B2 microglobulin levels (above normal), longest diameter of the largest involved node (>6 cm), bone marrow involvement, hemoglobulin <12 g/dL, and age >60 years. Based on these factors, the 3-year overall survival and progression-free survival (PFS) rates were 99 and 91 % for low-risk disease (0 factor), 96 and 69 % for intermediate-risk disease (1–2 factors), and 84 and 51 % for high-risk disease (3–5 factors).

Treatment Strategies and Their Variations

Case (1). Several options exist for the management of stage II low-risk FLIPI and intermediate-risk FLIPI2. With this patient, we discussed definitive treatment with radiotherapy or management with immunotherapy. The consensus among his oncologists was definitive treatment with involved-site radiotherapy to a dose of 24 Gy in 12 fractions, which the patient agreed to pursue.

Case (2). The patient was tired of chemotherapy but had symptomatic disease. Palliative radiotherapy of 4 Gy in two fractions of 2 Gy/fraction was offered to the patient.

Early-Stage Disease

The diagnosis of stages I and II FL is rare; consequently, few prospective clinical studies have been conducted to determine the most successful approach to treatment. Historically, definitive management with radiotherapy has been the recommended standard of care based on large historical retrospective cohorts (Table 3.1). However, the National LymphoCare study, a multicenter, longitudinal observational study that included patients from both academic and community practices, demonstrated that there was great variety in how patients with early-stage FL were being managed [3, 8]. Approaches included observation alone (29 %), radiation therapy alone (23 %), rituximab alone or with chemotherapy (35 %), and rituximab followed by radiation therapy (8 %). Although similar excellent outcomes were seen during the short median follow-up of just less than 5 years, the cohort represents a heterogenous group of patients, with only 62 % staged with a PET-CT scan [3, 8].

Radiation therapy has been the standard treatment of early-stage FL for over 50 years based on large single-institution retrospective studies. Table 3.1 lists an assortment of these studies and their outcomes [9–12]. The largest studies of approximately 200 patients included those conducted by the British Columbia Cancer Agency, Stanford University (California), Princess Margaret Hospital (Toronto, Ontario), and British National Lymphoma Investigation, which all demonstrated 10-year PFS rates of 44–53 % and 10-year overall survival rates of 58–66 % using radiation doses between 20 and 50 Gy and extended-field radiation therapy (EFRT) as well as involved-field radiation therapy (IFRT)

Table 3.1 Literature review of definitive treatment of stage I/II follicular lymphoma with radiotherapy alone

Institution	No. of patients	Median follow-up (years)	Percentage of patients with stage I disease	Percentage of patients with stage II disease	10-year progression-free survival	10-year overall survival	Radiotherapy dose (Gy)	Radiotherapy field
University of Florida [9]	72	8.5	75 %	25 %	59 %	46 %	20–50	EFRT/IFRT
Stanford University [10]	177	7.7	41 %	59 %	44 %	64 %	35–50	TLI/EFRT/IFRT
British Columbia Cancer Agency [11]	237	7.3	76 %	24 %	49 %	66 %	20–40	EFRT/INRT + 5 cm
Princess Margaret [12]	460	10.6	74 %	26 %	52 %	62 %	16–48	IFRT

Abbreviations: *EFRT* extended-field radiation therapy, *IFRT* involved-field radiation therapy, *TLI* total lymphoid irradiation, *INRT* involved-node radiation therapy designs. Considering the significant upstaging with PET-CT scans, it is likely that some stage I/II patients treated before the use of PET-CT had stage III/IV disease. Therefore, outcomes might be improved for patients evaluated during the PET-CT era.

Radiation dose has been evaluated across several single-institution databases to understand the doses needed for definitive treatment of patients with FL. In 2011, a published randomized study from the United Kingdom compared 24 Gy in 12 fractions to 40–45 Gy in 20–23 fractions among patients with indolent NHL, including those with advanced-stage disease and those treated with chemotherapy [13]. With a median follow-up of 5.6 years, overall PFS was 55 %, and no difference was seen in freedom from local progression (79 % vs 76 %, $p = 0.68$). Additionally, no difference in overall survival was seen at 5 years (73 % vs 74 %, $p = 0.84$). Among patients treated with radiotherapy alone, no difference was seen in PFS; 54 % in the high-dose arm and 64 % in the low-dose arm were alive without a recurrence at 5 years. Furthermore, a randomized study comparing 24 Gy in 12 fractions with 4 Gy in two fractions among patients with indolent histologies demonstrated that when the intent was cure, local control improved with 24 Gy ($p = 0.0051$) [14].

Radiation treatment field design has included EFRT, IFRT, and generous involved-node radiation therapy (INRT) with up to a 5-cm margin [11]. Although no randomized studies have been conducted to directly compare larger fields with smaller fields, Campbell et al. reported no significant difference in 10-year disease-specific survival (85 % vs 78 %, $p = 0.14$) or PFS (48 % vs 50 %, $p = 0.50$) between involved regional radiotherapy and radiotherapy to the involved node + 5 cm.

Owing to advances in imaging technique since two-dimensional imaging, such as PET-CT imaging, the International Lymphoma Radiation Oncology Group (ILROG) recently developed new guidelines for radiation field design for the management of lymphoma called involved-site radiotherapy (ISRT) [15]. ISRT utilizes modern radiation techniques and incorporates the current concepts of volumes as reported by the International Commission on Radiation Units (ICRU) report 83. The current guidelines for indolent nodal NHL and extranodal NHL have been published [15, 16].

Advanced-Stage Disease

Advanced-stage FL is typically managed with active surveillance, immunotherapy, chemotherapy, or radioimmunotherapy. Curative treatment with total lymphoid irradiation (TLI) has been reported, but long-term toxicities and a high relapse rate have made it more or less obsolete [17, 18].

Radiotherapy, however, can play an extremely important palliative role in patients with advanced FL owing to the radiation sensitivity of FL. Table 3.2 includes several studies that have evaluated palliative low-dose radiotherapy with doses of 4 Gy delivered in two fractions

Table 3.2 Literature review of palliative treatment of advanced indolent non-Hodgkin lymphoma with 4 Gy

Institution	No. of patients	Radiation therapy dose (Gy)	Complete response (%)	Partial response (%)	Median time to local progression (months)
Centre hospitalier universitaire vaudois [19]	43	4	28	35	21
Princess Margaret Hospital [20]	54	4	49	32	19
The Netherlands Cancer Institute [21]	109	4	61	31	25
Brigham and Women's Hospital and Dana-Farber Institute [22]	127	4	57	25	14

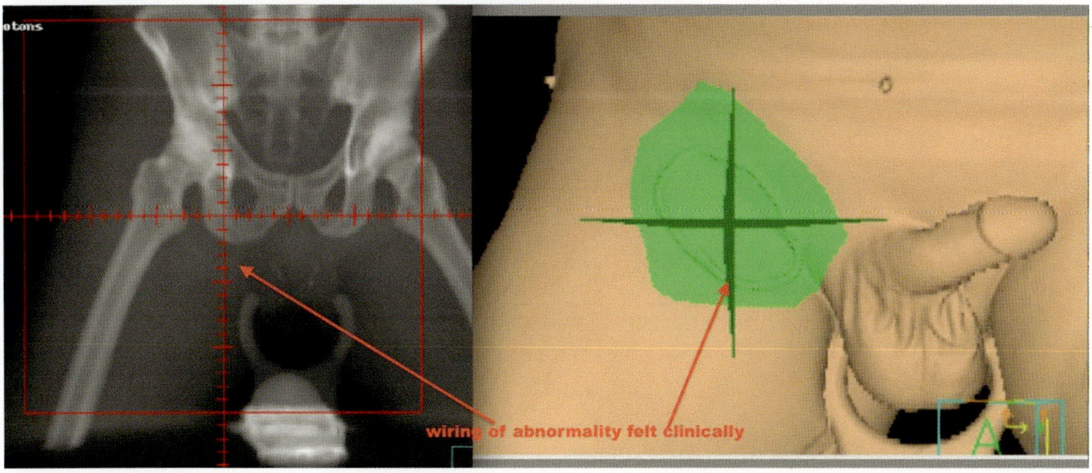

Fig. 3.3 Showing patient set up on the digitally reconstructed radiograph (DRR) as well as the skin rendering from the CT scan simulation

(2 Gy/fraction) in patients with advanced-stage disease [19–22]. Response rates of 60–96 % have been reported with an average median time to local progression of 18 months. Considering the low rate of acute side effects expected with these low doses, 2 Gy delivered twice is an excellent treatment option for patients with symptomatic disease, including the chemorefractory variety.

Post Images, Contours, Margins Determination, Planning Method, and Images of the Plan

Case (1). The patient was simulated in a blue bag to maintain a frog-leg position. A CT simulation was performed. The ISRT guidelines were followed. The gross tumor volume (GTV) was contoured on the CT images with the assistance of the PET-CT scan. A 1.5-cm margin was added to the gross disease to create the clinical target volume (CTV). The CTV was expanded by a 1.5-cm margin to create the planning target volume (PTV). Obviously the PTV has to be changed on case-by-case basis depending on the site treated taking into consideration the internal and external uncertainties of each treated site.

Treatment planning to a dose of 24 Gy in 12 treatments using 16-MeV electron appositional field was used; the plan was developed in an effort to cover 95 % of the PTV with 100 % of the dose (Fig. 3.2). *Doses to the organs at risk, which in this case is the testis, were taken into consideration; we used a clamshell to protect the testis from scattered radiation; obviously the clamshell does not protect it from internal scatter* (Figs. 3.3 and 3.4). *We placed a thermoluminescent detector inside the clamshell on the testis skin to measure the actual dose, and it was 2 cGy per treatment.*

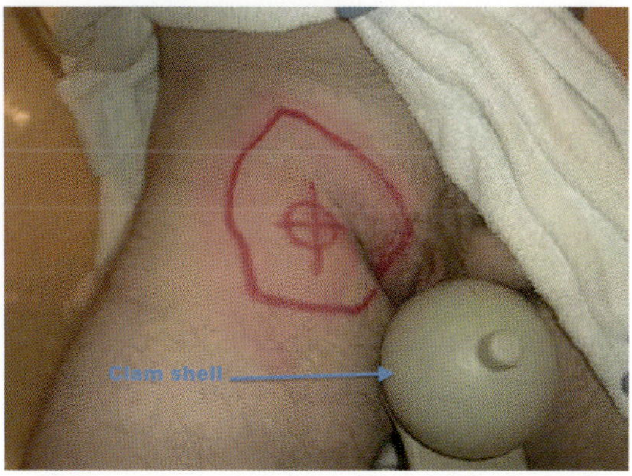

Fig. 3.4 Patient set up with frog-leg position, showing the field and the clamshell used to protect the testis from scattered radiation

Long-term survival is common among patients with indolent NHL, so late toxicities, such as second cancers and cardiovascular problems, must be considered when evaluating a treatment plan.

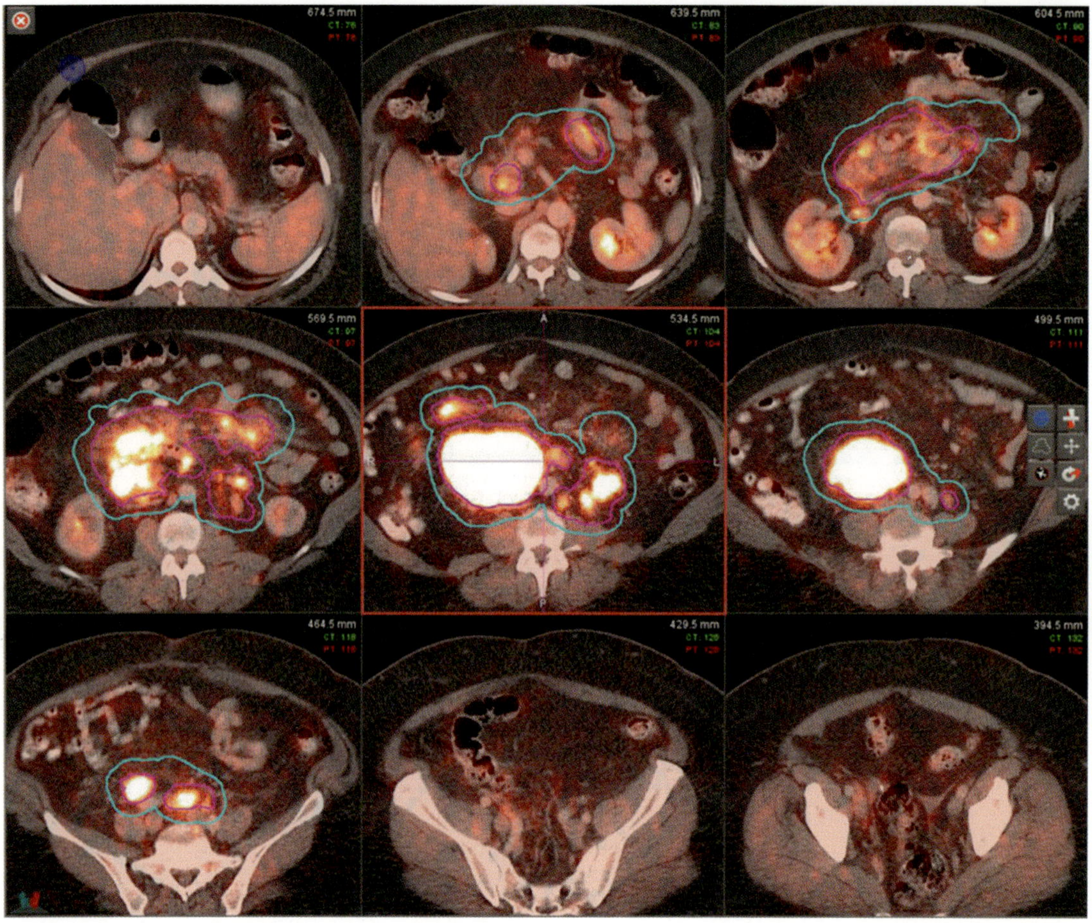

Fig. 3.5 Treatment targets for the patient described in Case 2 who received palliative treatment. The gross tumor volume is in *pink*, and the planning target volume is in *light blue*

However, based on the typical age at diagnosis, it is unlikely that late toxicities will be as problematic as they are among young Hodgkin lymphoma patients.

Case (2). *For this palliative treatment, the patient was placed in a comfortable position on the treatment table with her arms at her sides while she underwent a three-dimensional CT scan for simulation. The GTV included the sites of disease thought to cause the patient's symptoms. Non-symptomatic disease that separates from the main target volume was not included as this was a palliative treatment. A PTV margin of 1 cm was added to the GTV, which is standard at our institution for this disease site.* Figure 3.5a, b *shows the targets. For this patient, we developed a simple 3 Dimensional Conformal Radiation Therapy (3DCRT) anterior-posterior/posterior-anterior treatment plan. Considering the low dose of radiotherapy delivered, no organs at risk were considered.*

References

1. Siegel R, Ma J, Zou Z, Jemal A. Cancer statistics, 2014. CA Cancer J Clin. 2014;64(1):9–29.
2. Solal-Celigny P, Roy P, Colombat P, White J, Armitage JO, Arranz-Saez R, et al. Follicular lymphoma international prognostic index. Blood. 2004;104(5):1258–65.
3. Friedberg JW, Taylor MD, Cerhan JR, Flowers CR, Dillon H, Farber CM, et al. Follicular lymphoma in the United States: first report of the national LymphoCare study. J Clin Oncol. 2009;27(8):1202–8.

4. Campo E, Swerdlow SH, Harris NL, Pileri S, Stein H, Jaffe ES. The 2008 WHO classification of lymphoid neoplasms and beyond: evolving concepts and practical applications. Blood. 2011;117(19):5019–32.
5. Eshoa C, Perkins S, Kampalath B, Shidham V, Juckett M, Chang CC. Decreased CD10 expression in grade III and in interfollicular infiltrates of follicular lymphomas. Am J Clin Pathol. 2001;115(6):862–7.
6. Wirth A, Foo M, Seymour JF, Macmanus MP, Hicks RJ. Impact of [18f] fluorodeoxyglucose positron emission tomography on staging and management of early-stage follicular non-hodgkin lymphoma. Int J Radiat Oncol Biol Phys. 2008;71(1):213–9.
7. Federico M, Bellei M, Marcheselli L, Luminari S, Lopez-Guillermo A, Vitolo U, et al. Follicular lymphoma international prognostic index 2: a new prognostic index for follicular lymphoma developed by the international follicular lymphoma prognostic factor project. J Clin Oncol. 2009;27(27):4555–62.
8. Friedberg JW, Byrtek M, Link BK, Flowers C, Taylor M, Hainsworth J, et al. Effectiveness of first-line management strategies for stage I follicular lymphoma: analysis of the National LymphoCare Study. J Clin Oncol. 2012;30(27):3368–75.
9. Kamath SS, Marcus Jr RB, Lynch JW, Mendenhall NP. The impact of radiotherapy dose and other treatment-related and clinical factors on in-field control in stage I and II non-Hodgkin's lymphoma. Int J Radiat Oncol Biol Phys. 1999;44(3):563–8.
10. Mac Manus MP, Hoppe RT. Is radiotherapy curative for stage I and II low-grade follicular lymphoma? Results of a long-term follow-up study of patients treated at Stanford University. J Clin Oncol. 1996;14(4):1282–90.
11. Campbell BA, Voss N, Woods R, Gascoyne RD, Morris J, Pickles T, et al. Long-term outcomes for patients with limited stage follicular lymphoma: involved regional radiotherapy versus involved node radiotherapy. Cancer. 2010;116(16):3797–806.
12. Gospodarowicz MK, Bush RS, Brown TC, Chua T. Prognostic factors in nodular lymphomas: a multivariate analysis based on the Princess Margaret Hospital experience. Int J Radiat Oncol Biol Phys. 1984;10(4):489–97.
13. Lowry L, Smith P, Qian W, Falk S, Benstead K, Illidge T, et al. Reduced dose radiotherapy for local control in non-Hodgkin lymphoma: a randomised phase III trial. Radiother Oncol. 2011;100(1):86–92.
14. Hoskin PJ, Kirkwood AA, Popova B, Smith P, Robinson M, Gallop-Evans E, et al. 4 Gy versus 24 Gy radiotherapy for patients with indolent lymphoma (FORT): a randomised phase 3 non-inferiority trial. Lancet Oncol. 2014;15(4):457–63.
15. Illidge T, Specht L, Yahalom J, Aleman B, Berthelsen AK, Constine L, et al. Modern radiation therapy for nodal non-Hodgkin lymphoma-target definition and dose guidelines from the International Lymphoma Radiation Oncology Group. Int J Radiat Oncol Biol Phys. 2014;89(1):49–58.
16. Yahalom J, Illidge T, Specht L, Hoppe R, Li Y, Tsang R, et al. Modern radiotherapy for extra-nodal lymphoma – field and dose guidelines from the International Lymphoma Radiation Oncology Group (ILROG). Int J Radiat Oncol Biol Phys. 2015;92:11–31.
17. Paryani SB, Hoppe RT, Cox RS, Colby TV, Kaplan HS. The role of radiation therapy in the management of stage III follicular lymphomas. J Clin Oncol. 1984;2(7):841–8.
18. De Los Santos JF, Mendenhall NP, Lynch Jr JW. Is comprehensive lymphatic irradiation for low-grade non-Hodgkin's lymphoma curative therapy? Long-term experience at a single institution. Int J Radiat Oncol Biol Phys. 1997;38(1):3–8.
19. Rossier C, Schick U, Miralbell R, Mirimanoff RO, Weber DC, Ozsahin M. Low-dose radiotherapy in indolent lymphoma. Int J Radiat Oncol Biol Phys. 2011;81(3):e1–6.
20. Chan EK, Fung S, Gospodarowicz M, Hodgson D, Wells W, Sun A, et al. Palliation by low-dose local radiation therapy for indolent non-Hodgkin lymphoma. Int J Radiat Oncol Biol Phys. 2011;81(5):e781–6.
21. Haas RL, Poortmans P, de Jong D, Aleman BM, Dewit LG, Verheij M, et al. High response rates and lasting remissions after low-dose involved field radiotherapy in indolent lymphomas. J Clin Oncol. 2003;21(13):2474–80.
22. Russo AL, Chen Y-H, Martin NE, Vinjamoori A, Luthy SK, Freedman A, et al. Low-dose involved-field radiation in the treatment of non-Hodgkin lymphoma: predictors of response and treatment failure. Int J Radiat Oncol Biol Phys. 2013;86(1):121–7.

Extranodal Marginal Zone Lymphoma

4

Umberto Ricardi, Andrea Riccardo Filippi, Cristina Piva, and Mario Levis

Abstract

Extranodal marginal zone lymphomas (EN-MZLs) comprise about 25 % of all non-Hodgkin lymphomas (NHL). The wide range of presentations of EN-MZL, involving virtually any organ, poses several challenges. The heterogeneity of the disease also explains the uncertainty and lack of consistency in radiotherapy approaches between centers and clinicians. EN-MZL often presents with localized/organ-confined disease, and RT is generally the primary curative modality. High local control rates can be achieved with relatively modest radiation doses, and local control often translates to cure.

In this chapter, we shortly present two clinical cases of the most common EN-MZL subtypes (gastric and ocular adnexa MZL), discussing diagnosis, staging, and therapeutic strategies, with a special focus on the role of radiotherapy. Current recommendations in terms of optimal dose, volumes, and techniques are also presented. Few tables summarize the results of the largest series reporting on the outcome following radiotherapy, and figures illustrate imaging features as well as contouring and planning examples.

Introduction

Indolent nonfollicular B-cell lymphoma (INFBCL) subtype has been classified in the World Health Organization (WHO) system among the mature B-cell neoplasms and includes nodal marginal zone lymphoma (NMZL), splenic marginal zone lymphoma (SMZL), extranodal marginal zone lymphoma (EN-MZL) of mucosa-associated lymphoid tissue (MALT), lymphoplasmacytic lymphoma (LPL), and small lymphocytic lymphoma (SLL) [79]. Marginal zone MALT lymphoma is the most frequent subtype among all marginal zone lymphomas (MZLs), accounting for 7 % of non-Hodgkin lymphoma (NHL); NMZL and SMZL represent only 2 % and 1 % of NHL, respectively [3, 54].

U. Ricardi (✉) • A.R. Filippi • C. Piva • M. Levis
Department of Oncology, University of Torino, Via Genova 3, Torino 10125, Italy
e-mail: umberto.ricardi@unito.it; andreariccardo.filippi@unito.it; cristinapiva83@gmail.com; mariolevis82@gmail.com

B.S. Dabaja, A.K. Ng (eds.), *Radiation Therapy in Hematologic Malignancies*,
DOI 10.1007/978-3-319-42615-0_4

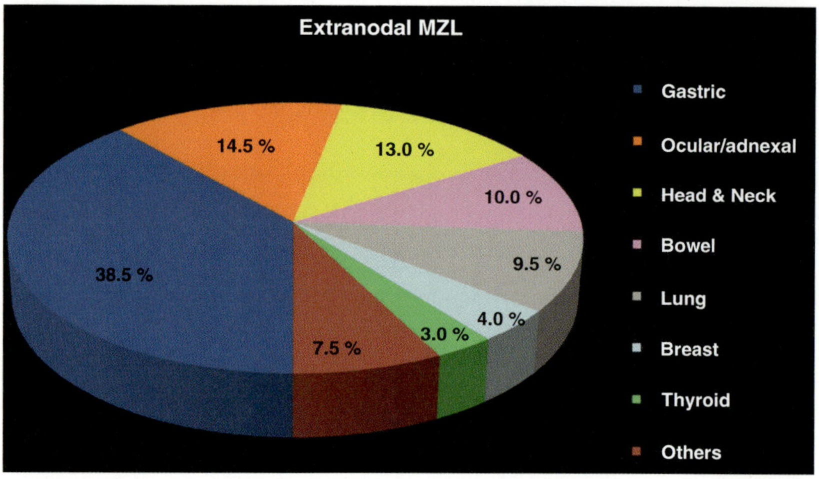

Fig. 4.1 Frequency rates of extranodal marginal zone lymphomas (MZL) according to site (excluding the skin and spleen), SEER data (Khalil et al. [40])

MALT lymphoma is a distinct B-cell lymphoma that develops in extranodal sites. MALT lymphoma differs from its splenic and nodal counterparts because it arises in organs (e.g., stomach, ocular adnexal, and lung) that normally lack lymphoid tissue but accumulate B cells in response to chronic infections or autoimmune processes. The most common extranodal MALT lymphoma involves the gastrointestinal tract (about 50 % of MALT lymphomas), followed by non-gastric sites such as the ocular adnexa (12 %), lung (10 %), skin (9 %), salivary glands (6 %), thyroid (4 %), and breast (2 %) [82]. Frequency rates of extranodal marginal zone lymphomas according to site are reported in Fig. 4.1 [40].

In this chapter, illustrative cases of a gastric and ocular MALT lymphoma, the most common EN-MZL, are presented followed by a discussion of the appropriate evaluation and management, with a focus on the role of radiotherapy.

Gastric Marginal Zone B-Cell Lymphomas (MALT Lymphomas)

The gastrointestinal tract is the most frequent site of extranodal lymphoma, and the stomach is involved in up to two-thirds of the cases [99]. Indeed, 30–45 % of all extranodal lymphomas are detected in the stomach [96]. Primary gastric lymphoma is a rare disease, representing nearly 2–8 % of all stomach tumors [56, 95]. Virtually all gastric lymphomas arise from B cells [95], as T-cell gastric lymphoma is extremely rare [64]. Marginal zone MALT lymphoma accounts for nearly 50 % of gastric lymphomas [59, 64]. Gastric MALT lymphoma is characterized by a dense lymphoid infiltrate mainly composed of small-size lymphocytes that invade and destroy gastric glands, configuring the so-called lymph epithelial lesion which is pathognomonic of lymphoma [37].

A recent systematic review including data of 2000 patients found that gastric MALT lymphoma occurs over a wide age range, with a mean of 57 years at diagnosis, and is slightly more prevalent in males (male–female ratio = 1.27:1) [97].

Clinical Case

A 61-year-old man was in his usual state of health until June 2002 when he began to suffer dyspepsia. At that time, he didn't report any other symptoms, like drenching night sweats, fevers, weight loss, or pruritus. An upper endoscopy demonstrated the presence of gastric macroscopic lesions, and biopsies showed a diagnosis of gastric MALT lymphoma with associated *Helicobacter pylori* (*H. pylori*) infection. Further assessment including a complete physical examination; routine laboratory tests; computed

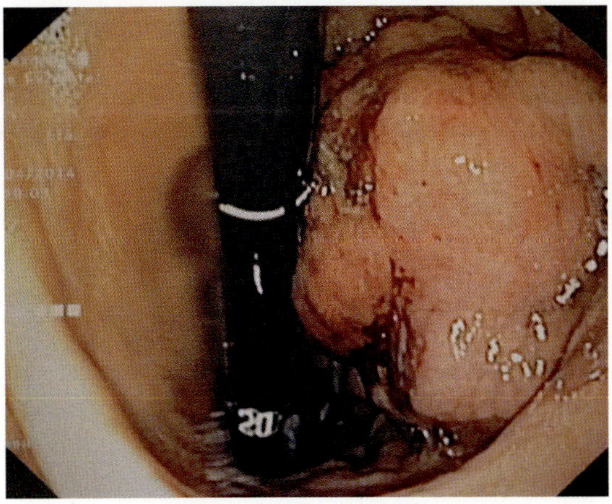

Fig. 4.2 Endoscopic finding with a well-visible massive gastric MZL lesion

tomography (CT) of the chest; abdomen, and pelvis; endoscopic ultrasonography; and bone marrow biopsy were performed and demonstrated a disease confined to one extranodal site. Therefore, the patient fell classically into a stage I disease. He underwent antibiotic eradication with resolution of the macroscopic lesion and negativity of *H. pylori* infection but persistence of MALT areas in the stomach. He repeated antibiotic therapy with endoscopic persistence of MALT areas in the stomach. For this reason, chemotherapy with six cycles of chlorambucil was administered. An upper endoscopy showed minimal residual disease, and patient started clinical-endoscopic follow-up with stable disease for many years. At August 2013 an endoscopy showed a progression of disease with evidence of new macroscopic MALT lesions in almost all the stomach (Fig. 4.2) and *H. pylori* negativity. A positron emission tomography (PET)/CT confirmed increased uptake to the whole stomach.

Clinical-Endoscopic Presentation

The clinical presentation of gastric lymphoma is poorly specific because symptoms range from vague dyspepsia, including epigastric pain or discomfort, to, less frequently, symptoms such as gastrointestinal bleeding or persistent vomiting [64, 99]. Classic B symptoms (fever, night sweats, weight loss) are extremely rare. A gastric MALT lymphoma is often diagnosed following an upper endoscopy performed for dyspepsia.

Similarly, several different nonspecific endoscopic patterns have been described. Although it may appear at endoscopy as a clear malignant lesion (giant ulcer, vegetant mass, etc.) as shown in Fig. 4.2, gastric MALT lymphoma is frequently characterized by erosions, small nodules, thickening of gastric folds – generally suggesting a benign condition – or even by apparently normal gastric mucosa [99].

Pathology and *Helicobacter pylori* Infection

The histologic diagnosis can be challenging due to the heterogeneity of cells within the tumor specimen, but the presence of lymph epithelial lesions (invasion of neoplastic cells into individual glands) is a strong indicator of gastric MALT lymphoma. Once the diagnosis is confirmed, the next task is to establish the *H. pylori* status [99]. Gastric MALT lymphoma is uniquely associated with *H. pylori* infection (present in 90% of cases). A variety of detection methods are available, including identification in the histologic specimen, a biopsy urease test, a urea breath test, a stool antigen test, and serology. Upon establishment of the diagnosis, it is then worthwhile to perform a FISH evaluation for a t(11;18)(q21;q21) [4]. This translocation is recurrent in MALT lymphomas and produces a fusion between the AIP2 gene and the MLT/MALT1 gene, generating a chimeric protein that promotes cell survival and proliferation via activation of the transcription factor NF-k. This translocation can be detected in 30–40% of gastric MALT lymphoma cases and has clinical significance. Patients harboring t(11;18) are more likely to have widely disseminated disease, more likely to be *H. pylori* negative, and less likely to respond to *H. pylori* eradication [39]. In one series, only 2 of 44 patients with t(11;18) responded to eradication therapy and both later relapsed. The t(1;14)(p22;q32) translocation is also found in gastric MALT lymphoma but less frequently (~4 % of cases). This translocation results in deregulation of the BCL10 gene with subsequent activation of NF-k B. Gastric MALT lymphoma with t(1;14) is also unlikely to respond to eradication therapy [93].

Diagnosis and Staging

Although gastric MALT lymphoma has a typical indolent course, with a low disease-related morbidity and mortality, an accurate staging procedure is considered mandatory [14, 69]. Gastric MALT lymphoma presents as localized disease in 90 % of cases; advanced stages (III–IV) at diagnosis usually present with localization in both lymph nodes and other organs, particularly the bone marrow, lungs, and liver [2]. A comprehensive staging procedure includes a complete physical examination; routine laboratory tests; CT of the chest, abdomen, and pelvis; endoscopic ultrasonography; as well as bone marrow biopsy. Endoscopic ultrasound allows to accurately assessing both gastric wall infiltration and regional lymph node involvement [12, 38, 57]. The depth of invasion into the different layers of the gastric wall is predictive of lymphoma remission following therapy [57]. The role of PET scan in such a setting is still unclear [8].

Treatment and Outcome

The mainstay of treatment for *H. pylori*-positive patients is a combination of proton pump inhibitors (PPI) and antibiotics [7, 90]. Treatment with amoxicillin, clarithromycin, and PPIs results in eradication rates of 90 %. An alternative regimen of metronidazole, clarithromycin, and PPIs achieves the same result. Initial treatment with chemotherapy, surgery, or radiotherapy (alone or in combination) has not been shown to be superior to antibiotic treatment [66]. Locally advanced disease that has infiltrated the muscularis mucosa, serosa, or perigastric lymph nodes has a significantly lower response rate (RR). Such cases and *H. pylori* eradication failures require alternative approaches; however, there is no consensus on how to manage these patients. In some centers, *H. pylori*-negative patients at diagnosis also receive eradication therapy and high-dose PPIs as frontline therapy. Alternative treatment options include oral chlorambucil, radiation therapy (RT), or rituximab, without convincing evidence on the superiority of one of these strategies over the others due to the lack of prospective randomized trials. The role of surgery has been questioned, as a more conservative local approach (low-dose radiotherapy) may obtain similar results while improving quality of life. A prospective observational study of all histological subtypes of NHL of the gastrointestinal tract (GIT NHL 01/1992) included 185 patients with stage I or II gastric lymphoma; 106 of these patients underwent nonsurgical treatment, i.e., radiotherapy and/or chemotherapy. The subsequent, second prospective observational study (GITNHL02/1996) included 393 patients with localized primary gastric lymphoma who were treated with radiotherapy and/or chemotherapy only or additional surgery in the time interval 1996–2003. The survival rate at 42 months for patients treated with surgery was 86 % compared with 91 % for patients without surgery. In both these nonrandomized studies, there was no disadvantage for an organ-preserving treatment, while quality of life was certainly better in non-operated patients. Patients with advanced-stage disease (10 %) should be treated according to the same principles as for other advanced-stage indolent B-cell lymphomas (single-agent rituximab, R-CVP, R-CHOP, R-fludarabine, etc.), without evidence in favor of one regimen over the others [39].

Role of Radiation Therapy

The efficacy of radiation therapy (RT) has been shown in several studies, with excellent results in terms of complete response rate (nearly 100 %) and long-term durability [5, 71, 91]. Historically, total abdominal radiation (20 Gy in 3–4 weeks) with a boost to the stomach, para-aortic lymph nodes, and spleen (20 Gy in 2–3 weeks) was given on the basis that the pattern of spread, i.e., to the peritoneum, was similar to its solid tumor counterpart, with 5-year survival rates quoted of 70–95% for stage I disease [1, 87]. In recent years radiation fields were progressively reduced: from the data of 72 patients who underwent radical surgery between 1991 and 2001, retrospectively reviewed by Park et al. [60], gastric MALT lymphoma emerged as localized gastric disease in the majority of cases. Of the 72 patients analyzed, 45 (62.5 %) had low-grade MALT lymphoma, and 67 % of low-grade tumors were confined to the mucosa and submucosa. Lymph node involvement was identified in 24.4 % of the low-grade MALT patients (and 63.0 % of the high-grade MLS patients). In the low-grade group, lymph node involvement was limited to the perigastric lymph nodes in all cases except for one. Thus, a rational radiation clinical treatment volume is the stomach itself and local perigastric nodes [1] (Fig. 4.3). In the experience of Princess Margaret Hospital in Toronto, RT was used in 167 patients with extranodal MALT lymphomas (involving the stomach in 25 patients). The median dose to non-orbital sites was 30 Gy (range 17.5–35 Gy). The median follow-up was 7.4 years (range 0.67–16.2 years) with a 10-year relapse-free survival of 92 % [31].

Radiotherapy Techniques

The optimal dose and technique of RT are currently not well defined. As already mentioned, the target volume should be limited to the stomach and perigastric nodes. In combination with reduced radiation doses, a smaller volume leads to equivalent disease control with less acute and late side effects. Excellent results were achieved after a median dose of 30 Gy in 15–20 fractions [42, 71, 87, 91]. Table 4.1 summarizes the most important experiences regarding the

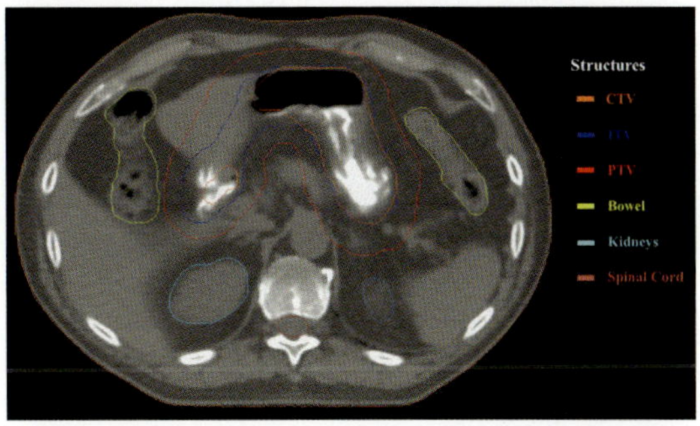

Fig. 4.3 Target delineation in our clinical case. A 4D-CT simulation was acquired to take into account gastric movements and displacement of organ at risk during respiratory phases

Table 4.1 Results of radiotherapy in patients with gastric MALT lymphoma

Reference, year	No. of patients	Treatment	RR (%)	EFS (%)	Survival (%)
Schechter et al. 1998 [71]	17	RT to the stomach and adjacent lymph nodes: 30 Gy/20 fr (range 28.5–43.5 Gy)	ND	27 months 100	27-month OS 100
Yahalom et al. 2002 [91]	51	RT to the stomach and adjacent nodes: median 30 Gy	CR 96	4-year FFTF 89	4-year OS 83 4-year CSS 100
Tsang et al. 2003 [84]	10	RT to the stomach and local nodes: 20–35 Gy	100	5 years 100	5-year OS 100
Koch et al. 2005 [42]	144	Whole abdominal RT: 30 Gy ± 10 Gy boost	ND	42-month FFP 88	42-month OS 93
Avilés et al. 2005 [5]	78	Whole abdominal RT : 30 Gy ± 10 Gy boost	CR 100	10-year FFP 52	10-year OS 75
Vrieling et al. 2008 [87]	56	Stomach + whole abdominal RT : 20 Gy + 20 Gy boost	CR 95	ND	5-year OS 74 10-year OS 63 10-year CSS 94
Wirth et al. 2013 [89]	102	RT to the stomach and involved nodes (61 pts) or whole abdominal RT (41 pts): median 40 Gy	CR 96	10-year FFTF 88	10-year OS 70

RR response rate, *EFS* event-free survival rate, *ND* not determined, *OS* overall survival rate, *CR* complete remission, *FFTF* freedom from treatment failure, *CSS* cancer-specific survival rate, *FFP* freedom from progression role of radiotherapy in gastric MALT lymphoma. A recent UK dose–response study that included extranodal lymphoma (although potential differences in efficacy at different anatomical sites have not been reported) suggested a dose of 24 Gy in 12 fractions [46]. This dose level is now accepted as a standard in most centers [22].

Improvements in target visualization (4D-CT scans) and radiation techniques and delivery (multi-fields 3D conformal-RT and intensity-modulated radiation therapy, IMRT) have further optimized gastric radiotherapy. Early reports suggested that 4D-CT and IMRT improve the definition of treatment volumes. Della Biancia et al. [18] analyzed 15 patients, categorized into three types depending on the geometric relationship between the planning target volume (PTV) and the kidneys. AP/PA and four-field three-dimensional conformal radiation therapy (3DCRT) plans were generated for each patient. IMRT was planned for four patients with a challenging geometric relationship. For patients without an overlap between PTV and kidneys, no benefit was shown for 3DCRT over AP/PA. However, for patients with PTVs in close proximity to the kidneys or with a high degree of overlap, the four-field 3DCRT plans were superior, reducing the volume of the left kidney receiving 15 Gy. In the selected cases, IMRT led to a further decrease in the left kidney dose as well as in the mean liver dose. This study showed that geometric relationships between the target and the kidneys should be taken into account when choosing the best beam arrangement. Van der Geld et al. [86] also showed that a reduction in kidney dose was evident with IMRT; the authors also evaluated the potential benefit of respiration-gated radiotherapy techniques, showing no differences. More recently, Watanabe et al. [88] demonstrated that both intrafractional gastric motion and interfractional variability of the stomach shape were considerable during RT and thus recommended regular verification of gastric movement and shape before and during RT in order to individualize treatment volume. Matoba et al. [50] compared a treatment planning approach using 4D-CT (plan A) and a conventional planning with a uniform margin (plan B), using dose-volume histograms of the planning target volume and the organ at risk, as well as the dose coverage of the clinical target volume (CTV) assessed by weekly online cone-beam CT during the treatment course. The mean PTV of plan A was significantly smaller than that of plan B ($p=0.008$). The mean doses to the liver and heart in plan A were significantly lower than those in plan B ($p=0.02$ and 0.03, respectively). The reductions of V(20Gy) of each kidney in plan A compared with those in plan B were $4.8 \pm 2.4\,\%$ in the right kidney and $16.3 \pm 10.4\,\%$ in the left. There was no significant difference in the dose coverage of the CTV between the plans during the treatment course. They concluded that treatment planning using 4D-CT for gastric MALT lymphoma was useful for minimizing the dose to organs at risk. In summary, in combination with treating the patient in a fasting state (to minimize stomach distension and movement), with oral contrast medium (Gastrografin), modern radiation techniques allow a homogeneous dose delivery to the stomach and perigastric lymph nodes while sparing the surrounding normal tissues such as the kidneys and liver.

In our patient exclusive RT was utilized after progression of disease in August 2013. A CT simulation after 6 h of fasting and using oral contrast with barium sulfate was performed with patient in supine position and arms above the head. We utilized a 4D-CT to document stomach movement with free-breathing respiratory motion. The CTV encompassed the entire stomach, while the internal target volume (ITV) corresponded to CTV enlarged to account for the movement of the stomach during the respiratory phases. An isotropic margin of 10 mm was added to ITV to obtain the PTV (Fig. 4.3). A total dose of 30 Gy in 20 fractions was delivered using image-guided volumetric radiation therapy (IGRT-VMAT), as shown in Fig. 4.4. Treatment was well tolerated without any significant toxicity. PET-CT scan (Fig. 4.5) and upper endoscopy, both performed 3 months after the end of treatment, showed a complete response of the MALT lymphoma, still persisting 20 months later.

Toxicity of Radiation Therapy

Acute toxicities are usually manageable during treatment and typically include anorexia, nausea, and vomiting. In the past, radiotherapy was often omitted because of concerns regarding the risk of perforation, hemorrhage, or late effects such as persistent renal damage. Mittal et al. [53], in a critical review of published studies in which an increased rate of gastric perforation had been described, identified that only one of the 75 gastric perforations reported (1 %) had truly occurred during or after radiotherapy. On the other hand, the risk of gastric perforation at the time of diagnosis, but before treatment, was 4 % (25 of 626 patients). It has to be noted that of the 25 patients with a gastric perforation before the starting of treatment, 16 had aggressive lymphomas and the other 9 NHL of the stomach without further subclassification. Thus an aggressive histology is probably a risk factor for perforation; the GIT NHL 01/1992 study reported no radiation-induced perforation or gastrointestinal hemorrhage among 185 patients with MALT lymphoma.

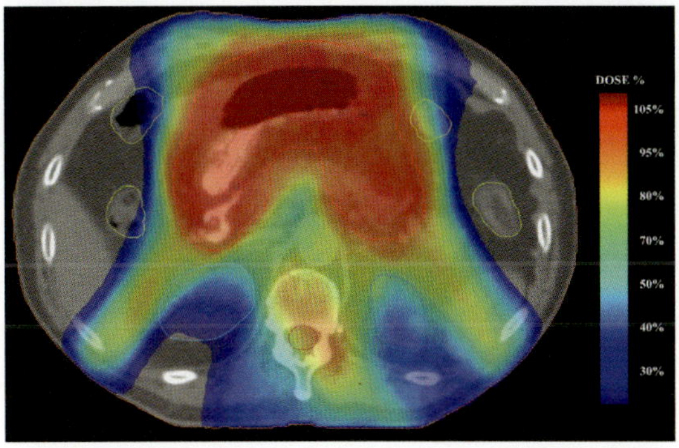

Fig. 4.4 IMRT/VMAT dose distribution generated for the RT plan. The intensive modulation plays an important role in obtaining good-quality plan for this type of case and allows a good sparing of organs at risk (e.g., kidneys, outlined with *blue lines*)

The risk of clinically significant renal damage or hypertension as a complication of primary radiotherapy of gastric lymphoma is very low. Maor et al. [48] studied 27 patients with gastric lymphoma in stage I or II, who had received at least 24 Gy of radiation to at least one third of the left kidney (unusual with current radiation volumes and dose). Only two patients developed mild hypertension (150/90 mmHg) after high-dose renal irradiation (irradiation of half, or all, of the left kidney with 40 Gy).

Summary

Radiation therapy is highly effective in the treatment of gastric MZL with excellent results in terms of complete response rate and long-term durability. A planning procedure with 4D-CT is

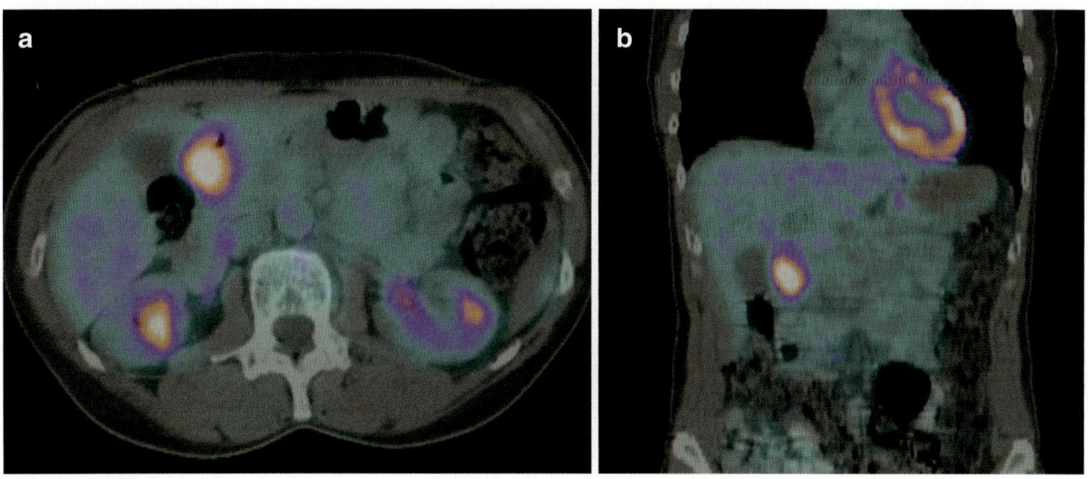

Fig. 4.5 Complete response at PET-CT scan 3 months after the end of radiation therapy (**a**) axial (**b**) coronal

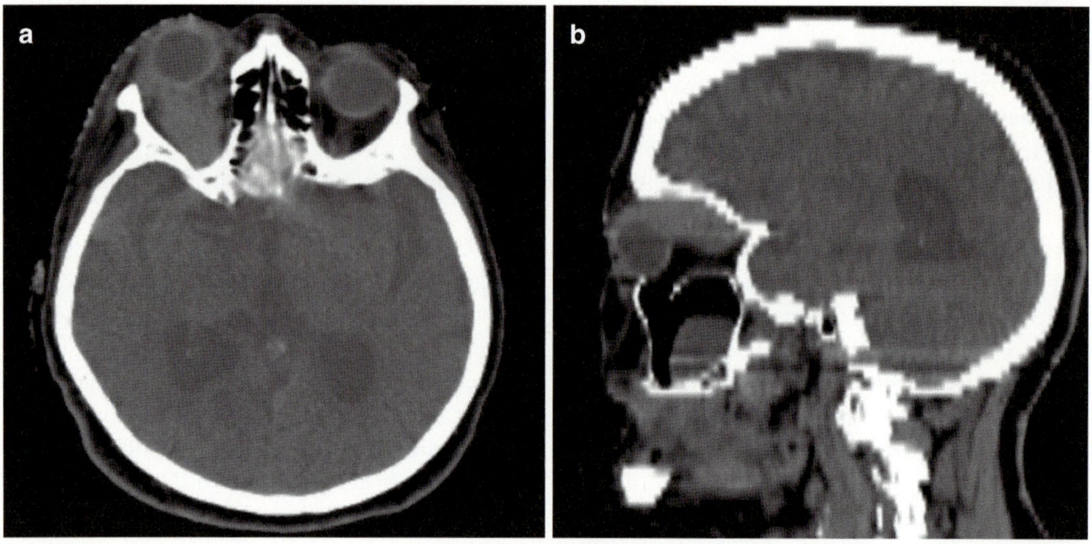

Fig. 4.6 Axial (**a**) and sagittal (**b**) view of the left orbital lesion at the MRI scan

highly recommended to account for gastric movements during the respiratory phases. GTV volume should include gross disease (if present and evaluable at CT and PET-CT scan); CTV should encompass the entire gastric volume and perigastric lymph nodes, if visible. ITV is determined in the case of 4D-CT planning. PTV volume is influenced by setup variation; we advise an isotropic expansion of 5–10 mm over the final ITV. We suggest to consider a total dose range between 24 and 30 Gy. Modern radiation techniques, including 3DCRT and IMRT, are recommended to reduce radiation of the kidneys and liver and keep the dose as low as reasonably achievable.

Ocular Adnexal Marginal Zone B-Cell Lymphomas (MALT Lymphomas)

Lymphomas of the ocular adnexa are a heterogeneous group accounting for approximately 1–2 % of all non-Hodgkin lymphomas and approximately 7–8 % of extranodal lymphomas [6, 28]. Ocular adnexa include the orbit, extraocular muscles, conjunctiva, eyelids, lacrimal gland, and apparatus. The incidence of ocular adnexal lymphoma (OAL) has increased by 6.3 % annually in the period from 1975 to 2001, more rapidly than non-Hodgkin lymphomas at other extranodal sites (Moslehi et al. [55]). Ninety-five percent to 100 % of reported cases of OAL are B-cell neoplasms, and the majority are low grade. Extranodal marginal zone lymphoma of MALT type is the most common histologic subtype of primary OAL, constituting about 35–80 % of cases [51].

Clinical Case

A 68-year-old woman was in her usual state of health until July 2014 when she first appreciated a swelling on the left eyelid. At that time, she didn't report any symptoms, like drenching night sweats, fevers, weight loss, or pruritus. After an ophthalmologic examination, an orbit CT demonstrated a dimensional enlargement of the left lacrimal gland. A magnetic resonance imaging (MRI) confirmed a superior-lateral mass of the left orbit that originated from the lacrimal gland and that caused deviation of the superior and lateral rectus muscles (Fig. 4.6). She underwent an incisional biopsy with diagnosis of ocular adnexal MALT lymphoma (OAML). Further assessment including a complete history and physical examination, routine laboratory studies, serum protein electrophoresis, serum LDH, β2-microglobulin, chest x-ray, and CT of the chest, abdomen, and pelvis were performed. Furthermore, she was evaluated for a *Chlamydophila psittaci* (Cp) infection resulting negative.

Clinical Presentation

OAML are mostly seen in the fifth to seventh decade of life (median age, 65 years), with female predominance (male–female = 1:1.5/2). In contrast, studies in Korean populations reveal a significantly younger age (median, 46 years) at the time of diagnosis, with male rather than female predominance [15, 94].

The most frequent site of origin is the orbit (40 %), followed by conjunctiva (35–40 %), lacrimal gland (10–15 %), and eyelid (10 %) [55]. Bilateral involvement occurs in 10–15 % of cases (80 % simultaneous, 20 % sequential events).

Conjunctival lesions typically present as mobile pink infiltrates in the substantia propria ("salmon-pink patch"), causing conjunctival swelling, redness, and irritation. Orbital lymphoid proliferations are characterized by a palpable, firm, or rubbery mass causing progressive proptosis, occasionally associated with periorbital edema, decreased visual acuity, motility disturbances, and diplopia. The median interval between the onset of symptoms and time of diagnosis is variable, ranging from 1 month to 10 years (median, 7 months). This delay can be attributed to the slow evolution of symptoms, especially in conjunctival lymphomas, which may masquerade as chronic conjunctivitis and frequently show an impressive initial response to topical steroids. Steroids may mask the clinical presentation and render pathologic diagnosis more difficult, frequently resulting in a need for repeat biopsy to establish the diagnosis [76].

Pathology and *Chlamydophila psittaci* Infection

In the clinical case, the final pathology demonstrated OAML. OAML show similar histology and immunophenotype to MALT lymphoma in other sites. Tumor cells typically express IgM, and less often IgA or IgG, and show light chain restriction. The tumor cells of MALT lymphoma are CD20+, CD79a+, CD5−, CD10−, CD23−, CD43±, and CD11c±(weak). Infrequent cases are CD5+. The lymphoma cells express the marginal zone cell-associated antigens CD21 and CD35. Staining for CD21 and CD35 also typically reveals expanded mesh works of follicular dendritic cells corresponding to colonized follicles [79]. The most frequent translocation in OAML, observed in 15–40 % of patients, is t(11;18)(q21;q21). The t(14;18)(q32;q21), t(1;14)(p22;q34), and t(3;14)(p14;q32) translocations are found in up to 38 %, less than 5 % and 20 % of patients, respectively [76].

Cp is the etiologic agent of psittacosis, an infection caused by exposure to infected animals [11, 61]. Cp infection is detected in tumor tissue of 11 % of B-cell lymphomas [24]. The most important Cp-related tumor is OAML of the ocular adnexae, with prevalence rates between 47 and 80 % in countries like Austria, Germany, Italy, and Korea [25].

Diagnosis and Staging

The initial evaluation of patients with OAL requires careful ophthalmologic examination and adequate tissue sampling for histopathologic diagnosis. Further assessment for accurate staging and therapy planning includes a complete history and physical examination, routine laboratory studies; serum protein electrophoresis; serum LDH; β2-microglobulin; chest x-ray; CT of the chest, abdomen, and pelvis; and bone marrow biopsy (controversial). CT and MRI with contrast enhancement are the primary imaging tools in the evaluation of ocular adnexal proliferations (Fig. 4.6). They aid in the assessment of location, size, and degree of infiltration; however, they cannot reliably distinguish between benign and malignant processes. Typical imaging appearance of a lymphoid lesion is a unifocal, homogeneous, well-circumscribed lesion of isodensity to slight hyper-density, with mild to moderate contrast enhancement, and smooth, distinct borders, molding into adjacent tissues and displacing rather than infiltrating orbital structures [78].

Traditional staging of OAL has used the Ann Arbor system [13]. However, the limitations of this system for staging extranodal non-Hodgkin lymphomas, such as OAL, have long been recognized, as these show different dissemination patterns from nodal lymphomas. Under the auspices of the American Joint Committee on Cancer, a new TNM-based staging system has been developed to overcome the shortcomings of the Ann Arbor System [17].

The majority (85–90 %) of patients with OAML present with localized disease (stage I). Nodal involvement is reported in approximately 5 % of patients. In various case series, 10–15 % of patients have disseminated disease (stage IV) at initial presentation, including bone marrow involvement in approximately 5–8 % [76].

Our patient presented with disease confined to one extranodal site, and therefore, she fell classically into a stage I disease.

Treatment and Outcome

In the determination of optimal therapy, several factors must be taken into account: (1) extension of disease, within and outside the periocular region, (2) prognostic factors related to the patient and the disease, and (3) additional consideration of the functional impact of the treatment on the eye. Several standard treatment modalities are available for OAL, including surgical excision, RT, chemotherapy (single agent or combination regimens), and immunotherapy. Newer options such as radioimmunotherapy, "wait-and-see" policy, and doxycycline antibiotic therapy have been recently proposed and tested in small studies.

Surgical biopsy, mandatory to determine the histologic subtype of OAL, can be incisional or excisional, especially for localized and/or encapsulated lesions of the conjunctiva or lacrimal gland. Although a number of studies have included patients treated with surgery alone, local relapse has been reported more commonly in these patients compared with those who also received RT [15, 20, 44]. Two studies from Japan evaluated a "watch-and-wait" policy or no initial adjuvant therapy after surgical removal of a MALT lymphoma of the ocular adnexa [47, 80]. In Tanimoto series, 36 patients with a median age of 63 years were followed for a median of 7.1 years. Of these, 17 patients progressed (47 %), but only 11 actually required treatment. All others were free of progression (19/36, 53 %). In another retrospective analysis, Mannami et al. observed 12 patients with stage I OAML for a median duration of 50 months. None of the patients progressed during this time period. This strategy remains controversial but may be appropriate in frail elderly patients with asymptomatic disease or in the setting of severe comorbidities that preclude an aggressive therapeutic approach. However, even in this population, local radiation therapy can usually be given [76].

There are limited data on chemotherapy for patients with OAML. A small number of single-center, retrospective case series have included patients treated with different chemotherapy regimens, such as COP/cyclophosphamide, vincristine, and prednisone (CVP); cyclophosphamide, Adriamycin, vincristine, and prednisone (CHOP); cyclophosphamide, vincristine, procarbazine, and prednisone (C-MOPP); and chlorambucil, either alone or in combination with other modalities [30, 52, 68, 70], but only few reports contain detailed response rates and outcomes [30, 67, 74, 81]. Chlorambucil, given in a variety of doses, schedules, and combinations, is the most frequently used chemotherapy agent and has a highly favorable toxicity profile, making it a suitable agent for the treatment of frail, elderly patients. Irrespective of chemotherapy regimens, complete responses are observed in 67–100 % of patients; however, long-term outcome data suggest that local recurrence is the predominant cause of treatment failure, occurring in up to 29 % of patients [76]. Several authors report successful salvage with RT in patients who experience local failure after initial treatment with chemotherapy [30, 74].

Phase 2 data by Conconi et al. [16], Raderer et al. [65], and Lossos et al. [45] using single-agent rituximab in previously untreated patients demonstrated overall response rates between 50 and 87 %, but median time to disease progression was less than 1 year. Only a few case reports using single-agent rituximab in patients with OAML have been published [9, 16, 27, 35]. They confirm the high activity of rituximab in both newly diagnosed and relapsed disease, but early recurrence is common, particularly in pretreated patients. An exciting new therapy has been developed in the form of the radioimmunoconjugate of 90Y ibritumomab tiuxetan, which links the specific anti-CD20 antibody to the radioactive moiety. Prospective clinical trial of 90Y ibritumomab tiuxetan for frontline treatment of stage IE indolent ocular adnexal lymphoma in 12 patients showed complete response in ten patients and partial response in the other two, with no cases of cataract, dry eye syndrome, or radiation retinopathy [21, 72].

Based on the association between Cp infection and OAML, Cp-eradicating antibiotic therapy has received attention as a novel treatment approach for this disease. Ferreri et al. [26] conducted a prospective phase 2 clinical trial of 27 patients (15 newly diagnosed and 12 relapsed) with OAML, using doxycycline 100 mg orally twice daily for 3 weeks. Cp infection was confirmed in 11 patients. Partial or complete lymphoma regression after antibiotic therapy was observed in 7 of 11 Cp-positive and 6 of 16 Cp-negative patients, with an overall response rate of 48 %. The 2 year failure free survival rate among patients treated with doxycycline was 66 %. Given the variable prevalence of Cp infection in patients with OAML, empiric antibiotic treatment without prior testing for chlamydial infection cannot be generally recommended [33]. To shed more light on the efficacy of antibiotics in the treatment of patients with OAML, Husain et al. [36] conducted a meta-analysis, identifying four studies with a total of 42 patients who had been treated with oral doxycycline. Objective documentation of response was available for only 3 of 20 patients who reportedly achieved some response, whereas other 20 patients had stable disease and 2 progressed during antibiotic therapy. After antibiotic therapy, seven patients developed disease recurrence, six of them within 12 months of follow-up. Prospective trials with standardized objective response criteria and longer follow-up will be necessary to further evaluate the role of antibiotics in the treatment of OAML in different geographic regions.

Role of Radiation Therapy

Radiation therapy is the treatment of choice for the majority of patients with localized OAML. Several retrospective studies, most of which include a variety of lymphoma subtypes, have documented the short- and long-term efficacy and side effects of this therapeutic modality [19, 34, 43, 44, 77, 81, 84, 85]. Overall, RT leads to very high local control rates of 85–100 %. These outstanding results have to be balanced against frequent treatment-related toxicities and a substantial risk of distant recurrence (10–25 %) over at least 10 years after treatment. Most series report long-term relapse-free or disease-free survival rates (DFS) in the range of 70–90 % [76]. The majority of relapses in these series was distant and tended to occur in other sites [32, 43]. In the study of Tran et al. [83], only one patient experienced extra-orbital relapse; the discrepancy in the rate of extra-orbital recurrence may reflect in part the difference in methods of the initial staging investigations as well as the intensity of follow-up screening investigations [49]. Several studies identified that disease subsite may be a significant prognostic factor with conjunctival lesions having an excellent outcome and lacrimal tumors doing more poorly [49, 58]. Synchronous bilateral disease is well recognized in MZL and is of uncertain prognostic significance. The prognostic impact of synchronous bilateral disease has varied across series, with some reports suggesting a higher rate of relapse in patients with bilateral orbital lymphoma presentations [32, 85]. Other studies do not report an elevated risk of relapse in this patient group [43, 49, 62]. In a more recent study, four patients with bilateral MZL (three with synchronous and one with metachronous disease) received bilateral orbital RT with curative intent, with no systemic relapses observed [83].

There is no universally accepted radiation schedule for patients with OAML, and controversy exists regarding the optimal radiation dose and fractionation. Several studies indicate that a dose of at least 25 Gy is required to provide optimal local control and minimize the rate of local failures in OAML [19, 84, 85]. Le et al. [43] found no differences in local or distal recurrence and survival after radiation with less than or equal to 34 Gy compared with higher doses; however, significant ophthalmologic toxicity with vision loss was observed after doses of more than or equal to 34 Gy. In the study of Rosado et al. [68], including 46 patients with stage I OAML, radiation therapy of 30–36 Gy (45 Gy in two patients) led to durable local control in 100 % of cases. More recently, Tran et al. [83] report the efficacy of low-dose RT and fractionation (total 24–25 Gy in 1.5–2 Gy fractions) in a retrospective analysis of 24 patients with orbital MZL, 22 of whom were stage IEA. Only one local failure occurred at the electron beam penumbra, attributed to marginal miss. Two further relapses, one in the contralateral orbit and one systemic relapse, occurred in patients with initial stage IEA disease. Five-year progression-free survival and overall survival were 81 % and 100 %, respectively. It is worth to mention that currently there is an effort to further lower the dose to as low as 4 Gy in two fractions. Fasola et al. [23] have recently reported on 27 sites with ocular involvement treated with 4 Gy leading to a 2-year freedom from regional relapse rate of 96 %, with only one patient who relapsed outside of the radiation field and who was rescued with another 4 Gy. These results are promising and might build a case to make this dose the standard of care in the future.

Radiotherapy Techniques

Radiotherapy techniques typically vary according to disease location in the orbit: tumors confined to superficial structures, such as the conjunctiva, eyelid, and lacrimal gland, can be approached with a direct electron beam using a lens-sparing device to avoid cataract formation, whereas retrobulbar tumors are treated with photon beam radiation. Questions regarding radiotherapy technique, including the required target volume (entire vs. partial orbital irradiation) for different subsites of disease, degree of protection from smaller fractions and lens shielding, and the use of bolus to improve efficacy, also need to be evaluated, as there are few data or little consensus available.

The first issue is whether the entire orbit needs to be irradiated in all cases. Pfeffer et al. [63] noted an increased risk of relapse when partial orbital irradiation was used, and Fung et al. [29] reported a posterior orbital relapse in a partially treated orbit. Several series reported the use of partial orbital shielding without an increase in relapse rates [49, 73, 85, 92]. In most series this has involved the use of anterior electron beam therapy for superficial anteriorly located lesions. It appears that anterior orbital irradiation is effective in patients with conjunctival and eyelid disease, but that partial orbital irradiation may lead to an increased relapse risk when the macroscopic disease extends even partly into the posterior orbital soft tissue [83]. The second issue relates to the use of lens shielding in order to reduce the incidence of cataract. Such shielding may be associated with inadvertent tumor underdosing and must be used with caution, to avoid an increased risk of local relapse. Several reports have highlighted this risk, with local relapses attributed to inadvertent partial shielding of tumor [29, 85]. However other reports would suggest that the careful use of lens shielding don’t lead to treatment failure [43, 49, 73, 83]. The third technical issue is whether to use bolus to ensure that conjunctival tumors or other very superficially located lesions receive the full dose of radiation. In at least three reports, local failure in superficial disease sites occurred with no mention of the use of bolus [73, 85, 92]. In contrast, Goda et al. [32] report that bolus was not used routinely in their cohort unless there was frank skin involvement, without an apparent increase in relapse rate. Table 4.2

Table 4.2 Results of radiotherapy as first-line treatment in patients with OAML

Reference, year	No. of patients	Stage I, %	Dose, Gy	CR, %	LR, %	DR, %	Survival, %	LRM, %
Stafford et al. 2001 [75]	40	85	15–54	98	2	25	5-year RFS 88 5-year OS 74 5-year DSS 100	0
Le et al. 2002 [43]	31	100	30–40	100	0	16	10-year PFS 71 10-year OS 73	3
Fung et al. 2003 [29]	48	81	30.6	100	8	25	10-year OS 81 10-year DSS 100	0
Hasegawa et al. 2003 [34]	20	95	30	100	5	20	10-year PFS 70 10-year DSS 100	0
Tsang et al. 2003 [84]	30	97	25	97	17	10	5-year DFS 74 5-year OS 97	ND
Uno et al. 2003 [85]	50	100	20–46	98	6	6	5-year OS 91	2
Lee et al. 2005 [44]	29	100	30–45	100	3	0	3-year EFS 93 3-year OS 100	0
Ejima et al. 2006 [19]	42	100	30–36	84	10	10	5-year PFS 77 5-year DSS 100	0
Suh et al. 2006 [77]	48	96	30.6	96	6	0	10-year DFS 93 10-year DSS 98	2
Tanimoto et al. 2007 [81]	58	94	30–40	83	9	2	10-year PFS 72 10-year OS 92	0
Nam et al. 2009 [58]	66	100	20–45	97	3	7.5	5-year RFS 92 5-year OS 96.4	ND
Goda et al. 2011 [32]	89	100	25	99	2	22.5	7-year OS 91 7-year DSS 96 % 7-year RFS 64 %	4
Tran et al. 2013 [83]	25	92	24–25	100	4	8	5-year PFS 81 5-year OS 100	0

OAML ocular adnexal MALT lymphoma, *CR* complete remission rate, *LR* local recurrence rate, *DR* distal recurrence rate, *LRM* lymphoma-related mortality, *RFS* relapse-free survival rate, *OS* overall survival rate, *DSS* disease-specific survival rate, *PFS* progression-free survival rate, *DFS* disease-free survival rate, *EFS* event-free survival rate, *ND* not determined

presents an overview on the most important retrospective studies regarding the role of radiotherapy in OAML.

In our patient, given the negativity of Cp infection, exclusive RT was utilized. The target volume included the entire orbit (Fig. 4.7a) that was treated with photon beam radiation using image-guided volumetric radiation therapy (IGRT-VMAT), as shown in Fig. 4.7b. A total dose of 24 Gy in 12 fractions was delivered without bolus and with slight cutaneous and conjunctival toxicity. The MRI scan performed 2 months after end of radiation showed a good partial response, and at the clinical evaluation, the patient had a complete resolution of the eyelid swelling.

Toxicity of Radiation Therapy

The rationale for using the lowest effective dose of radiation for orbital MZL is to reduce the incidence of both early and late toxicities. Immediate toxicity consists of mild to moderate cutaneous or conjunctival reactions. Long-term complications are observed in up to 50 % of patients, including cataract formation (30–50 %) and xerophthalmia (20–40 %) [75]. In addition to RT dose, cataractogenesis is influenced by numerous risk factors such as age, familial predisposition, diabetes mellitus, and drugs. A reduction in the incidence of cataracts from lens shielding has been documented in many but not all series evaluating this endpoint [10, 62].

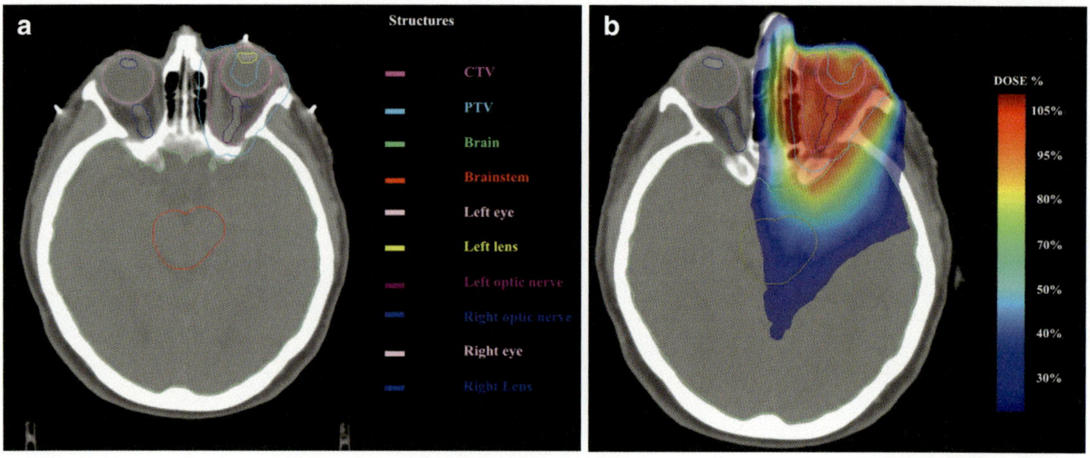

Fig. 4.7 IMRT/VMAT dose distribution generated for this case. Strong efforts were done to spare organs at risk as much as possible. (**a**) target and organs at risk (**b**) isodose distribution

Differences between series may reflect variations in the technical method of lens shielding. Aside from cataractogenesis, the most common late toxicity reported after orbital irradiation is xerophthalmia. Kennerdell et al. [41] reported the development of mild xerophthalmia in 26 of 54 patients with orbital lymphoma treated with low-dose RT, with 18 of 54 patients having chronic symptoms. In Tran et al. [83] study, nine patients (38 %) had grade 1 xerophthalmia, but most required the use of lubricating eye drops weekly or less often. Goda et al. [32], who used 2.5 Gy per fraction to a total of 25 Gy, reported a 32 % incidence of dry eye but with four patients having grade 2–3 xerophthalmia. Radiation doses of more than or equal to 36 Gy may result in deleterious ophthalmologic toxicity, such as ischemic retinopathy, optic atrophy, corneal ulceration, and neovascular glaucoma, associated with significant vision loss [75].

Summary

Radiation therapy is highly effective and plays a major role in the treatment of OAML. A complete staging with MRI of orbits and adjacent structures is recommended to better define the target volumes. CTV should encompass the entire orbit, including extra-orbital extension if suspected. Partial orbital irradiation should be left to particular cases and used with caution. We suggest a CTV to PTV expansion of 5 mm. A total dose of 24 Gy is considered safe and effective. Modern radiation techniques, including 3DCRT or IMRT, are recommended to reduce radiation of contralateral orbit. Bolus should be used in the case of conjunctival MZL; lens shielding should be used with caution to avoid target missing.

References

1. Aleman BM. Role of radiotherapy in the treatment of lymphomas of the gastrointestinal tract. Best Pract Res Clin Gastroenterol. 2010;24:27–34.
2. Andriani A, Zullo A, Di Raimondo F, et al. Clinical and endoscopic presentation of primary gastric lymphoma: a multicentre study. Aliment Pharmacol Ther. 2006;23:721–6.
3. Armitage JO, Weisenburger DD. New approach to classifying non-Hodgkin's lymphomas: clinical features of the major histologic subtypes. Non-Hodgkin's lymphoma classification project. J Clin Oncol. 1998;16:2780–95.
4. Auer IA, Gascoyne RD, Conners JM, et al. t(11;18)(q21;q21) is the most common translocation in MALT lymphomas. Ann Oncol. 1997;8:979–85.
5. Avilés A, Nambo MJ, Neri N, Talavera A, Cleto S. Mucosa-associated lymphoid tissue (MALT) lymphoma of the stomach: results of a controlled clinical trial. Med Oncol. 2005;22:57–62.

6. Bairey O, Kremer I, Rakowsky E, et al. Orbital and adnexal involvement in systemic non-Hodgkin's lymphoma. Cancer. 1994;73:2395–9.
7. Bayerdorffer E, Neubauer A, Rudolph B, et al. Regression of primary gastric lymphoma of mucosa-associated lymphoid tissue type after cure of Helicobacter pylori infection. MALT Lymphoma Study Group. Lancet. 1995;345(8965):1591–4.
8. Beal KP, Yeung HW, Yahalom J. FDG-PET scanning for detection and staging of extranodal marginal zone lymphomas of the MALT type: a report of 42 cases. Ann Oncol. 2005;16:473–80.
9. Benetatos L, Alymara V, Asproudis I, Bourantas KL. Rituximab as first line treatment for MALT lymphoma of extraocular muscles. Ann Hematol. 2006;85:625–6.
10. Bolek TW, Moyses HM, Marcus RBJ, et al. Radiotherapy in the management of orbital lymphoma. Int J Radiat Oncol Biol Phys. 1999;44:31–6.
11. Byrne GI, Ojcius DM. Chlamydia and apoptosis: life and death decisions of an intracellular pathogen. Nat Rev Microbiol. 2004;2(10):802–8.
12. Caletti G, Zinzani PL, Fusaroli P, et al. The importance of endoscopic ultrasonography in the management of low-grade gastric mucosa-associated lymphoid tissue lymphoma. Aliment Pharmacol Ther. 2002;16:1715–22.
13. Carbone PP, Kaplan HS, Musshoff K, et al. Report of the committee on Hodgkin's disease staging classification. Cancer Res. 1971;31:1860–1.
14. Cavalli F, Isaacson PG, Gascoyne RD, Zucca E. MALT lymphomas. Hematology Am Soc Hematol Educ Program. 2001:241–58.
15. Cho EY, Han JJ, Ree HJ, et al. Clinicopathologic analysis of ocular adnexal lymphomas: extranodal marginal zone B-cell lymphoma constitutes the vast majority of ocular lymphomas among Koreans and affects younger patients. Am J Hematol. 2003;73:87–96.
16. Conconi A, Martinelli G, Thieblemont C, et al. Clinical activity of rituximab in extranodal marginal zone B-cell lymphoma of MALT type. Blood. 2003;102:2741–5.
17. Coupland SE, White V, Rootman J, et al. TNM Staging of ocular adnexal lymphomas. In: Edge SE, Byrd DR, Carducci MA, et al., editors. AJCC Cancer staging manual. 7th ed. New York: Springer; 2009.
18. Della Biancia C, Hunt M, Furhang E, Wu E, Yahalom J. Radiation treatment planning techniques for lymphoma of the stomach. Int J Radiat Oncol Biol Phys. 2005;62:745–51.
19. Ejima Y, Sasaki R, Okamoto Y, et al. Ocular adnexal mucosa-associated lymphoid tissue lymphoma treated with radiotherapy. Radiother Oncol. 2006;78:6–9.
20. Esik O, Ikeda H, Mukai L, et al. A retrospective analysis of different modalities for treatment of primary orbital non-Hodgkin's lymphomas. Radiother Oncol. 1996;38:13–8.
21. Esmaeili B, McLaughlin P, Pro B, et al. Prospective trial of targeted radioimmunotherapy with Y-90 ibritumomab tiuxetan (Zevalin) for frontline treatment of early stage extranodal indolent ocular adnexal lymphoma. Ann Oncol. 2009;20:709–14.
22. Falk S. Lymphomas of the upper GI tract: the role of radiotherapy. Clin Oncol. 2012;24:352–7.
23. Fasola CE, Jones JC, Huang DD, Le QT, Hoppe RT, Donaldson SS. Low-dose radiation therapy (2 Gy × 2) in the treatment of orbital lymphoma. Int J Radiat Oncol Biol Phys. 2013;86(5):930–5. doi:10.1016/j.ijrobp.2013.04.035. Epub 2013 May 29.
24. Ferreri AJ, Dognini GP, Ponzoni M, et al. Chlamydia psittaci eradicating antibiotic therapy in patients with advanced-stage ocular adnexal MALT lymphoma. Ann Oncol. 2008;19(1):194–5.
25. Ferreri AJ, Govi S, Ponzoni M. Marginal zone lymphomas and infectious agents. Semin Cancer Biol. 2013;23(6):431–40.
26. Ferreri AJ, Ponzoni M, Dognini GP, et al. Bacteria-eradicating therapy for ocular adnexal MALT lymphoma: questions for an open international prospective trial. Ann Oncol. 2006;17:1721–2.
27. Ferreri AJ, Ponzoni M, Martinelli G, et al. Rituximab in patients with mucosal-associated lymphoid tissue-type lymphoma of the ocular adnexa. Haematologica. 2005;90:1578–9.
28. Freeman C, Berg JW, Cutler SJ. Occurrence and prognosis of extranodal lymphoma. Cancer. 1972;29:252–60.
29. Fung CY, Tarbell NJ, Lucarelli MJ, et al. Ocular adnexal lymphoma: clinical behavior of distinct World Health Organization classification subtypes. Int J Radiat Oncol Biol Phys. 2003;57:1382–91.
30. Galieni P, Polito E, Leccisotti A, et al. Localized orbital lymphoma. Haematologica. 1997;82:436–9.
31. Goda JS, Gospodarowicz M, Pintillie M, et al. Long-term outcome in localized extranodal mucosa-associated lymphoid tissue lymphomas treated with radiotherapy. Cancer. 2010;116:3815–24.
32. Goda JS, Le LW, Lapperrier NJ, et al. Localized orbital mucosa associated lymphoma tissue lymphoma managed with primary radiation therapy: efficacy and toxicity. Int J Radiat Oncol Biol Phys. 2011;81:e659–66.
33. Grünberger B, Hauff W, Lukas J, et al. 'Blind' antibiotic treatment targeting Chlamydia is not effective in patients with MALT lymphoma of the ocular adnexa. Ann Oncol. 2006;17:484–7.
34. Hasegawa M, Kojima M, Shioya M, et al. Treatment results of radiotherapy for malignant lymphoma of the orbit and histopathologic review according to the WHO classification. Int J Radiat Oncol Biol Phys. 2003;57:172–6.
35. Heinz C, Merz H, Nieschalk M, et al. Rituximab for the treatment of extranodal marginal zone B-cell lymphoma of the lacrimal gland. Br J Ophthalmol. 2007;91:1563–4.
36. Husain A, Roberts D, Pro B, et al. Meta-analyses of the association between Chlamydia psittaci and ocular adnexal lymphoma and the response of ocular adnexal lymphoma to antibiotics. Cancer. 2007;110:809–15.

37. Isaacson PG. Update on MALT lymphomas. Best Pract Res Clin Haematol. 2005;18:57–68.
38. Janssen J. The impact of EUS in primary gastric lymphoma. Best Pract Res Clin Gastroenterol. 2009;23: 671–8.
39. Kahl B, Yang D. Marginal zone lymphomas: management of nodal, splenic and MALT NHL. Hematology Am Soc Hematol Educ Program. 2008:359–64.
40. Khalil MO, Morton LM, Devesa SS, et al. Incidence of marginal zone lymphoma in the United States, 2001–2009 with a focus on primary anatomic site. Br J Haematol. 2014;165:67–77.
41. Kennerdell JS, Flores NE, Hartsock RJ. Low-dose radiotherapy for lymphoid lesions of the orbit and ocular adnexa. Ophthal Plast Reconstr Surg. 1999;15:129–33.
42. Koch P, Probst A, Berdel WE, et al. Treatment results in localized primary gastric lymphoma: data of patients registered within the German multicenter study (GIT NHL 02/96). J Clin Oncol. 2005;23(28): 7050–9.
43. Le QT, Eulau SM, George TI, et al. Primary radiotherapy for localized orbital MALT lymphoma. Int J Radiat Oncol Biol Phys. 2002;52:657–63.
44. Lee JY, Kim MK, Lee KH, et al. Extranodal marginal zone B-cell lymphomas of mucosa-associated lymphoid tissue-type of the orbit. Ann Hematol. 2005;84:12–8.
45. Lossos IS, Morgensztern D, Blaya M, et al. Rituximab for treatment of chemoimmunotherapy naive marginal zone lymphoma. Leuk Lymphoma. 2007;48: 1630–2.
46. Lowry L, Smith P, Qian W, et al. Reduced dose radiotherapy for local control in non-Hodgkin lymphoma: a randomised phase III trial. Radiother Oncol. 2011;100:86–92.
47. Mannami T, Yoshino T, Oshima K, et al. Clinical, histopathological and immunogenetic analysis of ocular adnexal lymphoproliferative disorders: characterization of MALT lymphoma and reactive lymphoid hyperplasia. Mod Pathol. 2001;14:641–9.
48. Maor MH, North LB, Cabanillas FF, et al. Outcomes of high-dose unilateral kidney irradiation in patients with gastric lymphoma. Int J Radiat Oncol Biol Phys. 1998;41:647–50.
49. Martinet S, Ozsahin M, Belkacemi Y, et al. Outcome and prognostic factors in orbital lymphoma: a Rare Cancer Network study on 90 consecutive patients treated with radiotherapy. Int J Radiat Oncol Biol Phys. 2003;55:892–8.
50. Matoba M, Oota K, Toyoda I, et al. Usefulness of 4D-CT for radiation treatment planning of gastric MZBCL/MALT. J Radiat Res. 2012;53:333–7.
51. McKelvie PA. Ocular adnexal lymphomas: a review. Adv Anat Pathol. 2010;17(4):251–61.
52. McKelvie PA, McNab A, Francis IC, et al. Ocular adnexal lymphoproliferative disease: a series of 73 cases. Clin Experiment Ophthalmol. 2001;29: 387–93.
53. Mittal B, Wasserman TH, Griffith RC. Non-Hodgkin's lymphoma of the stomach. Am J Gastroenterol. 1983;78:780–7.
54. Morton LM, Wang SS, Devesa SS, et al. Lymphoma incidence patterns by WHO subtype in the United States, 1992–2001. Blood. 2006;107:265–76.
55. Moslehi R, Devesa SS, Schairer C, et al. Rapidly increasing incidence of ocular non-Hodgkin lymphoma. J Natl Cancer Inst. 2006;98:936–9.
56. Nakamura S, Matsumoto T, Iida M, et al. Primary gastrointestinal lymphoma in Japan: a clinicopathologic analysis of 455 patients with special reference to its time trends. Cancer. 2003;97:2462–73.
57. Nakamura S, Matsumoto T, Suekane H, et al. Predictive value of endoscopic ultrasonography for regression of gastric low grade and high grade MALT lymphomas after eradication of Helicobacter pylori. Gut. 2001;48:454–60.
58. Nam H, Ahn YC, Kim YD, et al. Prognostic significance of anatomic subsites: results of radiation therapy for 66 patients with localized orbital marginal zone B cell lymphoma. Radiother Oncol. 2009;90: 236–41.
59. Neubauer A, Zucca E. Gastrointestinal tract lymphomas. In: Cavalli F, Stein H, Zucca E, editors. Extranodal lymphomas pathology and management. London: Informa Health Care; 2008. p. 233–43.
60. Park W, Chang SK, Yang WI, et al. Rationale for radiotherapy as a treatment modality in gastric mucosa-associated lymphoid tissue lymphoma. Int J Radiat Oncol Biol Phys. 2004;58:1480–6.
61. Peeling RW, Brunham RC. Chlamydiae as pathogens: new species and new issues. Emerg Infect Dis. 1996;2(4):307–19.
62. Pelloski CE, Wilder RB, Ha CS, et al. Clinical stage IEA-IIEA orbital lymphomas: outcomes in the era of modern staging and treatment. Radiother Oncol. 2001;59:145–51.
63. Pfeffer MR, Rabin T, Tsvang L, et al. Orbital lymphoma: is it necessary to treat the entire orbit? Int J Radiat Oncol Biol Phys. 2004;60:527–30.
64. Psyrri A, Papageorgiou S, Economopoulos T. Primary extranodal lymphomas of stomach: clinical presentation, diagnostic pitfalls and management. Ann Oncol. 2008;19:1992–9.
65. Raderer M, Jager G, Brugger S, et al. Rituximab for treatment of advanced extranodal marginal zone B cell lymphoma of the mucosa-associated lymphoid tissue lymphoma. Oncology. 2003;65: 306–10.
66. Reinartz G, Willich N, Koch P. Strahlentherapie bei primaren gastrointestinalen Lymphomen. Chir Gastroenterol. 2002;18:53–9.
67. Rigacci L, Nassi L, Puccioni M, et al. Rituximab and chlorambucil as first-line treatment for low grade ocular adnexal lymphomas. Ann Hematol. 2007;86:565–8.
68. Rosado MF, Byrne Jr GE, Ding F, et al. Ocular adnexal lymphoma: a clinicopathologic study of a large cohort

of patients with no evidence for an association with Chlamydia psittaci. Blood. 2006;107:467–72.
69. Ruskoné-Four Mestraux A, Fischbach W, Aleman BMP, et al. EGILS consensus report. Gastric extranodal marginal zone B-cell lymphoma of MALT. Gut. 2011;60:747–58.
70. Sasai K, Yamabe H, Dodo Y, et al. Non-Hodgkin's lymphoma of the ocular adnexa. Acta Oncol. 2001;40:485–90.
71. Schechter NR, Portlock CS, Yahalom J. Treatment of mucosa-associated lymphoid tissue lymphoma of the stomach with radiation alone. J Clin Oncol. 1998;16:1916–21.
72. Shome D, Esmaeli B. Targeted monoclonal antibody therapy and radioimmunotherapy for lymphoproliferative disorders of the ocular adnexa. Curr Opin Ophthalmol. 2008;19:414–21.
73. Son SH, Choi BO, Kim G, et al. Primary radiation therapy in patients with localized orbital marginal zone B-cell lymphoma of mucosa-associated lymphoid tissue (MALT Lymphoma). Int J Radiat Oncol Biol Phys. 2010;77:86–91.
74. Song EK, Kim SY, Kim TM, et al. Efficacy of chemotherapy as a first-line treatment in ocular adnexal extranodal marginal zone B-cell lymphoma. Ann Oncol. 2008;19:242–6.
75. Stafford SL, Kozelsky TF, Garrity JA, et al. Orbital lymphoma: radiotherapy outcome and complications. Radiother Oncol. 2001;59:139–44.
76. Stefanovic A, Lossos IS. Extranodal marginal zone lymphoma of the ocular adnexa. Blood. 2009;114(3):501–10.
77. Suh CO, Shim SJ, Lee SW, et al. Orbital marginal zone B-cell lymphoma of MALT: radiotherapy results and clinical behavior. Int J Radiat Oncol Biol Phys. 2006;65:228–33.
78. Sullivan TJ, Valenzuela AA. Imaging features of ocular adnexal lymphoproliferative disease. Eye. 2006;20:1189–95.
79. Swerdlow SH, Campo E, Harris NL, et al. World Health Organization classification of tumours of haematopoietic and lymphoid tissues. 4th ed. Lyon: IARC; 2008.
80. Tanimoto K, Kaneko A, Suzuki S, et al. Long-term follow-up results of no initial therapy for ocular adnexal MALT lymphoma. Ann Oncol. 2006;17:135–40.
81. Tanimoto K, Kaneko A, Suzuki S, et al. Primary ocular adnexal MALT lymphoma: a long-term follow-up study of 114 patients. Jpn J Clin Oncol. 2007;37:337–44.
82. Tarella C, Arcaini L, Baldini L, et al. Italian Society of Hematology, Italian Society of Experimental Hematology, and Italian Group for Bone Marrow Transplantation Guidelines for the management of indolent, nonfollicular B-cell lymphoma (marginal zone, lymphoplasmacytic, and small lymphocytic lymphoma). Clin Lymphoma Myeloma Leuk. 2015;15:75–85. doi:10.1016/j.clml.2014.07.002.
83. Tran K, Campbell BA, Fua T, et al. Efficacy of low dose radiotherapy for primary orbital marginal zone lymphoma. Leuk Lymphoma. 2013;54:491–6.
84. Tsang RW, Gospodarowicz MK, Pintilie M, et al. Localized mucosa-associated lymphoid tissue lymphoma treated with radiation therapy has excellent clinical outcome. J Clin Oncol. 2003;21:4157–64.
85. Uno T, Isobe K, Shikama N, et al. Radiotherapy for extranodal, marginal zone, B-cell lymphoma of mucosa-associated lymphoid tissue originating in the ocular adnexa: a multiinstitutional, retrospective review of 50 patients. Cancer. 2003;98:865–71.
86. Van der Geld YG, Senan S, van Sornsen de Koste JR, et al. A four-dimensional CT-based evaluation of techniques for gastric irradiation. Int J Radiat Oncol Biol Phys. 2007;69:903–9.
87. Vrieling C, de Jong D, Boot H, de Boer JP, Wegman F, Aleman BM. Long-term results of stomach-conserving therapy in gastric MALT lymphoma. Radiother Oncol. 2008;87:405–11.
88. Watanabe M, Isobe K, Takisima H, et al. Intrafractional gastric motion and interfractional stomach deformity during radiation therapy. Radiother Oncol. 2008;87: 425–31.
89. Wirth et al. Annal Oncl. 2013;24(5):1344–51.
90. Wotherspoon AC, Doglioni C, Diss TC, et al. Regression of primary low-grade B-cell gastric lymphoma of mucosa-associated lymphoid tissue type after eradication of Helicobacter pylori. Lancet. 1993;342:575–7.
91. Yahalom J, Schechter NR, Gonzales M, et al. H.Pylori-independant MALT lymphoma of the stomach: 10-year experience with 51 patients treated with radiation alone. Ann Oncol. 2002;13 Suppl 2:43.
92. Yamashita H, Nakagawa K, Asari T, et al. Radiotherapy for 41 patients with stages I and II MALT lymphoma: a retrospective study. Radiother Oncol. 2008;87: 412–7.
93. Ye H, Gong L, Liu H, et al. Strong BCL10 nuclear expression identifies gastric MALT lymphomas that do not respond to H. pylori eradication. Gut. 2006;55:137–8.
94. Yoon JS, Ma KT, Kim SJ, et al. Prognosis for patients in a Korean population with ocular adnexal lymphoproliferative lesions. Ophthal Plast Reconstr Surg. 2007;23:94–9.
95. Zucca E, Cavalli F. Extranodal lymphomas. Ann Oncol. 2000;11 Suppl 3:219–22.
96. Zucca E, Roggero E, Bertoni F, Cavalli F. Primary extranodal non-Hodgkin's lymphomas. Part 1: gastrointestinal, cutaneous and genitourinary lymphomas. Ann Oncol. 1997;8:727–37.
97. Zullo A, Hassan C, Andriani A, et al. Primary low-grade and high-grade gastric MALT-lymphoma presentation: a systematic review. J Clin Gastroenterol. 2010;44:340–4.
98. Zullo A, Hassan C, Cristofari F, Perri F, Morini S. Gastric low grade mucosal-associated lymphoid tissue lymphoma: Helicobacter pylori and beyond. World J Gastrointest Oncol. 2010;2:181–6.
99. Zullo C, Hassan C, Ridola L, et al. Gastric MALT lymphoma: old and new insights. Ann Gastroenterol. 2014;27:27–33.

Primary Mediastinal (Thymic) Large B-Cell Lymphoma

5

Andrea K. Ng

Abstract

Primary mediastinal (thymic) large B-cell lymphoma (PMBL) is a distinct entity that arises from the thymic B cell, with clinical and pathologic features that differ from diffuse large B-cell lymphoma (DLBCL). In the era of immunochemotherapy, a variety of chemotherapy regimens have been used for PMBL, including rituximab, cyclophosphamide, doxorubicin, vincristine, and prednisone (R-CHOP); rituximab, methotrexate, leucovorin, doxorubicin, cyclophosphamide, vincristine, prednisone, and bleomycin (R-MACOP-B); rituximab, etoposide, leucovorin, doxorubicin, cyclophosphamide, vincristine, prednisone, and bleomycin (R-VACOP-B); and infusional dose-adjusted etoposide, prednisone, vincristine, cyclophosphamide, and doxorubicin (EPOCH)-rituximab. The role of radiotherapy for PMBL is evolving. Phase II studies have investigated the use of chemotherapy alone, and retrospective analyses have explored a PET-guided approach on the radiotherapy decision. The use of PET response to guide decision on radiation therapy in PMBL is currently explored by a prospective randomized trial conducted by the International Extranodal Lymphoma Study Group (IELSG-37). While awaiting level I evidence, adjuvant radiotherapy should be strongly considered in patients with initial bulky disease or in those with a less than complete response to chemotherapy. Radiation therapy also plays an important role as part of salvage therapy in patients with relapsed or refractory disease after chemotherapy.

A.K. Ng, MD, MPH
Department of Radiation Oncology, Dana-Farber Cancer Institute, Brigham and Women's Hospital, Harvard Medical School, 75 Francis Street, ASB1-L2, Boston, MA 02115, USA
e-mail: ang@lroc.harvard.edu

B.S. Dabaja, A.K. Ng (eds.), *Radiation Therapy in Hematologic Malignancies*,
DOI 10.1007/978-3-319-42615-0_5

Clinical Presentation and Pathology

Case 1

A 38-year-old man presented with dyspnea on exertion while playing basketball. Chest x-ray revealed mediastinal widening. Chest computed tomography (CT) confirmed a 9.5×7.4×4.8 cm anterior mediastinal mass. A Chamberlain procedure was performed, and pathology showed primary mediastinal (thymic) large B-cell lymphoma. Immunohistochemical studies showed that the neoplastic cells were CD20-positive B cells, which co-express CD45, Bcl-2, Bcl-6, and CD30 (subset, weak) and were negative for CD5, CD10, CD15, and EMA. Fluorescence in situ hybridization (FISH) analysis showed no evidence of MYC, BCL2, and BCL6 rearrangement. The Ki-67 proliferative index was approximately 50%.

Case 2

A 26-year-old woman presented to the emergency room with a several-day history of facial and lower neck swelling, cough, chest pressure, and voice changes. A chest CT revealed a 10.2×5.0×4.8 cm anterior mediastinal mass with mild narrowing of the trachea, compression of the upper esophagus, and moderate narrowing of the right jugular vein and superior vena cava (Fig. 5.1). *A left neck biopsy showed primary mediastinal (thymic) large B-cell lymphoma with similar morphologic, immunohistochemical, and cytogenetic findings as Case 1. The Ki-67 proliferative index was approximately 80% in this case.*

Primary mediastinal (thymic) large B-cell lymphoma (PMBL) accounts for approximately 5% of all cases of non-Hodgkin lymphoma. The

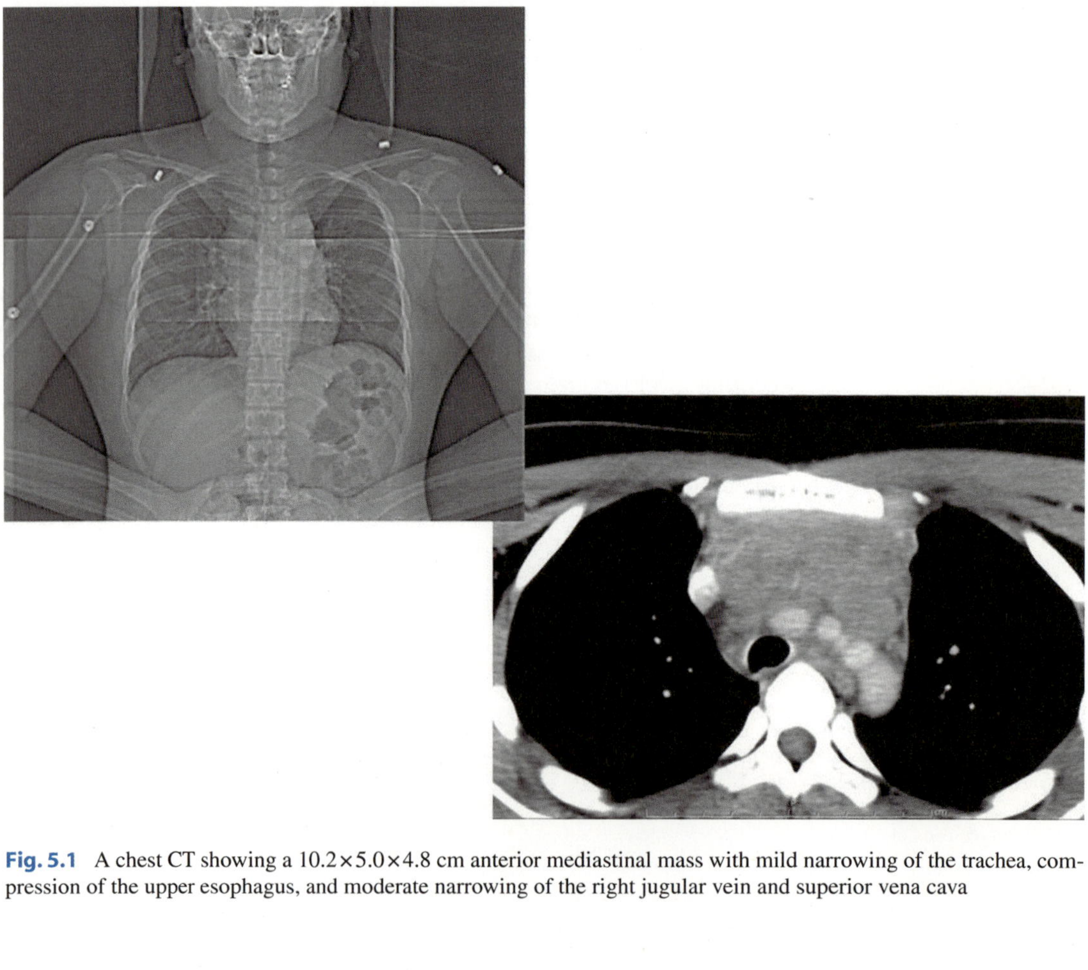

Fig. 5.1 A chest CT showing a 10.2×5.0×4.8 cm anterior mediastinal mass with mild narrowing of the trachea, compression of the upper esophagus, and moderate narrowing of the right jugular vein and superior vena cava

median age at presentation is in the third to fourth decades, with a female predominance [1, 2]. The majority of cases present with bulky disease localized to the anterior mediastinum, often with associated pleural and pericardial effusions. Superior vena cava syndrome is a common clinical presentation. Although PMCL are largely localized at diagnosis, relapses tend to occur in extranodal organs such as the gastrointestinal tract, kidneys, adrenals, liver, and ovaries.

The postulated cell of origin of PMBL is thymic B cell. Although previously classified as a subtype of diffuse large B-cell lymphoma, in the World Health Organization (WHO) classification, PMBL is considered a distinct entity [3]. Morphologically, immunophenotypically, and according to gene expression profiling studies, PMBL is thought to be more closely related to classical Hodgkin lymphoma [4, 5]. The malignant cells of PMBL express B-cell markers such as CD19 and CD20 but lack CD5 and CD10 expression. Expression of CD30 is often present but is weak. More recently, the pathogenesis of PMBL has been associated with the Janus Kinase-Signal Transducer and Activator of Transcription (JAK-STAT) and nuclear factor kappa-b (NF-kb) signaling pathways, and overexpression of PD-1 ligands has been identified, findings that may guide the development of new therapeutic targets for PMBL [6–8].

Staging and Prognostic Factors

Imaging

Case 1

Positron emission tomography-computed tomography (PET-CT) was performed, showing a large superior anterior mediastinal mass with intense fluorodeoxyglucose (FDG) uptake with a standardized uptake value (SUV) max of 15.4 (Fig. 5.2).

Case 2

PET-CT was performed, showing FDG-avid disease involving the left supraclavicular region (SUV max 8.2) and the anterior mediastinum extending from the thoracic inlet to the level of the aortic root with an SUV max of 14 (Fig. 5.3).

Blood work in both cases included complete blood count (CBC) with differential, serum lactate dehydrogenase (LDH), blood urea nitrogen (BUN), and creatinine; electrolytes were all within normal limits. Human immunodeficiency (HIV) and *hepatitis B and C serologies were negative. Bone marrow biopsies were performed in both cases, both showing no evidence of marrow involvement.*

The staging workup for PMBL is similar to that for diffuse large B-cell lymphoma. Relevant history and physical examination include documentation of signs and symptoms that may be related to the mediastinal disease including chest pain, shortness of breath, cough, voice changes, facial or neck swelling, and chest wall masses. Imaging studies include PET-CT and optional chest CT with contrast which may aide subsequent radiation treatment planning. Although bone marrow involvement is rare in PMBL, bone marrow biopsy should be performed especially in the absence of evidence of bone/bone marrow involvement on PET-CT [9].

Modifications to the Ann Arbor staging system were recently made in the Lugano Classification for the staging of lymphoma [9]. The designation of "X" for bulky disease was eliminated, and instead, it was recommended that the largest tumor diameter be recorded. This may be especially pertinent to PMBL, which tend to present with bulky disease. In addition, specifically for non-Hodgkin's lymphoma, the designation of "B" symptoms was eliminated.

The overall prognosis of patients with PMBL has been shown to be more favorable than patients with diffuse large cell lymphoma [10]. The international prognostic index (IPI) and the subsequent revised IPI [11], developed for patients with aggressive non-Hodgkin lymphoma treated with anthracycline-based chemotherapy, can be extrapolated for use in patients with PMBL, although available data suggest that age-adjusted IPI may not be predictive of overall survival in patients with PMBL [10, 12]. In a recent study focusing on 123 patients with PMBL treated with rituximab, cyclophosphamide, doxorubicin, vincristine, and

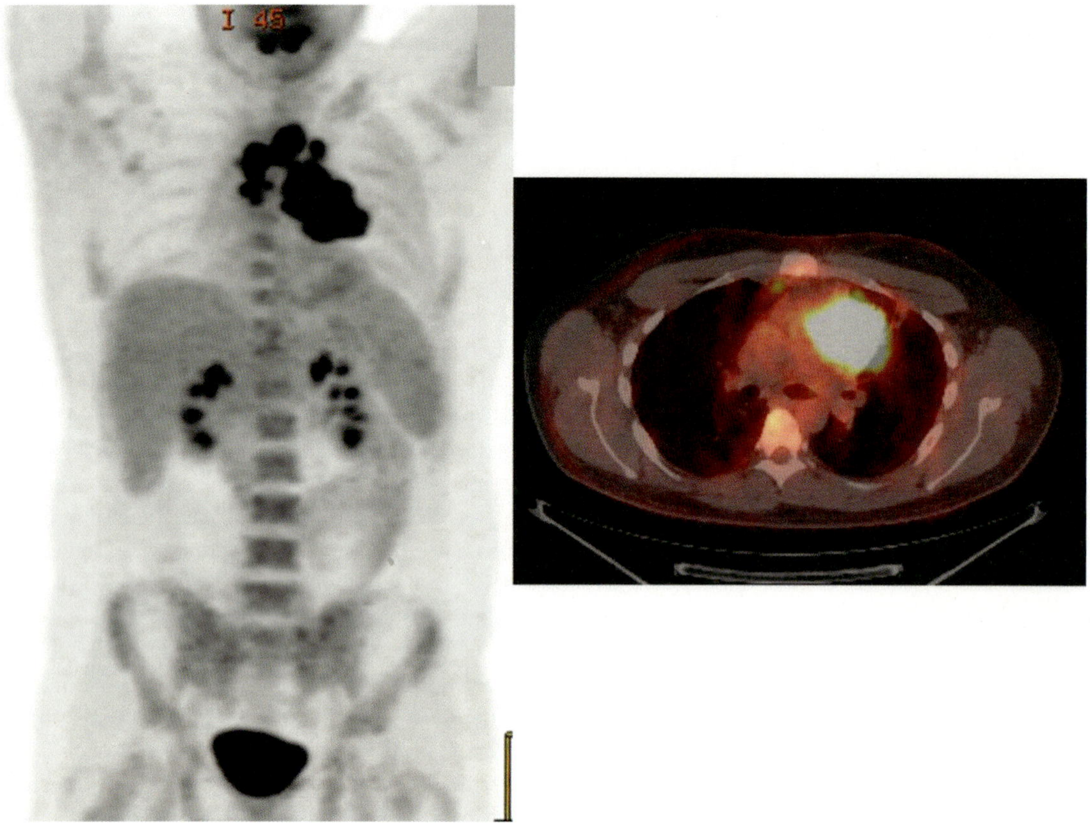

Fig. 5.2 Positron emission tomography-computed tomography (PET-CT) showing a large superior anterior mediastinal mass with intense fluorodeoxyglucose (FDG) uptake with a standardized uptake value (SUV) max of 15.4

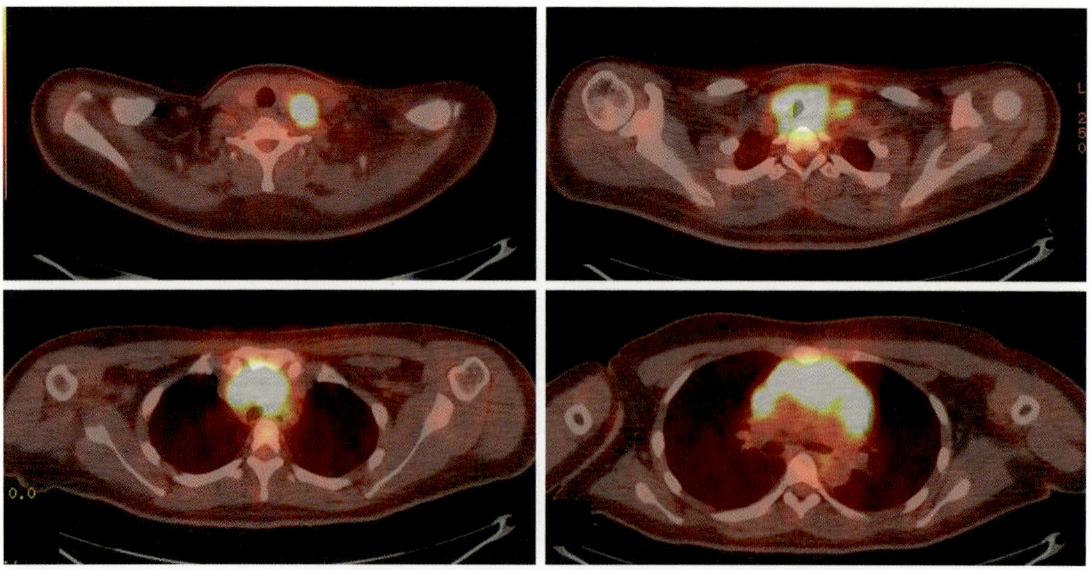

Fig. 5.3 PET-CT showing FDG-avid disease involving the left supraclavicular region (SUV max 8.2) and the anterior mediastinum extending from the thoracic inlet to the level of the aortic root with an SUV max of 14

prednisone (R-CHOP) chemotherapy, the presence of pleural or pericardial effusion at diagnosis was the only factor that independently predicted for primary refractory disease or early relapse within 12 months [13].

Treatment

Case 1

The patient was initiated on R-CHOP chemotherapy. Restaging PET-CT after 3 cycles of chemotherapy showed a partial response with a Deauville score of 4 (Fig. 5.4a). *The patient completed 3 additional cycles of chemotherapy, and restaging PET-CT performed 4 weeks after the chemotherapy showed further response with a Deauville score of 2* (Fig. 5.4b). *The patient was then referred for radiation therapy.*

Radiation Treatment

The patient was simulated in an arm-down position with a Vac-LoK bag for immobilization and a face mask to keep the neck in an extended position. CT simulation was performed using a three-dimensional scan and deep-inspiration breath-hold technique. The planning CT was fused with the pre-chemotherapy PET-CT, and the clinical target volume (CTV) was determined according to

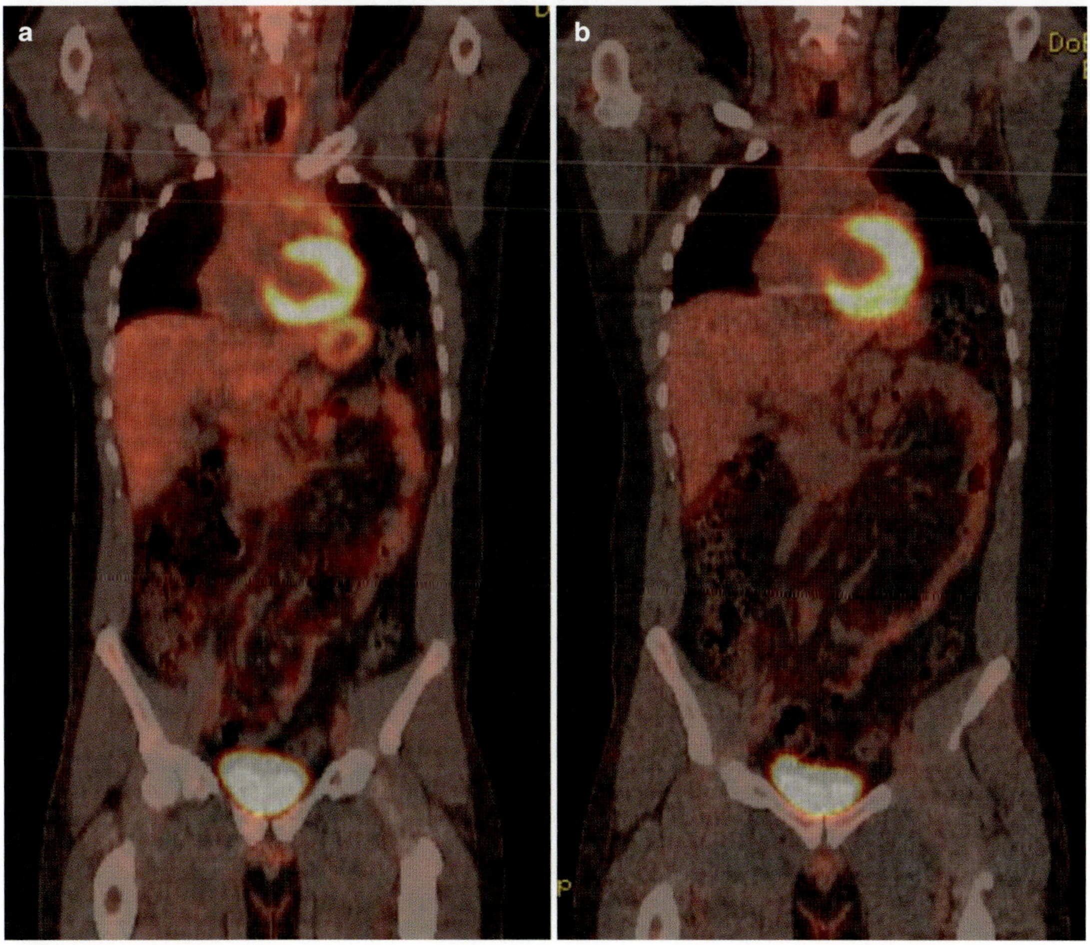

Fig. 5.4 (**a**) Restaging PET-CT after 3 cycles of chemotherapy showing a partial response with a Deauville score of 4 (**a**). (**b**) After 3 additional cycles of chemotherapy, restaging PET-CT performed 4 weeks after the chemotherapy showing further response with a Deauville score of 2

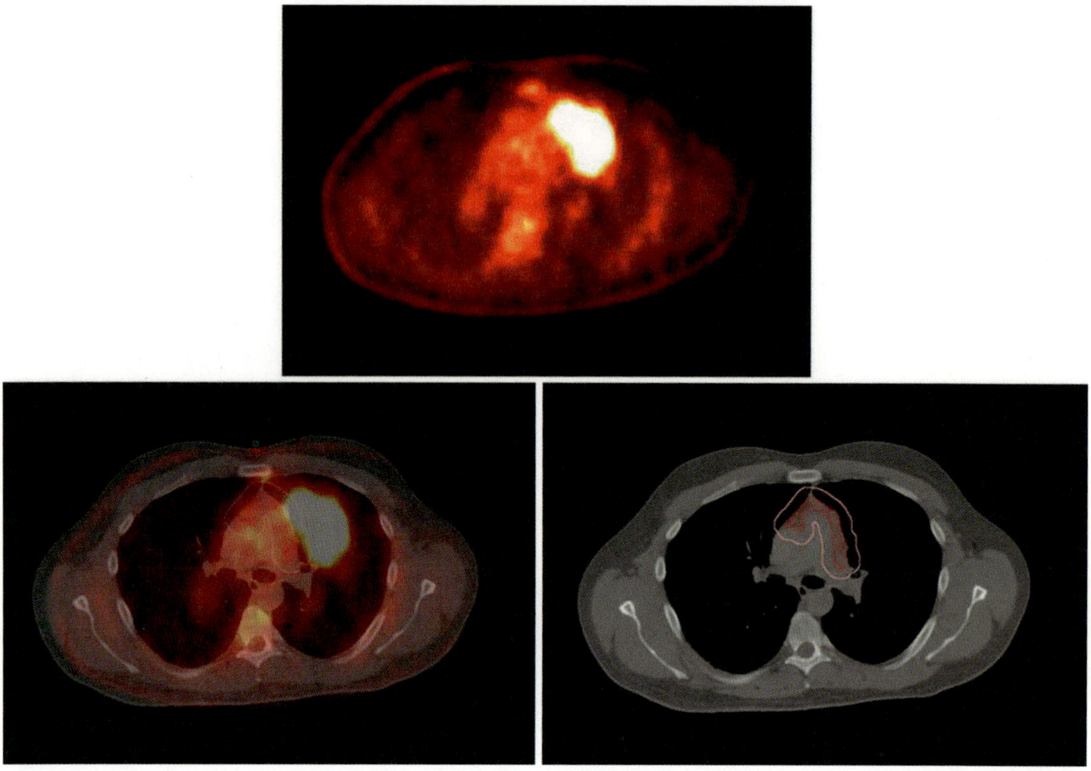

Fig. 5.5 CTV including the initially involved disease extent but excluding the previously displaced, uninvolved normal structures (lungs, major vessels, heart, bones, muscles).

the International Lymphoma Radiation Oncology Group and involved site radiation therapy (ISRT) guidelines [14, 15]. *The CTV included the initially involved disease extent but excluded the previously displaced, uninvolved normal structures (lungs, major vessels, heart, bones, muscles)* (Fig. 5.5). *An expansion to internal target volume (ITV) was not performed because breath-hold technique was used. A 1-cm CTV to planning target volume (PTV) expansion was used to account for daily setup errors. A primarily anterior-posterior/posterior-anterior beam arrangement intensity-modulated radiation therapy (IMRT) approach was used* (Fig. 5.6a), *in order to reduce low doses to large volume of lungs. Since no lateral beams were used, the patient was simulated and treated in an arm-down position (which is especially important in cases of female patients in which an arm-up position will bring more breast tissue into the radiation field). This IMRT technique is referred to as the butterfly technique* [16]. *A total dose of 30 Gy in 15 fractions was prescribed. The dose volume histogram (DVH) is shown in* Fig. 5.6b. *The mean heart dose (MHD) was 11.5 Gy, and the mean lung dose (MLD) was 9.1 Gy. The lung V5 and V20 were 42 % and 20 %, respectively.*

Case 2

The patient was started on dose-adjusted etoposide, doxorubicin, and cyclophosphamide with vincristine, prednisone, and rituximab (DA-EPOCH-R) with prompt resolution of the facial and neck swelling. Restaging PET-CT after 3 cycles of chemotherapy showed a complete metabolic response (Deauville 2) (Fig. 5.7). *The patient received a total of 6 cycles of DA-EPOCH-R, and restaging PET-CT 1 month post-chemotherapy showed continued complete response. Radiation oncology was not consulted*

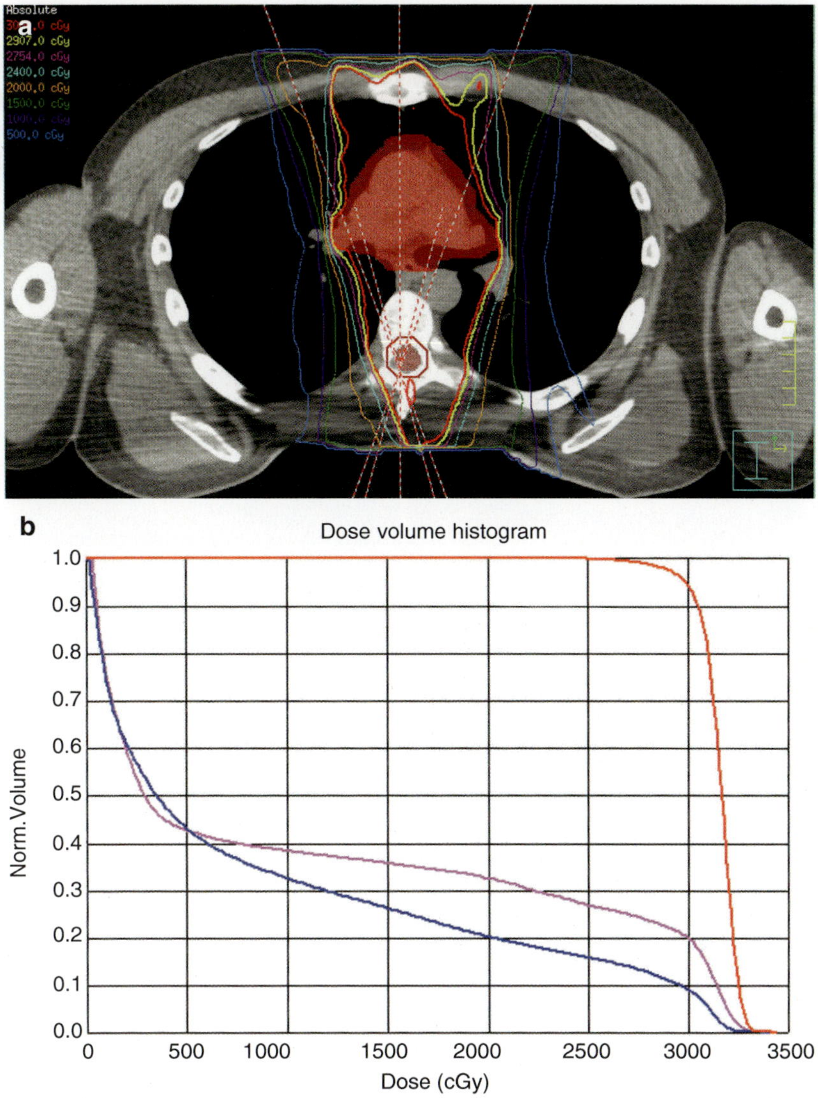

ROI Statistics

Line Type	ROI	Trial or Record	Min.	Max.	Mean	Std. Dev.
—	Heart	Aprvd BSD	30.9	3432.3	1151.9	1281.6
—	Total Lung	Aprvd BSD	6.2	3369.2	914.6	1067.3
—	pPTV 30.6	Aprvd BSD	1535.8	3432.3	3148.6	105.5

Fig. 5.6 (**a**) Axial view showing IMRT planning with anteroposterior beam arrangement used. (**b**) Dose volume histogram

as complete remission was achieved and there were also concerns with late toxicity of mediastinal irradiation in a young woman.

At 5 months posttreatment, the patient presented with recurrent symptoms of chest pressure and cough. Chest CT showed a left-sided anterior mediastinal mass (Fig. 5.8). *A CT-guided biopsy revealed relapsed PMBL. PET-CT showed that the recurrent FDG-avid disease was limited to the mediastinum, with no other sites of disease*

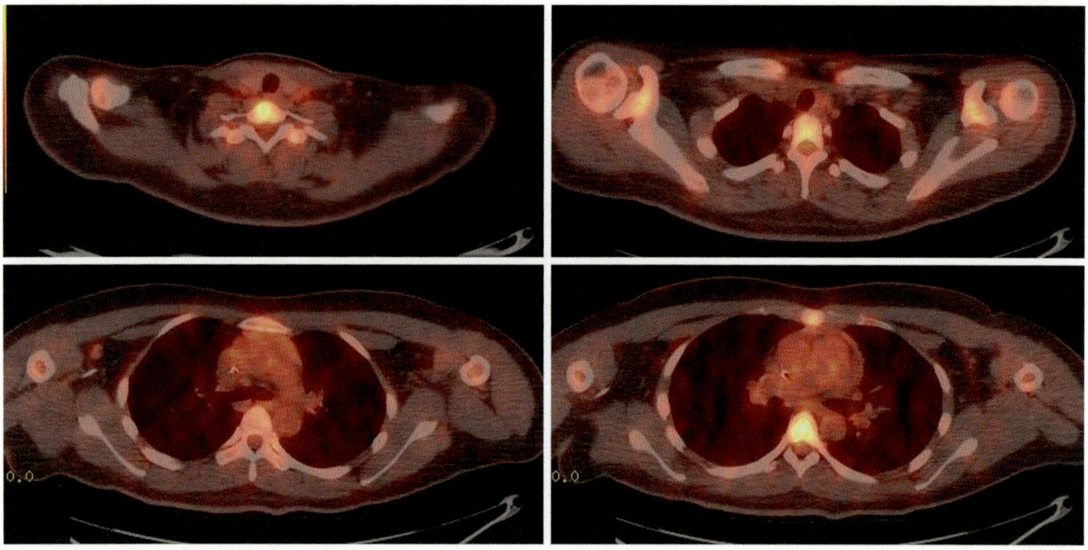

Fig. 5.7 Restaging PET-CT after 3 cycles of chemotherapy showing a complete metabolic response (Deauville 2)

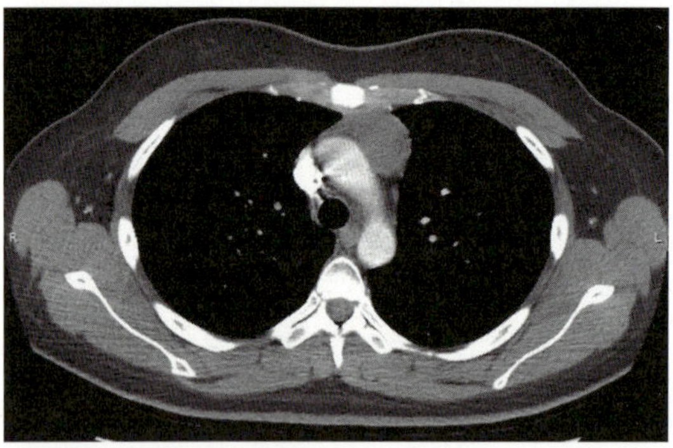

Fig. 5.8 Chest CT showing a left-sided anterior mediastinal mass

involvement. The patient underwent salvage chemotherapy with R-ifosfamide, carboplatin, etoposide (ICE) x 2 without improvement on PET-CT. The patient was then referred for radiation therapy.

Radiation Treatment

The same immobilization and breath-hold techniques as Case 1 were used in this case. The planning CT, with IV contrast, was fused with the PET-CT that showed the refractory disease after 2 cycles of salvage R-ICE chemotherapy. The CTV was the same as the gross target volume (GTV), and similar to Case 1, a 1-cm CTV to PTV expansion was used (Fig. 5.9). *Given the chemotherapy refractoriness of the disease, a total dose of 50.4 Gy in 28 fractions to the PTV was prescribed, with plan for an autologous stem cell transplantation post-radiation therapy. An initial AP-PA approach was used to a dose of 39.6 Gy in 1.8 Gy fractions, followed by oblique fields off the spinal cord for an additional 10.8 Gy* (Fig. 5.10). *The DVHs are shown in* Fig. 5.11. *The MHD and MLD were 13.0 Gy and 13.2 Gy, respectively. The lung V5 and V20 were 47.2 % and 22.5 %, respectively.*

The optimal treatment for PMBL is controversial. In the era of chemoimmunotherapy, the addition of rituximab to CHOP-based chemotherapy for PMBL has been shown to significantly improve event-free survival rates from approximately 50–80 % [17, 18]. A variety of multi-agent chemotherapy regimen has been used for the treatment of PMBL, including R-CHOP; rituximab, methotrexate, leucovorin, doxorubicin, cyclophosphamide, vincristine, prednisone, and bleomycin (R-MACOP-B); rituximab, etoposide, leucovorin, doxorubicin, cyclophosphamide, vincristine, prednisone, and bleomycin (R-VACOP-B); and infusional dose-

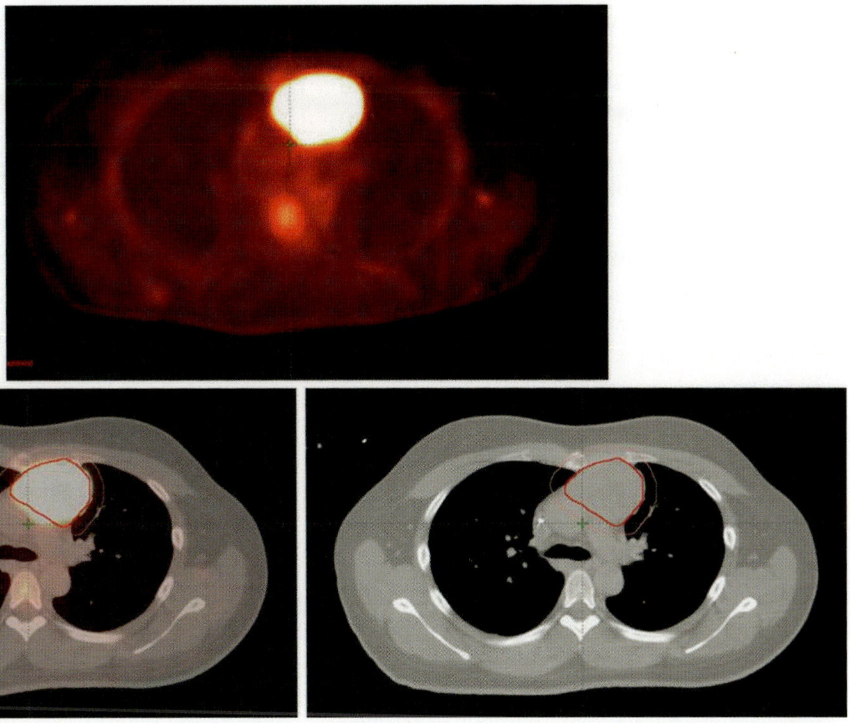

Fig. 5.9 The planning CT, with IV contrast, was fused with the PET-CT showing refractory disease after 2 cycles of salvage R-ICE chemotherapy. The CTV was the same as the gross target volume (GTV), and, similar to Case 1, a 1-cm CTV to PTV expansion was used

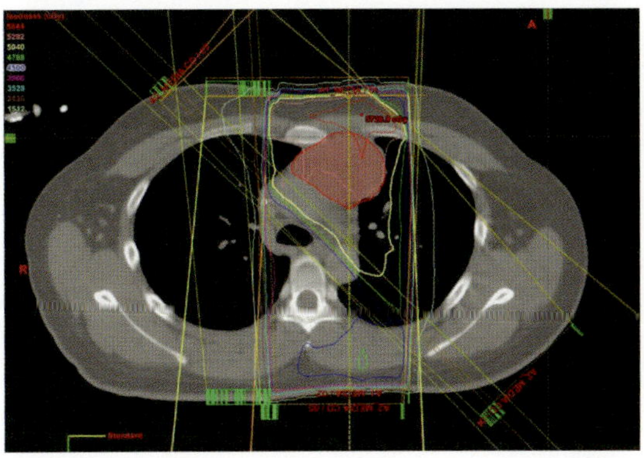

Fig. 5.10 An initial AP-PA approach to a dose of 39.6 Gy in 1.8 Gy fractions, followed by oblique fields off the spinal cord for an additional 10.8 Gy

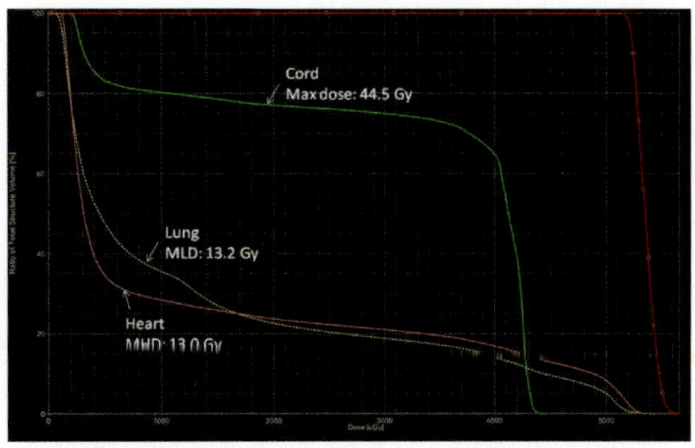

Fig. 5.11 The DVHs are shown

adjusted etoposide, prednisone, vincristine, cyclophosphamide, and doxorubicin (EPOCH)-rituximab therapy [19–22]. When used in conjunction with radiotherapy, excellent treatment outcome with an approximately 90 % disease-free survival can be achieved [20, 21].

The role of adjuvant radiation therapy is evolving. Phase II studies have explored chemotherapy regimens including dose-dense R-CHOP x 3 followed by ICE [23] and DA-EPOCH-R [22] without radiation therapy, showing promising results. A retrospective series from British Columbia explored a PET-guided approach on the radiation therapy decision, and among the 35 of 59 (59 %) patients who achieved PET-negative disease at the end of chemotherapy, 33 did not receive radiation therapy. In these PET-negative patients, there were 6 relapses (4 in the mediastinum), yielding a 5-year time to progression of 78 %, which did not differ significantly from patients with residual PET-positive disease who received radiotherapy, leading to the authors' conclusion that PET guidance may reduce radiotherapy use while maintaining good outcome. A recent Italian study showed similar disease-free survival rates between 23 patients with PET-negative disease after chemotherapy and did not receive radiation therapy versus 51 patients with PET-positive disease after chemotherapy and treated with radiation therapy (90 % vs. 90.7 %) [24]. The use of PET response to guide decision on radiation therapy in PMBL is currently explored by a prospective randomized trial conducted by the International Extranodal Lymphoma Study Group (IELSG-37). In this study, patients with PMBL without evidence of extranodal disease outside of the chest are treated with at least 6 cycles of rituximab and anthracycline-based chemotherapy. PET-CT is performed 5–6 weeks post-chemotherapy, and patients with complete metabolic response are randomized to 30 Gy of mediastinal irradiation versus observation.

In the first case, the decision to add radiotherapy was based on the initial bulk of the disease and the initially slow response to chemotherapy. Given an excellent response was ultimately achieved at the end of chemotherapy, the clinical target volume defined according to the ISRT was limited in nature. The modest radiation volume and dose of 30 Gy, along with deep-inspiration breath-hold technique, significantly reduce the amount of heart and lungs in the treatment field.

In patients with relapsed PMBL, response to salvage chemotherapy is inferior to that of diffuse large B-cell lymphoma [25], as illustrated in Case 2. Radiotherapy plays an integral part in the salvage treatment of this patient given the localized nature of her relapsed/refractory disease in an attempt to achieve a minimal disease state prior to the autologous stem cell transplantation. As the disease was refractory to the salvage chemotherapy, a higher dose of 50 Gy was used [26]. With pre-transplant chest radiotherapy, it is anticipated that the patient will likely experience increased risk of pneumonitis and esophagitis during the transplant. The long-term risk of breast cancer with chest radiotherapy in young women is often raised as a concern. However, it is important to note that this is entirely based on long-term data from women with Hodgkin lymphoma treated with historical mantle field radiation therapy. In this particular case, the foremost priority is control of her refractory lymphoma. Her long-term breast cancer risk, were she to survive the lymphoma, will likely be attenuated by the chemotherapy effect on her ovarian function [27, 28].

PMBL is an entity with distinctive underlying biology, clinical presentation, response to initial and salvage treatment, patterns of relapse, and overall prognosis. In the era of effective immunochemotherapy and PET assessment of response to systemic therapy, the role of radiation therapy is unclear and is currently being addressed by the IELSG-37 trial. An important goal in the management of PMBL is maximizing cure upfront, given the known poor response of the disease to salvage therapy. With modern radiotherapy doses and techniques, radiation exposure to organs at risk can be kept to a minimum thus reducing treatment-related toxicity.

References

1. Nguyen LN, Ha CS, Hess M, et al. The outcome of combined-modality treatments for stage I and II primary large B-cell lymphoma of the mediastinum. Int J Radiat Oncol Biol Phys. 2000;47(5):1281–5.
2. Cazals-Hatem D, Lepage E, Brice P, et al. Primary mediastinal large B-cell lymphoma. A clinicopathologic study of 141 cases compared with 916 nonmediastinal large B-cell lymphomas, a GELA ("Groupe d'Etude des Lymphomes de l'Adulte") study. Am J Surg Pathol. 1996;20(7):877–88.
3. Campo E, Swerdlow SH, Harris NL, Pileri S, Stein H, Jaffe ES. The 2008 WHO classification of lymphoid neoplasms and beyond: evolving concepts and practical applications. Blood. 2011;117(19):5019–32.
4. Savage KJ, Monti S, Kutok JL, et al. The molecular signature of mediastinal large B-cell lymphoma differs from that of other diffuse large B-cell lymphomas

and shares features with classical Hodgkin lymphoma. Blood. 2003;102(12):3871–9.
5. Rosenwald A, Wright G, Leroy K, et al. Molecular diagnosis of primary mediastinal B cell lymphoma identifies a clinically favorable subgroup of diffuse large B cell lymphoma related to Hodgkin lymphoma. J Exp Med. 2003;198(6):851–62.
6. Twa DD, Chan FC, Ben-Neriah S, et al. Genomic rearrangements involving programmed death ligands are recurrent in primary mediastinal large B-cell lymphoma. Blood. 2014;123(13):2062–5.
7. Steidl C, Gascoyne RD. The molecular pathogenesis of primary mediastinal large B-cell lymphoma. Blood. 2011;118(10):2659–69.
8. Gunawardana J, Chan FC, Telenius A, et al. Recurrent somatic mutations of PTPN1 in primary mediastinal B cell lymphoma and Hodgkin lymphoma. Nat Genet. 2014;46(4):329–35.
9. Cheson BD, Fisher RI, Barrington SF, et al. Recommendations for initial evaluation, staging, and response assessment of Hodgkin and non-Hodgkin lymphoma: the Lugano classification. J Clin Oncol. 2014;32(27):3059–68.
10. Savage KJ, Al-Rajhi N, Voss N, et al. Favorable outcome of primary mediastinal large B-cell lymphoma in a single institution: the British Columbia experience. Ann Oncol. 2006;17(1):123–30.
11. Sehn LH, Berry B, Chhanabhai M, et al. The revised International Prognostic Index (R-IPI) is a better predictor of outcome than the standard IPI for patients with diffuse large B-cell lymphoma treated with R-CHOP. Blood. 2007;109(5):1857–61.
12. Hamlin PA, Portlock CS, Straus DJ, et al. Primary mediastinal large B-cell lymphoma: optimal therapy and prognostic factor analysis in 141 consecutive patients treated at Memorial Sloan Kettering from 1980 to 1999. Br J Haematol. 2005;130(5):691–9.
13. Aoki T, Izutsu K, Suzuki R, et al. Prognostic significance of pleural or pericardial effusion and the implication of optimal treatment in primary mediastinal large B-cell lymphoma: a multicenter retrospective study in Japan. Haematologica. 2014;99(12):1817–25.
14. Illidge T, Specht L, Yahalom J, et al. Modern radiation therapy for nodal non-Hodgkin lymphoma-target definition and dose guidelines from the International Lymphoma Radiation Oncology Group. Int J Radiat Oncol Biol Phys. 2014;89(1):49–58.
15. Specht L, Yahalom J, Illidge T, et al. Modern radiation therapy for Hodgkin lymphoma: field and dose guidelines from the international lymphoma radiation oncology group (ILROG). Int J Radiat Oncol Biol Phys. 2014;89(4):854–62.
16. Voong, et al. Radiat Oncol. 2014;9:94. http://www.ro-journal.com/content/9/1/94.
17. Rieger M, Osterborg A, Pettengell R, et al. Primary mediastinal B-cell lymphoma treated with CHOP-like chemotherapy with or without rituximab: results of the Mabthera International Trial Group study. Ann Oncol. 2011;22(3):664–70.
18. Vassilakopoulos TP, Pangalis GA, Katsigiannis A, et al. Rituximab, cyclophosphamide, doxorubicin, vincristine, and prednisone with or without radiotherapy in primary mediastinal large B-cell lymphoma: the emerging standard of care. Oncologist. 2012;17(2):239–49.
19. Avigdor A, Sirotkin T, Kedmi M, et al. The impact of R-VACOP-B and interim FDG-PET/CT on outcome in primary mediastinal large B cell lymphoma. Ann Hematol. 2014;93(8):1297–304.
20. Zinzani PL, Stefoni V, Finolezzi E, et al. Rituximab combined with MACOP-B or VACOP-B and radiation therapy in primary mediastinal large B-cell lymphoma: a retrospective study. Clin Lymphoma Myeloma. 2009;9(5):381–5.
21. Martelli M, Ceriani L, Zucca E, et al. [18F]fluorodeoxyglucose positron emission tomography predicts survival after chemoimmunotherapy for primary mediastinal large B-cell lymphoma: results of the International Extranodal Lymphoma Study Group IELSG-26 Study. J Clin Oncol. 2014;32(17):1769–75.
22. Dunleavy K, Pittaluga S, Maeda LS, et al. Dose-adjusted EPOCH-rituximab therapy in primary mediastinal B-cell lymphoma. N Engl J Med. 2013;368(15):1408–16.
23. Moskowitz AJ, Hamlin P, Maraguilia J, Meikle J, Zelenetz A. Sequential dose-Dende R-CHOP followed by ICE consolidation (MSKCC Protocol 01–142) without radiotherapy for patients with primary mediastinal large B-cell lymphoma. ASH Abstract. 2010:420.
24. Zinzani PL, Broccoli A, Casadei D, Stefoni V, Pellegrini C, Gandolfi L. The role of rituximab and positron emission tomography in the treatment of primary mediastinal large B-cell lymphoma: experience on 74 patients. Hematol Oncol. 2015;33:145–50.
25. Kuruvilla J, Pintilie M, Tsang R, Nagy T, Keating A, Crump M. Salvage chemotherapy and autologous stem cell transplantation are inferior for relapsed or refractory primary mediastinal large B-cell lymphoma compared with diffuse large B-cell lymphoma. Leuk Lymphoma. 2008;49(7):1329–36.
26. Tseng YD, Chen YH, Catalano P, Ng A. Rates and durability of response to salvage radiotherapy among patients with refractory or relapsed aggressive non-Hodgkin lymphoma. Int J Radiat Oncol Biol Phys. 2015;91(1):223–31.
27. van Leeuwen FE, Klokman WJ, Stovall M, et al. Roles of radiation dose, chemotherapy, and hormonal factors in breast cancer following Hodgkin's disease. J Natl Cancer Inst. 2003;95(13):971–80.
28. De Bruin ML, Sparidans J, van't Veer MB, et al. Breast cancer risk in female survivors of Hodgkin's lymphoma: lower risk after smaller radiation volumes. J Clin Oncol. 2009;27(26):4239–46.

Plasmacytoma and Multiple Myeloma

6

Richard Tsang

Abstract

In this chapter, two challenging cases of plasma cell neoplastic diseases are presented. The first is a solitary plasmacytoma, diagnosed in a setting of POEMS syndrome (Dispenzieri, Am J Hematol 89(2):214–223, 2004). This illustrates the potential curative nature of radiation therapy in this rare disease. The second case is the more common multiple myeloma, treated with systemic chemotherapy and autologous peripheral blood stem transplantation, but with unusual spread to the central nervous system. The case presentations will be followed by a discussion of the salient clinical evaluation and management in each case, with a focus on the role of radiation therapy and the sequencing of various therapies applied in these unusual and challenging clinical scenarios.

Clinical Presentation 1: Solitary Plasmacytoma of the Scapula in a Patient with POEMS Syndrome (*P*olyneuropathy, *O*rganomegaly, *E*ndocrinopathy, *M*onoclonal Plasma Cell Disorder, and *S*kin Abnormalities)

A 60-year-old woman presented with numbness and progressive weakness of her legs over 3–4 months. She also complained of some weight loss and blurriness of vision. When assessed by an ophthalmologist, she was diagnosed with papilledema, cause unidentified. She developed diabetes mellitus requiring an oral hypoglycemic. Her leg weakness progressed to the point where she was not able to walk, and her arms started to be weak too. She was found to have a thrombocytosis between 640 and 860×10^9/L. She had further weight loss of 30 lbs and had developed generalized edema affecting her body (anasarca). At this time, about 12 months after her initial symptoms, she was admitted to hospital for investigations and saw a hematologist who suspected POEMS syndrome and a plasma cell proliferative disorder. She had a significant past medical history of (1) IgA nephropathy with chronic renal failure 14 years previously and treated initially with hemodialysis for 5 years and then a renal allograft transplant. She was

R. Tsang, MD, FRCP(C)
Department of Radiation Oncology, University of Toronto, Princess Margaret Cancer Centre, 610 University Ave, Toronto, ON M5G 2M9, Canada
e-mail: Richard.tsang@rmp.uhn.on.ca

B.S. Dabaja, A.K. Ng (eds.), *Radiation Therapy in Hematologic Malignancies*,
DOI 10.1007/978-3-319-42615-0_6

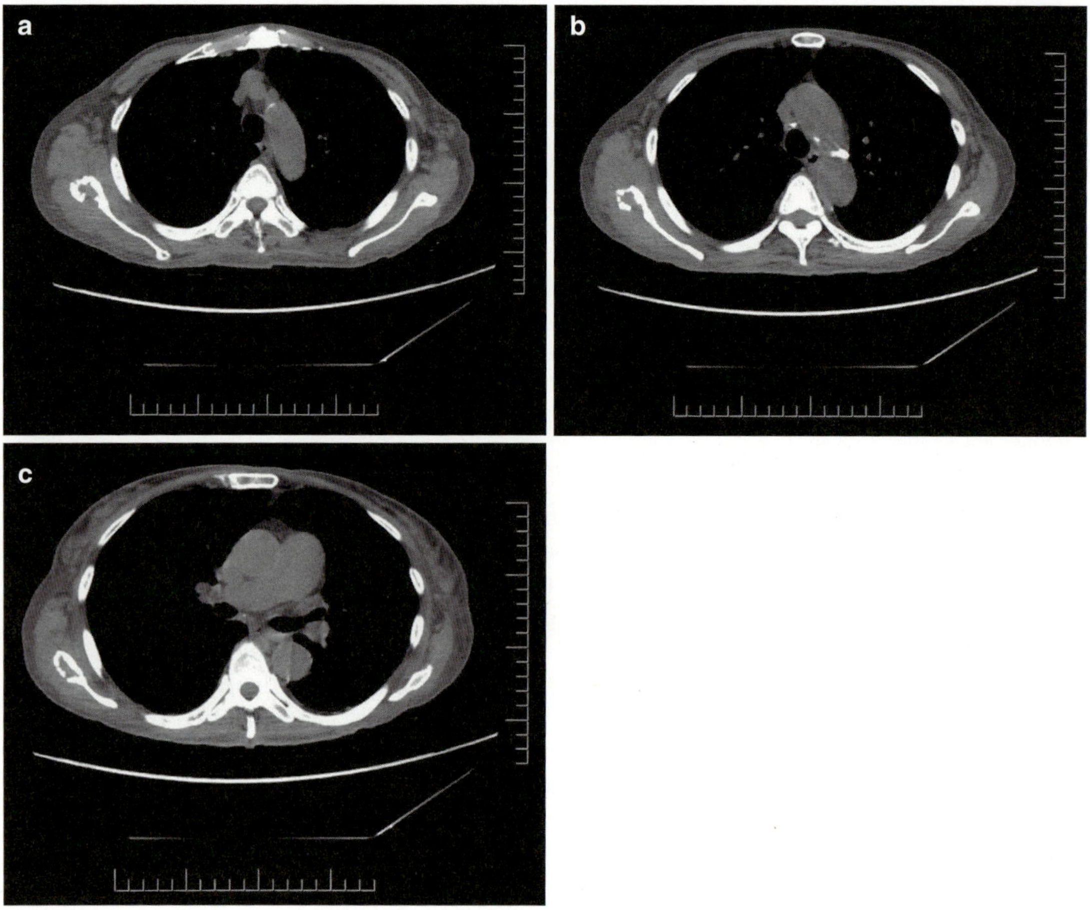

Fig. 6.1 (**a–c**) Axial CT scan slices showing a mixed sclerotic lytic lesion in the right scapula. There was associated soft tissue swelling in the surrounding musculature

maintained on immunosuppression with mycophenolate mofetil and tacrolimus. (2) Transient ischemic attack 1.5 years previously with complete occlusion of the right internal carotid artery on ultrasound, no sustained neurologic deficits.

Her clinical examination confirmed bilateral papilledema, a bilateral symmetrical sensory motor neuropathy of both arms and legs (worse in legs), a borderline enlarged right cervical lymph node (1.5 cm) but no other lymphadenopathy, moderate anasarca, and splenomegaly. She has no skin changes or other organomegaly noted. She denied bone pain. Her ECOG performance status was 4 because she was completely bedridden. Her investigations showed the following: normal hemoglobin and white cell count and platelets elevated as above. Albumin was low at 29 g/L. Serum creatinine, calcium, liver function tests, and $\beta_2$microglobulin were all normal. HIV test is negative. Electromyography testing confirmed a severe demyelinating sensorimotor polyradicular neuropathy. Her skeletal survey and CT and MR scans showed a 4 cm (transverse) × 7 cm (craniocaudal) lytic-sclerotic lesion in the right scapula (Figs. 6.1 and 6.2), with an associated soft tissue mass in the surrounding musculature. There were no skeletal abnormalities elsewhere. CT scan also confirmed splenomegaly and moderate ascites, but no generalized lymphadenopathy apart from the borderline right cervical lymph node. Blood and urine were negative for monoclonal proteins, and serum light chains were normal.

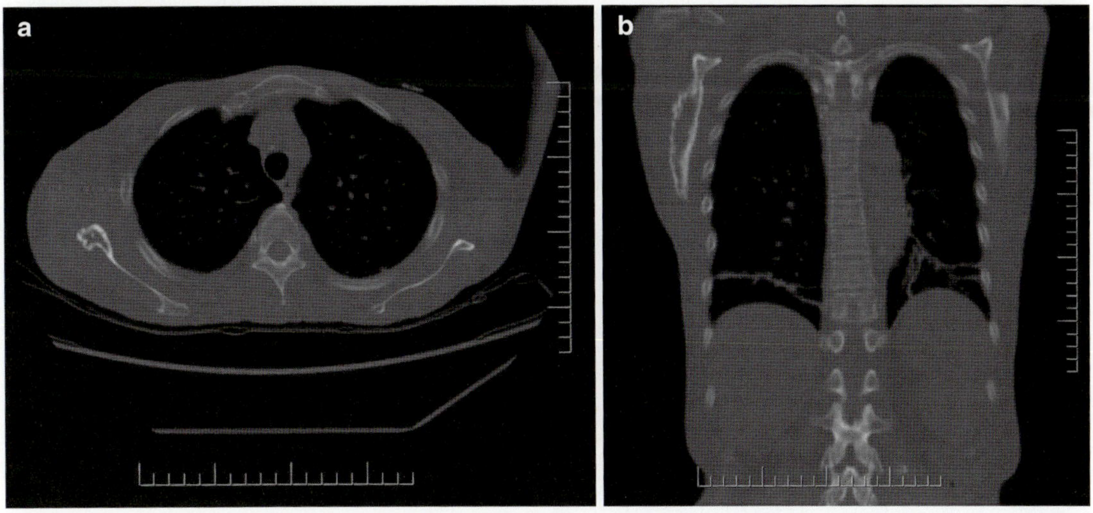

Fig. 6.2 Axial (**a**) and coronal (*right panel*) CT scan with bone windows, showing the partly sclerotic and partly lytic nature of the lesion. Note splenomegaly in the coronal CT (**b**)

Bone marrow biopsy shows mild hypercellularity, but plasma cells were normal (<5 %). There was no evidence of multiple myeloma. A biopsy of the right scapula mass showed plasmacytoma, with the abnormal plasma cells lambda restricted, and a low Ki-67 proliferation rate of 3 %. Biopsy of the right neck node revealed Castleman's disease, multicentric type. FDG-PET scan showed solitary uptake in the right scapula lesion, with SUV_{max} value 24.3 (Fig. 6.3). Subsequently she also had an elevation of serum vascular endothelial growth factor (VEGF) documented. She was diagnosed with POEMS syndrome, with a solitary plasmacytoma involving her right scapula. There was no evidence of multiple myeloma.

The Diagnosis of POEMS Syndrome and Solitary Plasmacytoma

POEMS syndrome is a rare condition with the acronym representing some (but not all) key paraneoplastic features of the syndrome: *p*olyneuropathy, *o*rganomegaly, *e*ndocrinopathy, *m*onoclonal plasma cell disorder, and *s*kin abnormalities. There are established diagnostic criteria with the mandatory ones being polyneuropathy and a monoclonal plasma cell disorder [1]. In addition, one of three major criteria and one of six minor criteria are required to secure the diagnosis [1]. In this case, the solitary plasmacytoma serves as one of the mandatory criteria, despite the absence of systemic multiple myeloma [1]. The co-diagnosis of Castleman's disease and a sclerotic bone lesion serves as major criteria. Bone lesion, if present in POEMS syndrome, is characteristically sclerotic [2], in contrast with solitary plasmacytoma without POEMS that is typically a purely lytic lesion. She also has a plethora of minor criteria conditions, characterized by splenomegaly (organomegaly), diabetes (endocrinopathy), thrombocytosis with prior thrombotic disease, papilledema, and edema. However she did not have characteristic features of skin changes such as hyperpigmentation or acrocyanosis [3] nor pulmonary manifestations [4]. Patients with POEMS syndrome have these disparate symptoms and signs, and it is quite common to have some typical features but not others, which is the reason why it is difficult to diagnose, in addition to its rarity (prevalence <0.5 per 100,000). Delays in establishing a diagnosis is unfortunately common with median time from onset of symptoms to diagnosis of 19 months in a series of 38 patients [5], similar to that observed in this case. The pathogenesis of POEMS is poorly understood, but it is known

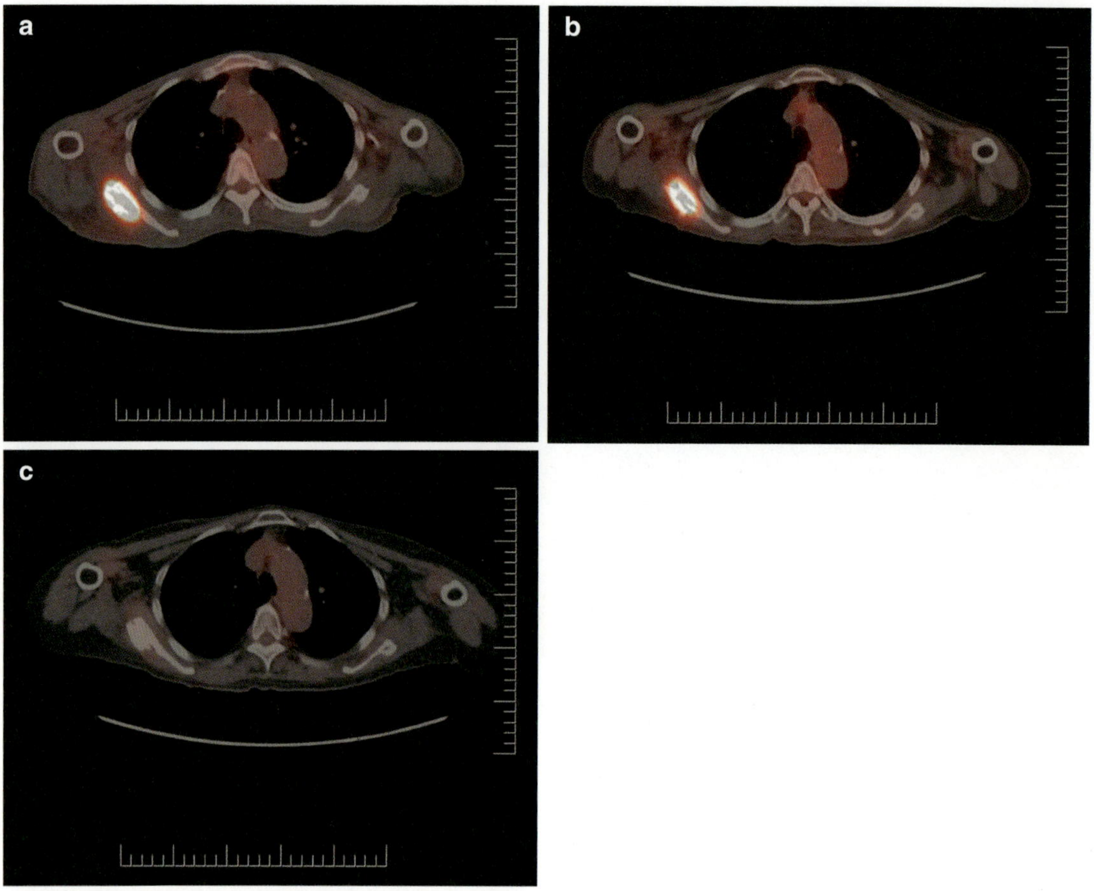

Fig. 6.3 PET/CT scan (axial slices) at initial diagnosis (**a**, *left*), 6 months (**b**, *middle*) and 16 months (**c**, *right*) after radiation treatment (35 Gy). The right scapula osteosclerotic solitary plasmacytoma is avid for FDG uptake with SUV_{max} of 24.3 prior to RT, decreasing to 10.7 at 6 months, and became normal (1.4) at 16 months, and metabolic local control was maintained at 4.5 years follow-up. However some sclerosis of the bone persisted

that treating the underlying monoclonal plasma cell disorder can result in improvement of the syndrome [1, 6, 7]. There is no documentation of IgA nephropathy to be associated with development of POEMS or plasma cell diseases, although one can speculate whether the immunosuppression might have a role in her developing the plasma cell neoplasia. It appears that elevated VEGF levels reflect the disease activity, but anti-VEGF therapy alone has not been successful suggesting that it is another manifestation of the disease rather than having a causative role [1].

The workup of a suspected diagnosis of solitary plasmacytoma is directed to exclude multiple myeloma. The following criteria must be satisfied: a biopsy-confirmed single lesion with negative skeletal imaging elsewhere, normal bone marrow biopsy (<10 % clonal plasma cells), and no myeloma-related organ dysfunction (normal blood counts, calcium and renal function) [8, 9]. A monoclonal protein can be present in blood or urine, but it is usually only minimally elevated. Solitary plasmacytomas present more commonly in the bone, and usual symptoms are pain, neurologic compromise (e.g., from vertebral lesion causing nerve or spinal cord compression), and sometimes pathologic fracture. It is unusual to be locally asymptomatic as in this case with the scapula lesion. Solitary plasmacytoma uncommonly presents in an extramedullary site (20 %), usually as a soft tissue mass in the head and neck

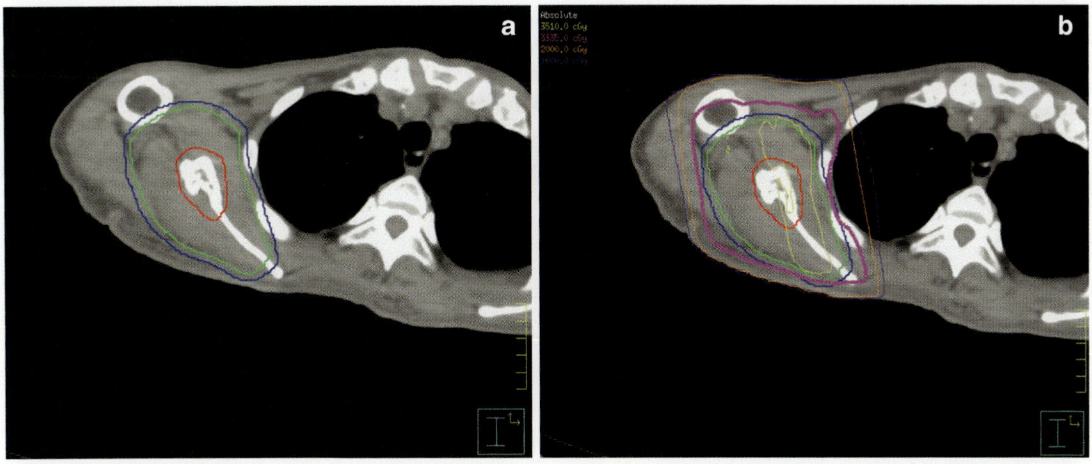

Fig. 6.4 Radiation treatment of right scapula plasmacytoma. (**a**) *Left panel*: Contours of the bony GTV (*red line*), CTV (*green line*), and PTV (*blue line*). (**b**) *Right panel*: Isodose distribution, with prescribed dose 35 Gy and the objective of PTV covered by the 95 % isodose line 33.25 Gy

areas [10]. After adequate local treatment, it is known that an extramedullary presentation is associated with a lesser probability of progression to multiple myeloma [10], in contrast with a bone presentation where the disease recurs as multiple myeloma with a high likelihood, usually within 5–10 years [9, 11].

Treatment Management

When the patient was assessed for radiation therapy, she was severely disabled and totally bedridden (ECOG performance status 4) due to her neuropathy and generalized edema. She required frequent care in hospital, and have not experienced any improvement following multiple pulse treatments with high-dose glucocorticoids and intravenous immunoglobulin treatment. It was elected to treat her with radiation therapy to the right scapula lesion, her only documented plasmacytoma. She received 35 Gy in 15 fractions (2.33 Gy fractions) over 3 weeks. This shorter regimen was chosen as she required inter-hospital transfer daily for her RT. Other acceptable regimens in common use are 40–45 Gy in conventional fractionation. However one of the largest multi-institutional reviews showed no evidence of dose response beyond 30 Gy in terms of local control, regardless of size of the tumor [11]. A 3D conformal treatment plan was used choosing beam angles and segmental fields to minimize lung exposure (Figs. 6.4 and 6.5). She tolerated RT well and was transferred to a rehabilitation facility following completion of radiation. At 6 months follow-up, she improved neurologically with recovery in her arms, but still unable to walk. Her edema resolved. Her serum VEGF level returned to normal. Repeat FDG PET/CT scan showed improvement in the scapula lesion, SUVmax decreased to 10.7 and no new lesions detected. Repeat bone marrow biopsy remained negative. One year following RT, she started to ambulate and was able to be discharged home. Repeat FDG PET/CT scans 16 months and 21 months post-RT showed complete metabolic response (no visual uptake in the right scapula), although CT scan continues to show some residual sclerosis at the local site. The patient functioned well apart from residual mild leg weakness.

Four years after RT, she experienced some worsening of her motor strength, and investigations revealed a recurrence of her POEMS syndrome with multiple FDG PET-avid spinal sclerotic lesions (Fig. 6.6) which were new, although small and asymptomatic. The scapula lesion remained controlled with no FDG uptake. She had elevation of serum VEGF (875 pg/ml).

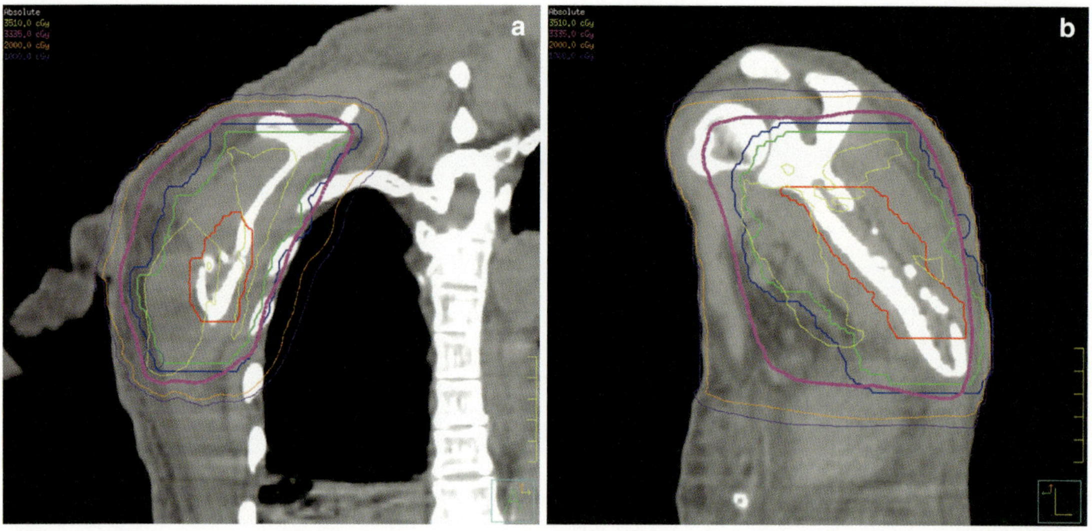

Fig. 6.5 RT treatment of right scapula plasmacytoma. Isodose distributions on CT coronal perspective (**a**) and sagittal perspective (**b**) and bone windows. The sclerotic lytic nature of the lesion is best appreciated on the sagittal image

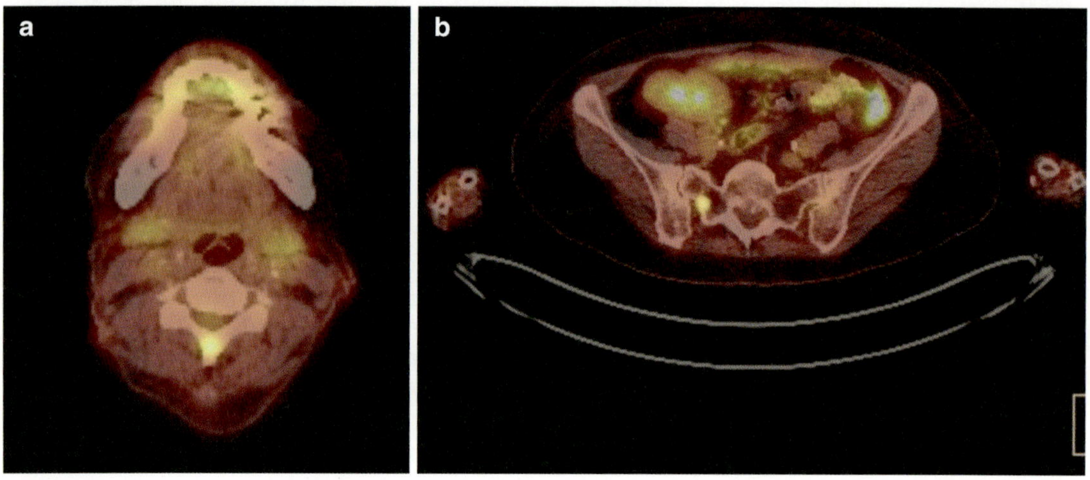

Fig. 6.6 PET/CT scan (axial slices) at time of relapse of disease, 4 years after radiation therapy to the plasmacytoma of the right scapula, showing multiple bone lesions in the spine, with FDG uptake at C5 spinous process (**a**) and right sacroiliac joint (**b**)

However her bone marrow biopsy remained negative for multiple myeloma, and she maintained absence of M-protein in blood and urine. After a brief course of chemotherapy with oral cyclophosphamide and prednisone, she received an autologous peripheral blood stem cell transplant with conditioning regimen consisting of melphalan 200 mg/M^2 and tolerated it well. Her further follow-up is awaited.

Discussion

Radiation therapy is the standard treatment for solitary plasmacytoma. In the presence of POEMS syndrome, provided that there is no evidence of a bone marrow plasma cell clone, radiation therapy is the best initial treatment, even for up to three isolated bone lesions. In one of the largest series of POEMS patients from the Mayo

Clinic ($n=146$), 38 patients (26%) satisfied this criteria and hence was found suitable for radiation therapy (RT) [5]. After median RT doses of 35–54 Gy (median 45 Gy), up to half of patients had clinical improvement or stability of POEMS-related symptoms, but most have some residual disability as in this case. With median follow-up of 43 months, the 4-year overall survival was 97%, although eventually 48% of patient required subsequent salvage therapy due to neurologic deterioration or worsened bone disease [5]. Most were treated with autologous stem cell transplantation, as in this case [12]. The expected 5-year progression-free survival is 75% with transplant [12]. The pretreatment disease features associated with a poor prognosis were pulmonary impairment with a DCLO <75% and elevated urinary total protein [5]. The case described in this report did not have these adverse features. Response to RT is also prognostic, not surprisingly, but as the case illustrates, residual sclerosis persist for many months to years after treatment, not indicative of disease, and this makes routine radiographs or CT scans difficult as a means to assess for residual disease. FDG PET is very helpful in this regard, but the response is very gradual as observed in this case, with a slow decrease in metabolic activity over a period of a year, with disappearance of metabolic activity only after 16 months from completion of RT. Local control has been maintained even when the patient progressed with multiple sclerotic lesions in her thoracic spine, as demonstrated by lack of FDG uptake in the scapula prior to her receiving the autologous stem cell transplant.

Although it is common practice to give a higher dose than 30–35 Gy for solitary plasmacytoma, with some historical data showing a lower local relapse rate of 6% with doses of ≥40 Gy, compared with 31% for lower doses [13], a large series from multiple institutions showed no evidence of improved local control with doses ranging 30–50 Gy, even for tumors >4 cm in maximum diameter [11]. In the case under discussion, a dose of 35 Gy in a slightly hypofractionated regimen have resulted in local control with a 4.5 years follow-up duration from RT. In general, a local control rate of 85–90% is expected from RT for solitary plasmacytoma. Gross target volume and clinical target volume require careful definition of the bone disease and soft tissue infiltration, if present, taking care to encompass adjacent bone which may contain microscopic disease; this can be done using an MRI and following the abnormal signal seen in the bone/bone marrow to include it in the CTV; this is based on the fact that myeloma is a marrow disease, and initially it starts by forming a tumor collection before it gets to produce the lytic lesion that can be seen on CT or to much lesser degree on a simple X-ray. As a general rule CTV is made by adding information from PET scan (avid sites) + MRI abnormal signal in the marrow + CT scan (typically lytic abnormality). In general PTV would vary depending on the site to be treated taking into consideration internal organ motion as well as daily setup, but generally no more than 2 cm is to be added if bone site is considered. Coverage of the whole bone is not required. In general regional nodes are not required to be covered as nodal failures are rare, with the exception that if the plasmacytoma was extramedullary and involve a lymphatic structure (e.g., Waldeyer's ring), the drainage lymph node region deemed at high risk of subclinical disease may be treated.

In summary this case illustrates the usefulness of definitive radiation therapy for solitary plasmacytoma, complicated by a rare debilitating paraneoplastic POEMS syndrome. Dramatic improvement in the POEMS syndrome was observed following RT, although this can take many months. Relapse of the disease with new bone lesions occurred and salvage treatment with an autologous peripheral blood stem cell transplant was required 4 years after the initial treatment.

Clinical Presentation 2: Relapse of Multiple Myeloma in the Central Nervous System

A 58-year-old man presented with a 2-month history of diffuse bone pain. He was traveling abroad and sought medical attention and was found to be anemic. By the time he returned home, he was

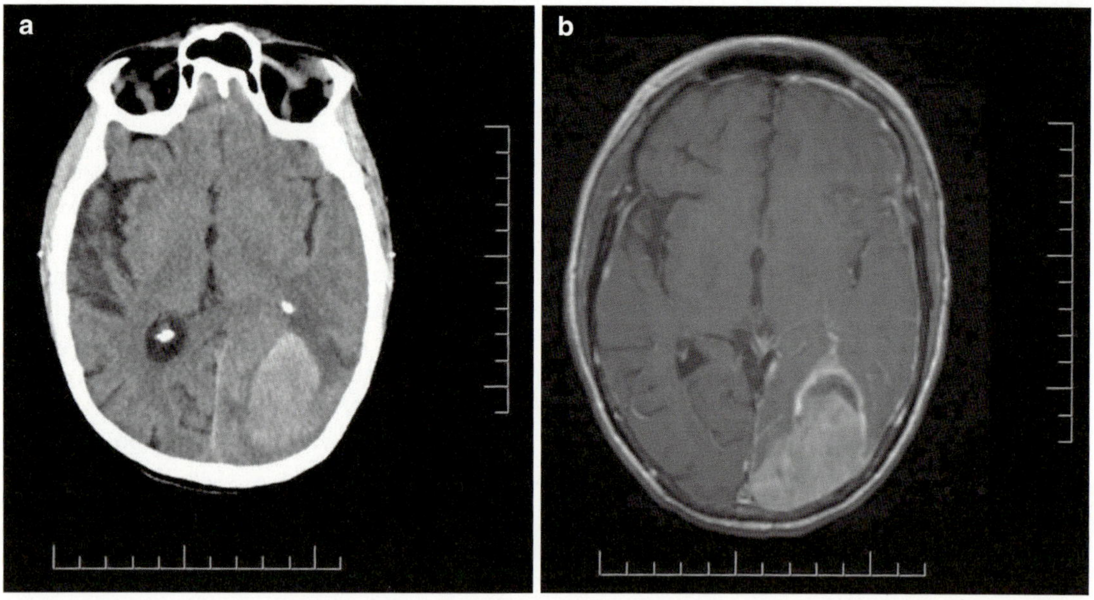

Fig. 6.7 Relapse of myeloma with an extramedullary plasmacytoma of the brain, with a left parietal-occipital mass on CT scan (**a**) and MR scan (**b**, T1 imaging). Mixed area of hemorrhage is evident within the mass. There was minimal midline shift

unwell with anorexia, fatigue, and worsening bone pain. He presented to emergency department and was hospitalized for investigations. He was found to be anemic (hemoglobin 89 g/L) and slightly hypercalcemic (2.66 mmol/L), with a high total protein and low albumin (29 g/L). He was in renal failure with serum creatinine 243 umol/L. Imaging with CT/MRI scans showed multiple lytic lesions throughout his skeleton. Serum protein electrophoresis shows a major M-spike of 73 g/L, an IgG kappa. Bone marrow biopsy showed 80 % infiltration with clonal plasma cells, kappa restricted. There were no adverse cytogenetics findings [such as t(4;14), t(14;16), del17p, etc.] by fluorescent in situ hybridization. His β_2 microglobulin was elevated to 14.3 mg/L. A diagnosis of multiple myeloma was established, and he had stage III disease according to the international staging system [14]. He was initiated on systemic chemotherapy with cyclophosphamide, bortezomib, and dexamethasone (CyBorD regimen) for five cycles, along with pamidronate on a monthly basis. He had improvement in his condition, and his M-protein dropped dramatically to <2 g/L. His bone pain resolved, and he did not require radiation therapy; however he did receive vertebral kyphoplasty to some of his lumbar vertebra. Six months following initial diagnosis, he received an autologous peripheral blood stem cell transplant with the conditioning regimen of melphalan 200 mg/M^2. Posttransplant he remained in complete remission of his myeloma and was started on maintenance lenalidomide 5 mg daily. He developed deep venous thrombosis and was started on anticoagulation treatment. Eight months after stem cell transplant, he started to have visual disturbance and also headaches and vomiting. He presented to the emergency department, and CT and MR scans show a large left occipital mass with hemorrhage (Fig. 6.7). A craniotomy was performed and tumor was resected, and the pathology showed plasmacytoma. Postoperative CT scan showed gross tumor removal was achieved (Fig. 6.8). A lumbar puncture showed that cerebrospinal fluid contained

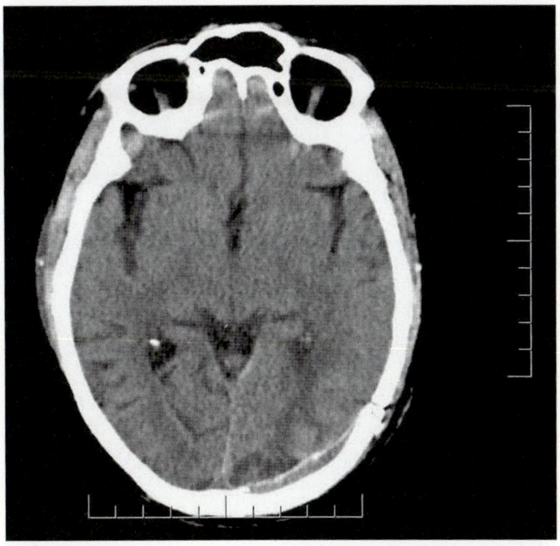

Fig. 6.8 CT scan postsurgical resection of the plasmacytoma of the brain. No residual gross disease was evident. There was minor postsurgical change along the dura in the left occipital area

numerous abnormal monoclonal plasma cells. His serum and urine M-protein remained very low, with no evidence of systemic myeloma on repeat bone marrow biopsy.

Treatment Management for CNS Disease

Central nervous system (CNS) involvement by myeloma is rare, although there are a number of case reports in recent years within the era of novel agents being commonly used in this disease with some prolongation of survival [15–17]. The development of CNS myeloma can be in the form of parenchymal brain disease and/or leptomeningeal involvement. Dura masses, often as a result of a lytic lesion in the skull bone, may be associated with a soft tissue mass which can compress or invade into the dura and should not be considered as true CNS disease. However, such dural involvement if obviously infiltrating through the dura and invading into brain or spread through the leptomeninges should be properly regarded as CNS disease. The CNS could be a relative sanctuary site for the novel agents in myeloma, such as the immunomodulatory drugs (thalidomide, lenalidomide) and the proteasome inhibitors (bortezomib, carfilzomib). In the case illustrated in this review, the patient has relapse of disease confined to the CNS with no detectable recurrence in the bone marrow. Therefore, following multidisciplinary review of treatment options, despite the expected poor prognosis, it was elected to give CNS-directed therapy with intrathecal (IT) chemotherapy to clear the CSF first, followed by consolidative craniospinal radiation. Through an intraventricular Ommaya reservoir inserted by neurosurgery, the patient proceeded with three doses of triple intrathecal chemotherapy with methotrexate 12 mg, cytarabine 40 mg, and hydrocortisone 15 mg, given over 2 weeks. His CSF became clear of plasma cells. Two additional IT treatments were given, and this was followed with craniospinal radiation therapy 30 Gy in 15 fractions to the brain, and the spinal dose was a slightly lower 24 Gy in 15 fractions. Lateral opposing fields were used to treat the brain and cervical spine, with a direct PA field (and segments) to the rest of the whole spine matched for divergence (Fig. 6.9). The junction was moved for a distance of 1 cm twice, after 5 and 10 fractions. Moderate doses were chosen as a trade-off between maintaining effectiveness for CNS control following clearance of the gross disease (in the brain with surgery and the CSF disease by IT chemotherapy) while attempting to limit toxicity for both acute (esophagus, bone marrow reserve), and late effects. The dose-volume histogram with target dose of 30 Gy to the brain is shown in (Fig. 6.10). The patient had completed therapy and further follow-up is awaited.

Discussion

In general the predominate role of radiation therapy in patients with multiple myeloma is for bone pain due to lytic bone disease, if it had not been well controlled on systemic chemotherapy, and for any neurologic compromise due to spinal cord or nerve root compression in the vertebral column or base of skull [8]. Palliative regimens

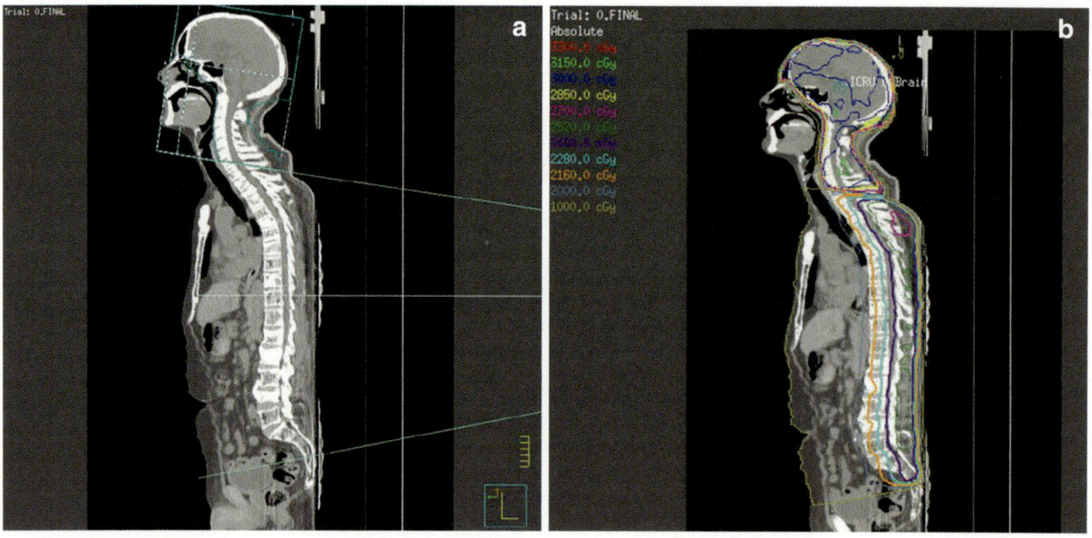

Fig. 6.9 Craniospinal radiation treatment. Lateral opposing fields treat the brain and cervical spine, with collimator rotation to match the divergent PA spinal field (**a**) and the isodose distribution (**b**) with the cranial dose 30 Gy and the spinal dose 24 Gy (given over 3 weeks)

of 10–30 Gy given over 1–3 weeks have been effective, and repeat treatments for the same bony site are seldom required [18]. It should be noted that for palliative bony sites, the target should be limited only to the gross disease noted on imaging with a margin. This is particularly important to avoid unnecessary radiation dose to the marrow causing myelosuppression and possible long-term myelofibrosis in a patient population where future systemic therapy is the mainstay of their treatment.

For spinal cord compression, a longer fractionated course (30 Gy in 10–15 fractions over 2 weeks) may give a better functional outcome than a shorter course [19] . Despite the incurable nature of multiple myeloma, even with 1–2 autologous stem cell transplantation procedures, the use of novel agents and the sequencing of different agents together with use of maintenance therapy have improved the survival rate of contemporarily treated patients [20]. Perhaps this explains the emergence of the more frequent observation of disease progressing to extramedullary sites such as the CNS, as a possible sanctuary site to chemotherapy [15–17]. Treating CNS disease is a challenge as these patients tend to be older (median age of patients with myeloma at diagnosis is over 60 years) and have been heavily pretreated, some with significant medical comorbidities and also complications of their myeloma treatment such as neuropathy or thrombotic disease (as in this case). Also there could be systemic relapse of the disease and also the complications of extensive lytic bone disease to be managed at the same time. In the case under discussion, the patient is relatively young (under 60) and has no systemic relapse of myeloma. There were both parenchymal and leptomeningeal diseases, and the tumor cells adopted a high proliferation rate by histologic assessment. Therefore the clinical decision was made to offer aggressive CNS-directed therapy to optimally control the CNS. From a review of a series of 37 patients with CNS myeloma, it appeared that approaches incorporating CNS radiation produced the best CNS control and also survival duration of >1 year [17]. Several of the "longer-term" survivors were treated with craniospinal radiation to doses of up to 30 Gy [17]. However one must keep in mind that the overall median survival expected is still short, in the range of 2–4 months, and only 9 (out of 37) patients survived for a duration of more than 1 year (median 17.1 months, range 1.1–5.6 years) in one series [17].

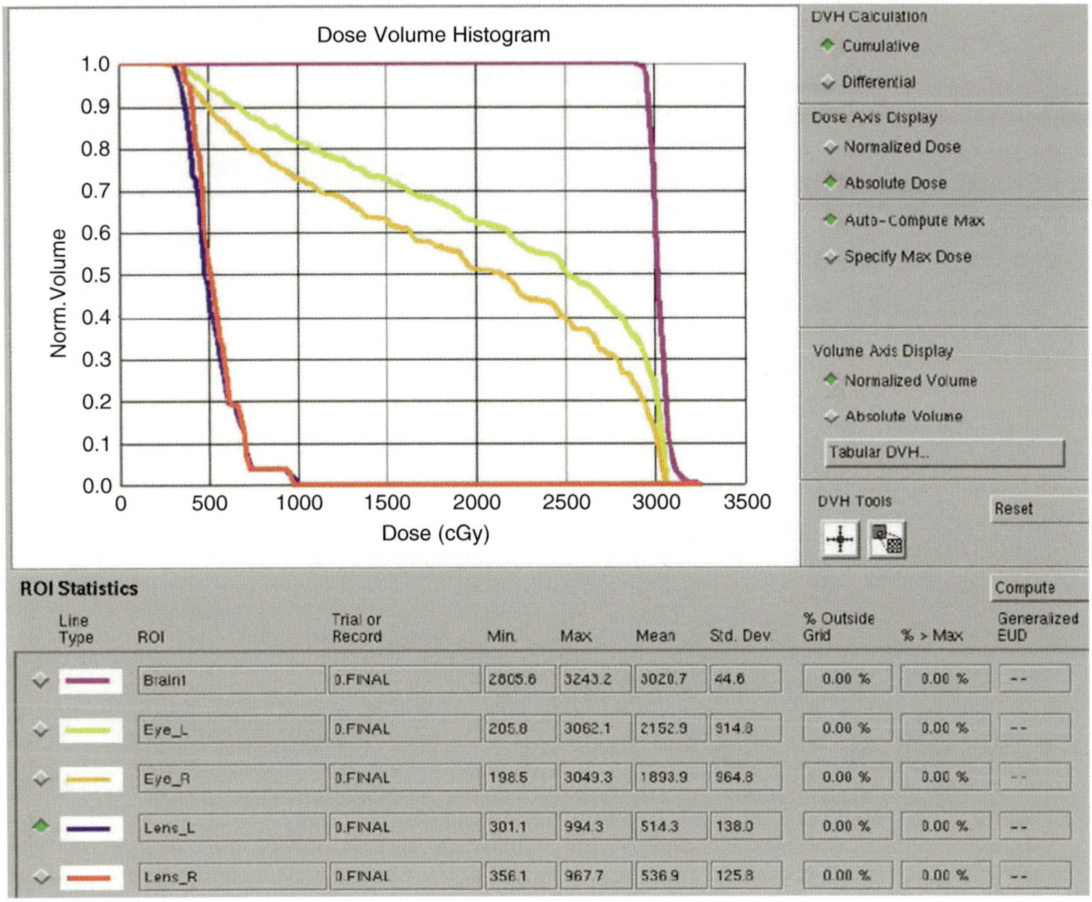

Fig. 6.10 Dose volume histogram showing brain target dose 30 Gy and the eye and lens doses

Conclusions

In summary, the two challenging cases presented in this report illustrated the effective use of radiation therapy in solitary plasmacytoma, under the rare circumstance of a paraneoplastic POEMS syndrome, and also an infrequent observation of multiple myeloma with spread to the central nervous system. While the usual and common use of palliative radiation therapy for bone disease is hardly considered "challenging," with the advent of effective novel systemic treatments for myeloma and patients living longer with their disease, unusual circumstance will continue to arise where radiation therapy may play an important role in management, as well as considerations with sequencing with other therapies and also devising overall treatment plans that are effective and yet safe.

References

1. Dispenzieri A. POEMS syndrome: 2014 update on diagnosis, risk-stratification, and management. Am J Hematol. 2014;89(2):214–23.
2. Glazebrook K, Guerra Bonilla FL, Johnson A, Leng S, Dispenzieri A. Computed tomography assessment of bone lesions in patients with POEMS syndrome. Eur Radiol. 2015;25(2):497–504.
3. Miest RY, Comfere NI, Dispenzieri A, Lohse CM, el-Azhary RA. Cutaneous manifestations in patients with POEMS syndrome. Int J Dermatol. 2013;52(11):1349–56.
4. Allam JS, Kennedy CC, Aksamit TR, Dispenzieri A. Pulmonary manifestations in patients with POEMS syndrome: a retrospective review of 137 patients. Chest. 2008;133(4):969–74.
5. Humeniuk MS, Gertz MA, Lacy MQ, Kyle RA, Witzig TE, Kumar SK, et al. Outcomes of patients with POEMS syndrome treated initially with radiation. Blood. 2013;122(1):68–73.

6. Chandrashekaran S, Dispenzieri A, Cha SS, Kennedy CC. Pulmonary morbidity improves after autologous stem cell transplantation in POEMS syndrome. Respir Med. 2015;109(1):122–30.
7. Karam C, Klein CJ, Dispenzieri A, Dyck PJ, Mandrekar J, D'Souza A, et al. Polyneuropathy improvement following autologous stem cell transplantation for POEMS syndrome. Neurology. 2015;84(19):1981–7.
8. Hodgson DC, Mikhael J, Tsang RW. Plasma cell myeloma and plasmacytoma. In: Halperin EC, Wazer DE, Perez CA, Brady LW, editors. Principles and practice of radiation oncology. 6th ed. Philadelphia: Lippincott Williams & Wilkins; 2013.
9. Tsang RW, Gospodarowicz MK, Pintilie M, Bezjak A, Wells W, Hodgson DC, et al. Solitary plasmacytoma treated with radiotherapy: impact of tumor size on outcome. Int J Radiat Oncol Biol Phys. 2001;50(1):113–20.
10. Bachar G, Goldstein D, Brown D, Tsang R, Lockwood G, Perez-Ordonez B, et al. Solitary extramedullary plasmacytoma of the head and neck--long-term outcome analysis of 68 cases. Head Neck. 2008;30(8):1012–9.
11. Ozsahin M, Tsang RW, Poortmans P, Belkacemi Y, Bolla M, Oner Dincbas F, et al. Outcomes and patterns of failure in solitary plasmacytoma: a multicenter Rare Cancer Network study of 258 patients. Int J Radiat Oncol Biol Phys. 2006;64(1):210–7.
12. D'Souza A, Lacy M, Gertz M, Kumar S, Buadi F, Hayman S, et al. Long-term outcomes after autologous stem cell transplantation for patients with POEMS syndrome (osteosclerotic myeloma): a single-center experience. Blood. 2012;120(1):56–62.
13. Mendenhall CM, Thar TL, Million RR. Solitary plasmacytoma of bone and soft tissue. Int J Radiat Oncol Biol Phys. 1980;6(11):1497–501.
14. Greipp PR, San Miguel J, Durie BG, Crowley JJ, Barlogie B, Blade J, et al. International staging system for multiple myeloma. J Clin Oncol Off J Am Soc Clin Oncol. 2005;23(15):3412–20.
15. Gangatharan SA, Carney DA, Prince HM, Wolf MM, Januszewicz EH, Ritchie DS, et al. Emergence of central nervous system myeloma in the era of novel agents. Hematol Oncol. 2012;30(4):170–4.
16. Gozzetti A, Cerase A, Lotti F, Rossi D, Palumbo A, Petrucci MT, et al. Extramedullary intracranial localization of multiple myeloma and treatment with novel agents: a retrospective survey of 50 patients. Cancer. 2012;118(6):1574–84.
17. Chen CI, Masih-Khan E, Jiang H, Rabea A, Cserti-Gazdewich C, Jimenez-Zepeda VH, et al. Central nervous system involvement with multiple myeloma: long term survival can be achieved with radiation, intrathecal chemotherapy, and immunomodulatory agents. Br J Haematol. 2013;162(4):483–8.
18. Leigh BR, Kurtts TA, Mack CF, Matzner MB, Shimm DS. Radiation therapy for the palliation of multiple myeloma. Int J Radiat Oncol Biol Phys. 1993;25(5):801–4.
19. Rades D, Hoskin PJ, Stalpers LJ, Schulte R, Poortmans P, Veninga T, et al. Short-course radiotherapy is not optimal for spinal cord compression due to myeloma. Int J Radiat Oncol Biol Phys. 2006;64(5):1452–7.
20. Kumar SK, Rajkumar SV, Dispenzieri A, Lacy MQ, Hayman SR, Buadi FK, et al. Improved survival in multiple myeloma and the impact of novel therapies. Blood. 2008;111(5):2516–20.

Role of Radiation in the Treatment of Leukemias: Lymphoblastic Lymphoma, Central Nervous System Disease, and Chloromas

7

Bouthaina Shbib Dabaja

Abstract

The role of radiation in the treatment of leukemia is becoming a crucial part of managing these patients. This is mainly the result of the improvement in the survival of patients affected by leukemia. Living longer made it possible for a local control offered by radiation to refind its way to the daily management of this disease.

We will discuss three of the most common scenarios where radiation is helpful in patients affected with leukemia.

Lymphoblastic Lymphoma: Clinical Presentation, Pathology, Treatment, and Role of Radiation

Case 1: *A 32-year-old man presented with increased shortness of breath and chest pain to the emergency room. A chest X-ray showed widening mediastinum* (Fig. 7.1); *a computed tomography (CT) scan showed a large anterior mediastinal mass extending superiorly to the level of the thyroid cartilage on the left side and inferiorly to the level of the anterior hemidiaphragms, along with matted adenopathy that is also present in the posterior mediastinum extending to the crura of the hemidiaphragms; and pleural effusion was noted on the left side* (Fig. 7.2).

A transthoracic core biopsy was done (Fig. 7.3), *and the diagnosis of T-lymphoblastic lymphoma was made. The pathology specimen revealed prominent population of aberrant T cells (75 % of total cells), which are positive for CD1a, surface CD3, CD4, CD7, CD8, and CD45 and negative for CD33.*

The proliferation index is approximately 80–90 % by Ki-67 stain. The rest of the workup included bone marrow biopsy and blood work to rule out blood involvement, and they both came back negative.

Clinical Presentation and Pathology

Lymphoblastic lymphoma (LBL) is mainly a T-cell neoplasm (90 %) [1] that resembles acute lymphoblastic lymphoma (ALL) with no or low risk for bone marrow involvement. It is grouped with ALL in the 2008 WHO classification [2]. The lack of bone marrow involvement (<25 % of

B.S. Dabaja, MD
Department of Radiation Oncology, University of Texas MD Anderson Cancer Center,
Holcombe Blvd, Houston, TX 77030, USA
e-mail: bdabaja@mdanderson.org

B.S. Dabaja, A.K. Ng (eds.), *Radiation Therapy in Hematologic Malignancies*,
DOI 10.1007/978-3-319-42615-0_7

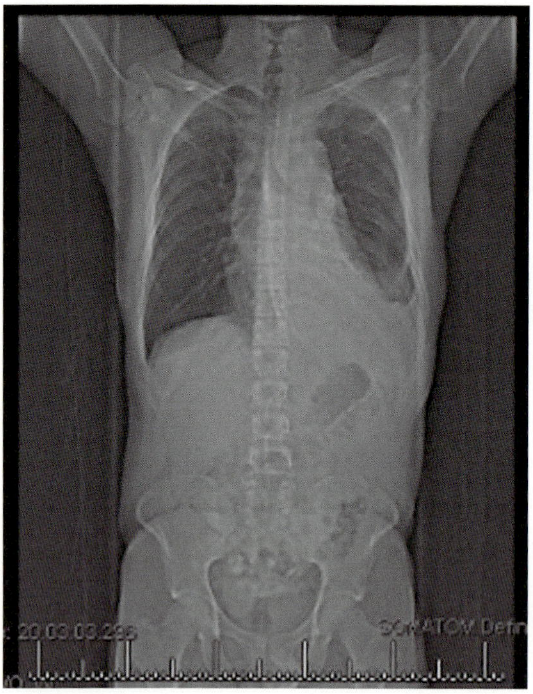

Fig. 7.1 Chest X-ray at presentation showing widening mediastinum

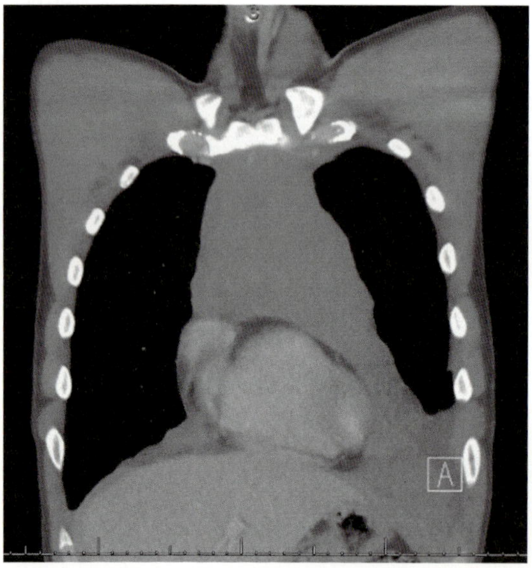

Fig. 7.2 CT chest at presentation showing the disease starting at the left neck to the lower mediastinum with pleural and pericardial effusion

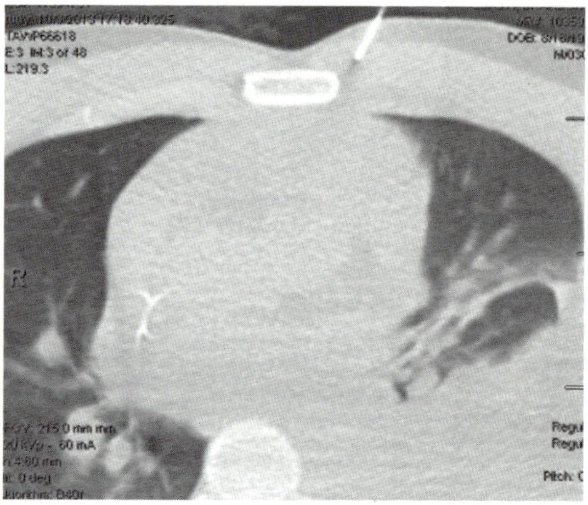

Fig. 7.3 Showing the biopsy taken from the mediastinal mass

blasts) along with a mediastinal mass originating from the thymus forms the unique presentation that makes this disease a distinct entity. Clinically, the hallmark is a mediastinal bulky disease in a young man, and the ratio of male to female is 2:1. Often, the mediastinal mass will grow to a size that will cause acute symptoms that will send the patient to the emergency room. Symptoms might include shortness of breath, chest pain, and superior vena cava syndrome. The mediastinal mass is often associated with a pleuropericardial effusion [3]. According to our institutional data, 70 % of patients present with stage III/IV, 70 % with mediastinal involvement, and only 9 % with CNS disease at presentation. Other groups reported up to 20 % CNS disease especially with no CNS prophylaxis. Other sites of involvement, although <10 %, includes the spleen/liver, kidney, bone, and skin.

Pathologically it is a neoplasm of immature T cells. This is also reflected by different stages of maturations seen. A recent study showed that the level of maturation could actually affect the clinical outcome. Early T-cell precursor (ETP) differentiation stage (recently immigrated cells from the bone marrow to the thymus and with a typical phenotype of CD1a−, CD8−, and CD5− and positivity for myeloid antigens) was associated with a lower remission rate as well as median survival compared to no ETP subtypes including thymic and mature subtypes [4].

For the patient in case 1, after completing workup including assessment of the heart and liver function, he was initiated on treatment as per

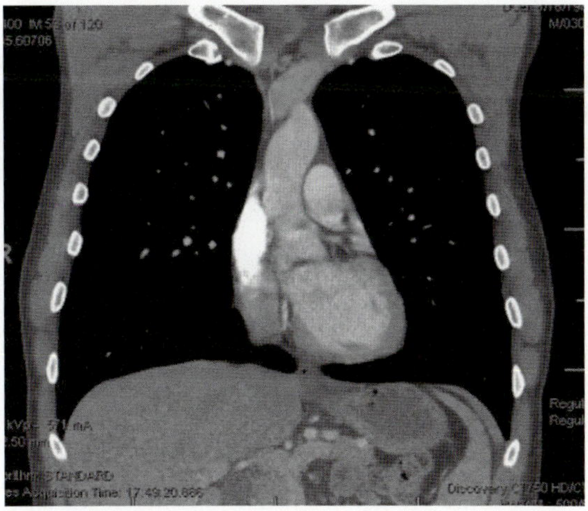

Fig. 7.4 Showing the complete remission at the end of chemotherapy

our institutional guidelines using leukemia-like regimen hyper-CVAD (hyper-cyclophosphamide, vincristine, doxorubicin, and dexamethasone) alternating with high-dose cytosine arabinoside (Ara-C) and methotrexate for a total of 8 cycles given usually over 4–5 months. There was no attempt to drain the pleural effusion. Every attempt was made to control and prevent tumor lysis syndrome. Concomitantly, the patient received central nervous system (CNS) prophylaxis using intrathecal chemotherapy with methotrexate on day 2, and Ara-C on days 7 and *8 of each cycle. An interim CT chest at the completion of 4 cycles showed almost complete disappearance of the mediastinal mass with a bone marrow still showing no evidence of disease. At the completion of chemotherapy and before starting maintenance therapy, the patient was referred for consolidation radiation therapy*; Fig. 7.4 *shows the status of the mediastinum at completion of his chemotherapy.*

Treatment of LBL with Chemotherapy

The cornerstone of treatment of LBL is leukemia-like regimens, which differ from one institution to another. The treatment regimens used are based on the successful experience in treating childhood leukemia. The German group regimen NHL-BFM 90 resulted in an outstanding 5-year event-free survival in children of 90 % [5]. Building on the pediatrics experience, the University of Texas MD Anderson Cancer Center reported a good outcome in adult leukemia using hyper-CVAD [6]. The same regimen was used for the treatment of patients with LBL with 91 % achieving complete remission and a 3-year progression-free and overall survival of 66 % and 70 %, respectively. Other investigators adopted different regimens, but it is widely accepted that more intensive regimens are superior, and it is also accepted that adding CNS prophylaxis decreases the risk of CNS relapse that could be as high as 26 % [7]. After completion of induction and consolidation chemotherapy, which in case 1 was 8 cycles of alternating hyper-CVAD and high MTX-Ara-C, patients will start maintenance therapy for 2 years consisting of intravenous POMP (6 mercaptopurine, methotrexate, vincristine, and prednisone).

The patient in case 1, as per our institutional policy, presented to the radiation oncology department to receive consolidation radiation therapy to the mediastinal area at the completion of his last chemotherapy cycle. It was insured that his blood counts have completely recovered with an absolute white blood cell count of >1500.

The patient was simulated in a supine position with arms down using an immobilization cradle to insure the reproducibility of the position of the neck in relation to the chest as well as the arms' positions in relation to the chest (Fig. 7.5). *The isocenter was placed 2 in. below the sternal notch. Computed tomography (CT) scan was obtained spanning from the mid head to the below the diaphragmatic crus to insure encapture of the entire lung (this is crucial as shown below for the daily verification of the treatment). At our institution and for all patients to be treated for thoracic targets, we do use deep inspiration breathhold (DIBH) technique. Patients are also treated on a 10°–15° incline board to displace mammary tissues in females inferolaterally and away from the radiation field. It also helps displace the heart inferoposteriorly and facilitate DIBH* [8]. *The patient in case 11* (Fig. 7.5) *was coached prior to the simulation for the breath-hold by watching a video showing the procedure in details. Respiration was monitored with a video-based, noninvasive system that includes an*

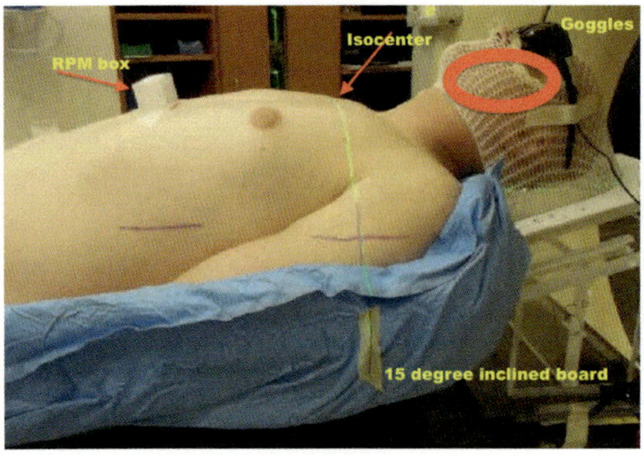

Fig. 7.5 Showing the details of the setup

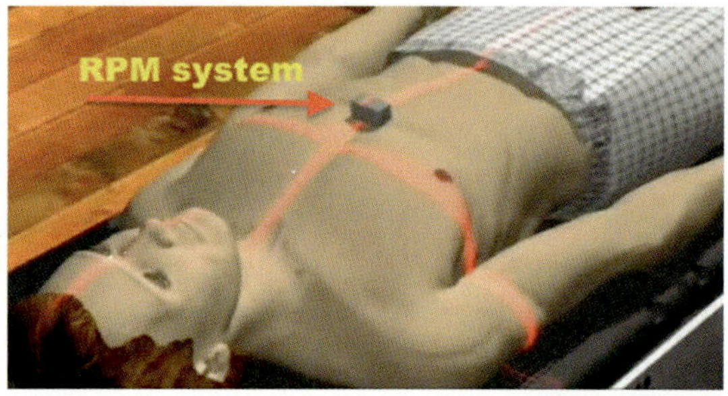

Fig. 7.6 Showing the RPM box placed on a cartoon illustration

infrared tracking camera and reflective marker (RPM [real-time position management] system (Fig. 7.6), *Varian Medical Systems, Palo Alto, CA). The patient performed DIBH and received feedback via video goggles to improve the stability and reproducibility of breath amplitude.*

At the time of treatment simulation, 3–4 breathhold-gated non-contrast CT scans were acquired with axial 2.5-mm slices. Imaging data were transmitted to a Pinnacle treatment planning system (Phillips Healthcare) where contouring of the tumor target and surrounding organs at risk as well as treatment planning was performed. Figure 7.7a–c *shows the clinical target volume (CTV, red) and planning target volume (PTV, green). Both contours were guided by fusing the CT simulation images with the initial contrast-enhanced CT.*

IMRT plans were generated with a Pinnacle treatment planning system. Coplanar 6-MV photons were used with 6 beams all anterior-posterior weighted according to our in in-house "butterfly" technique [9] (Fig. 7.8). *Involved-site radiation therapy was used for target delineation as per published guidelines from the International Lymphoma Radiation Oncology Group (ILROG)* [10].

Figure 7.9 *shows the IMRT plan generated. Only the mediastinal disease was included in the target volume. There was no attempt to chase the pleural or pericardial effusions. Additionally, the distal part of the mediastinum in the anterior aspect of heart was not included either in an effort to limit heart toxicity. The total dose was 30.6 Gy in 17 fractions. IMRT was delivered by a linear accelerator with step-and-shoot multi-leaf collimation. Low-dose CT on rails was used for daily image guidance (Varian Medical Systems)* (Fig. 7.10). *Both the lungs and heart structures were delineated on the treatment-planning scan to generate lung and heart dose-volume histogram (generated by the Pinnacle system)* (Fig. 7.9c).

Role of Radiation

The clinical presentation with a bulky mediastinal mass makes it appealing to address the local disease with radiation therapy to prevent local relapse. This is an approach that has been adopted in other disease subtypes where mediastinal diseases have a similar presentation, including Hodgkin's lymphoma and primary mediastinal large B-cell lymphoma. The evidence for the benefit of radiation in LBL comes mainly from subset analysis in large studies and several retrospective studies. The role of radiation was questioned based on a 47 % mediastinal relapse rate in a publication by Hoelzer et al. [11]. However, among the 45 treated patients, the rate of complete remission was 93 %; out of the 15 (30 %) patients who relapsed, 7 patients relapsed in the mediastinum. Arguably that means that 8 did not relapse in the mediastinum, and also arguably there are 30 patients who did not even relapse and the mediastinal area was controlled. The authors though did not conclude that radiation should not be used. On the contrary

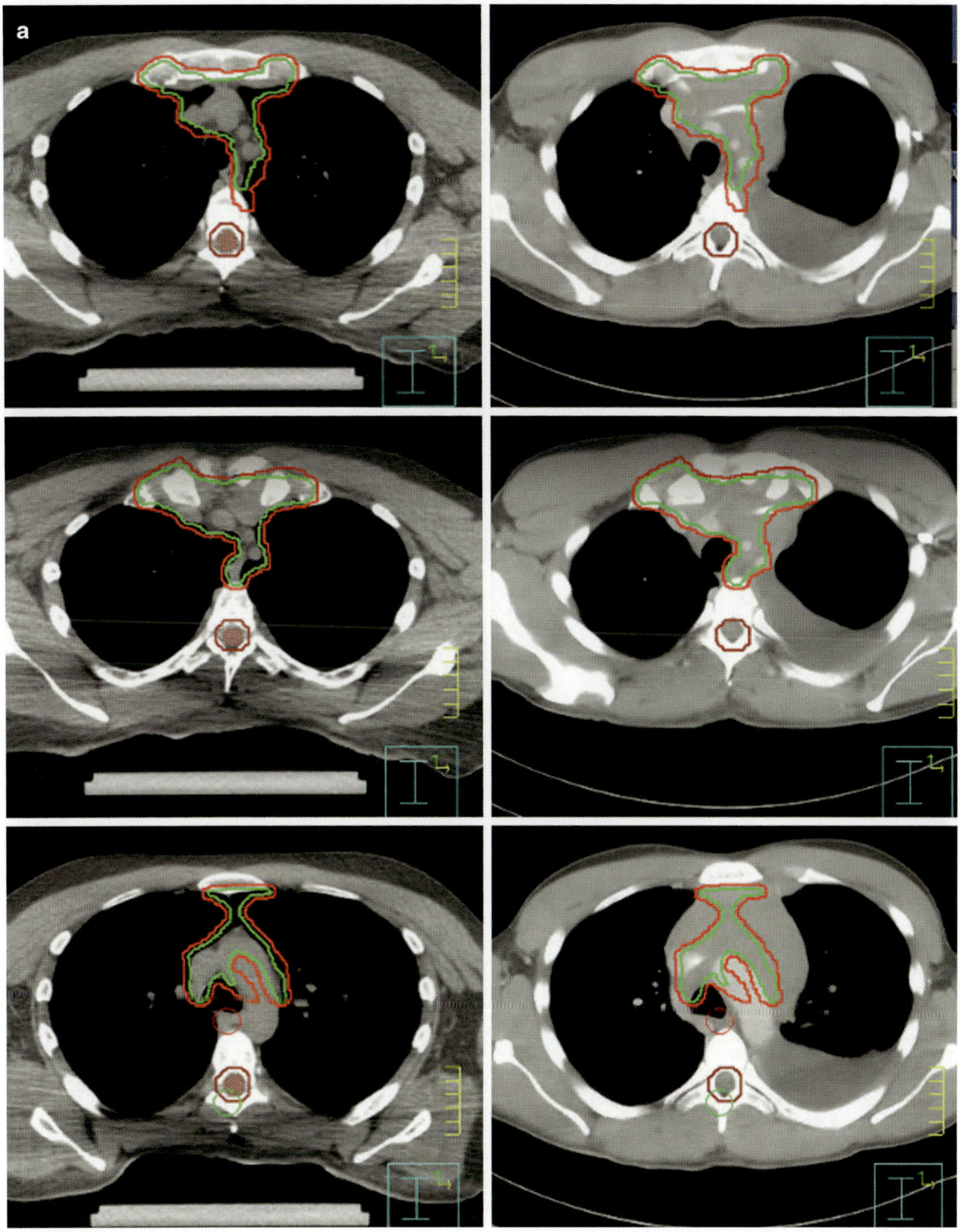

Fig. 7.7 (**a**, **b**) Showing the CTV (*green*) and PTV (*red*). (**c**) Showing the CTV (*green*) and PTV (*red*). Omitting the part where the mass hanging in front of the heart and avoiding the area of the pleural effusion

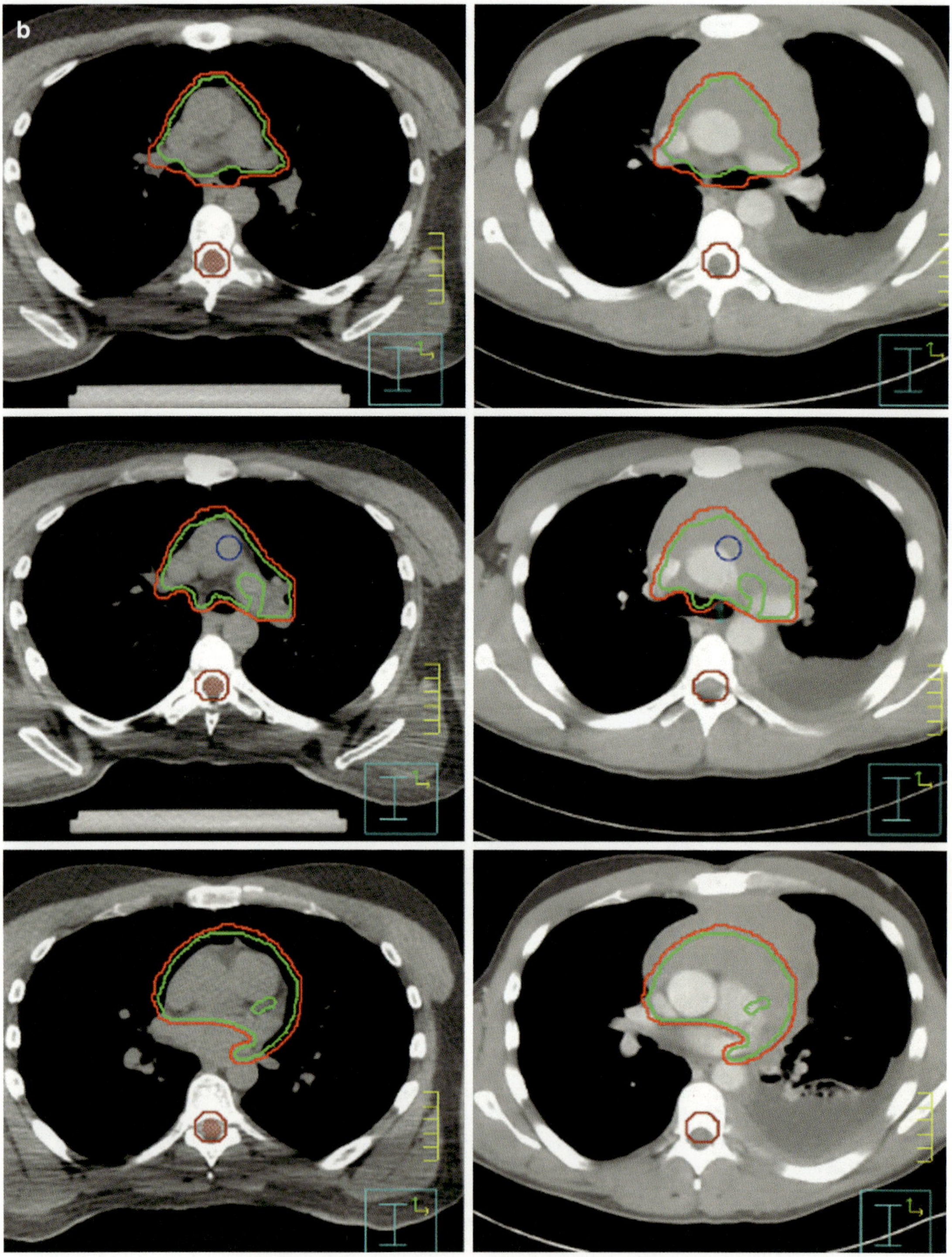

Fig. 7.7 (continued)

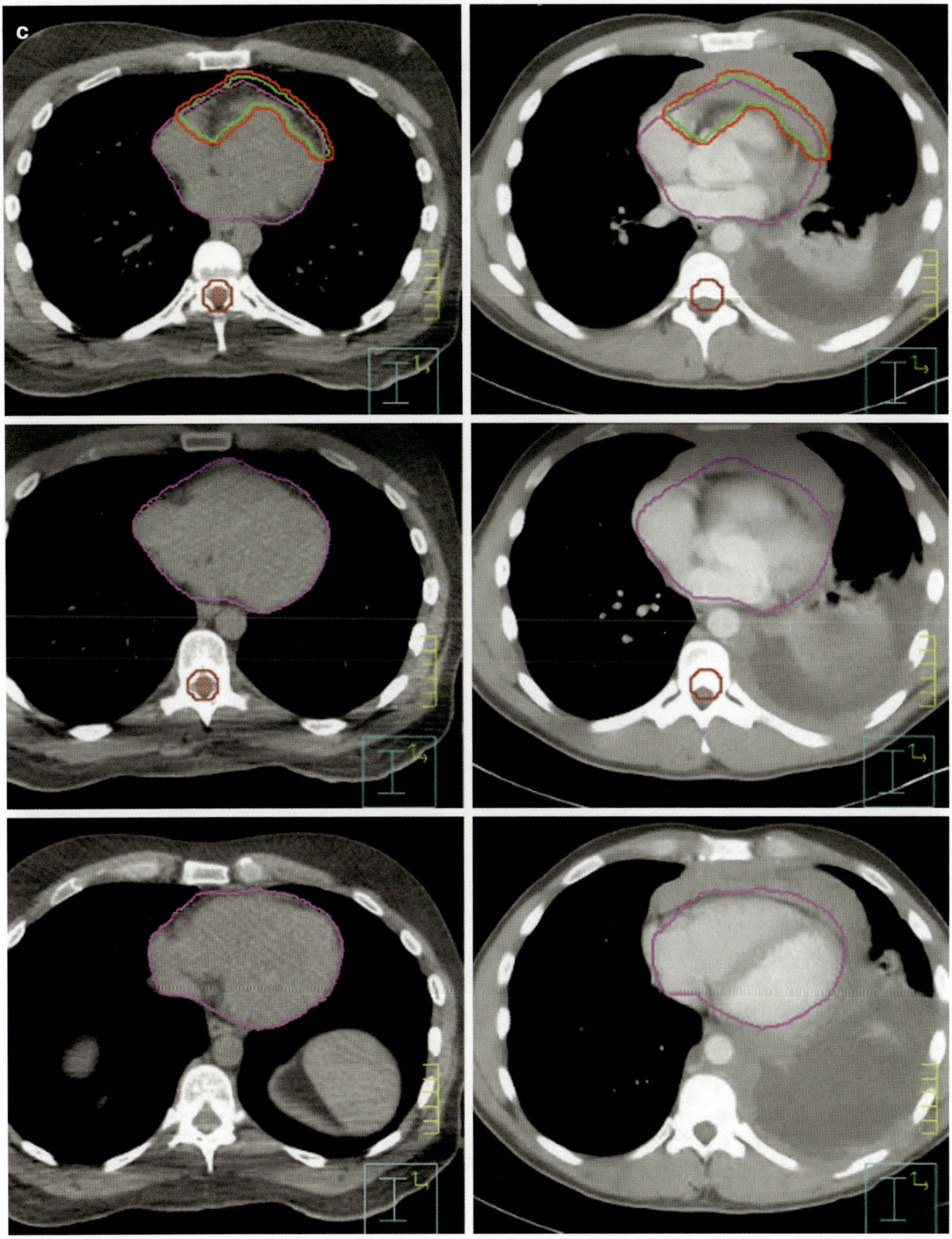

Fig. 7.7 (continued)

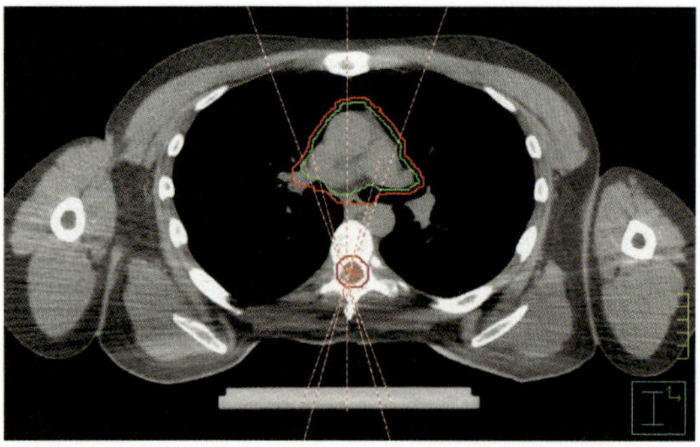

Fig. 7.8 Showing the beam arrangement used as per the butterfly technique

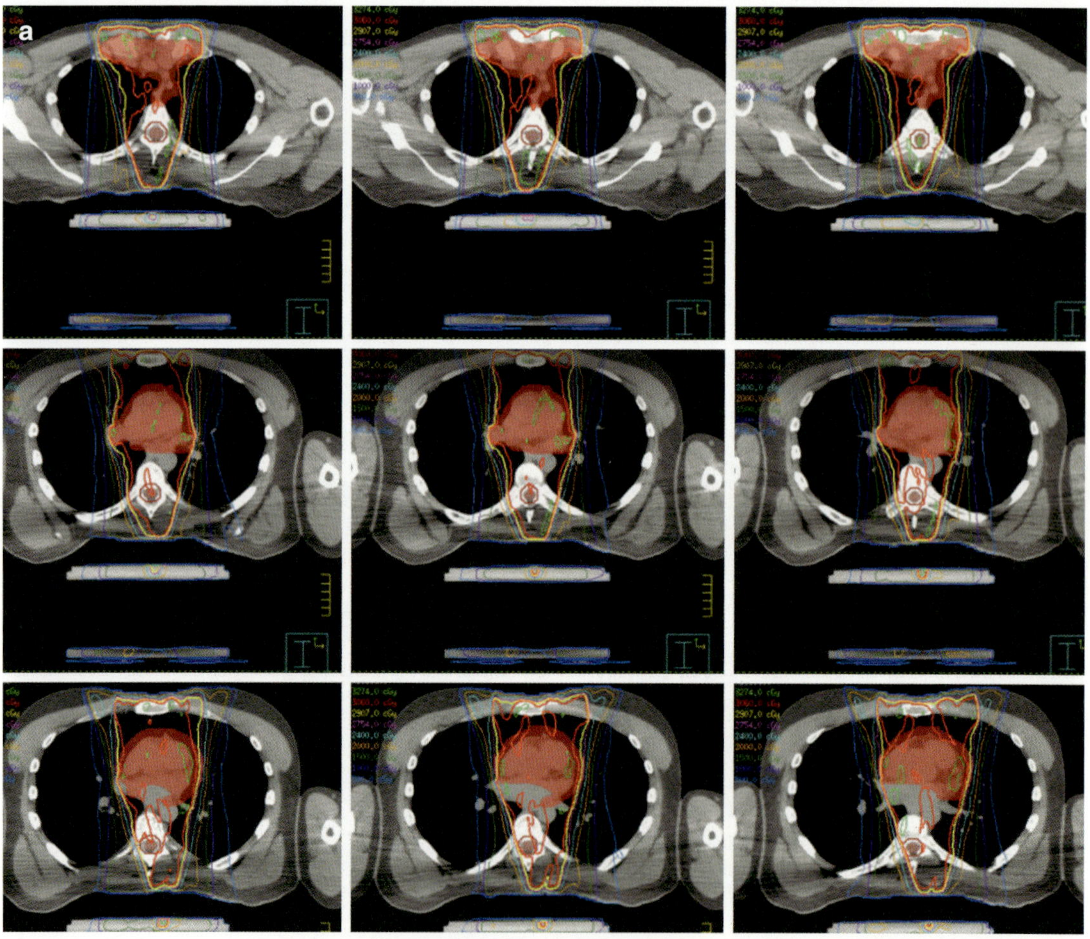

Fig. 7.9 (**a**) Showing the isodose lines sparing the lung from the low dose by only using anteroposterior beams. (**b**) Coronal view. (**c**) Showing the dose-volume histogram for case 1

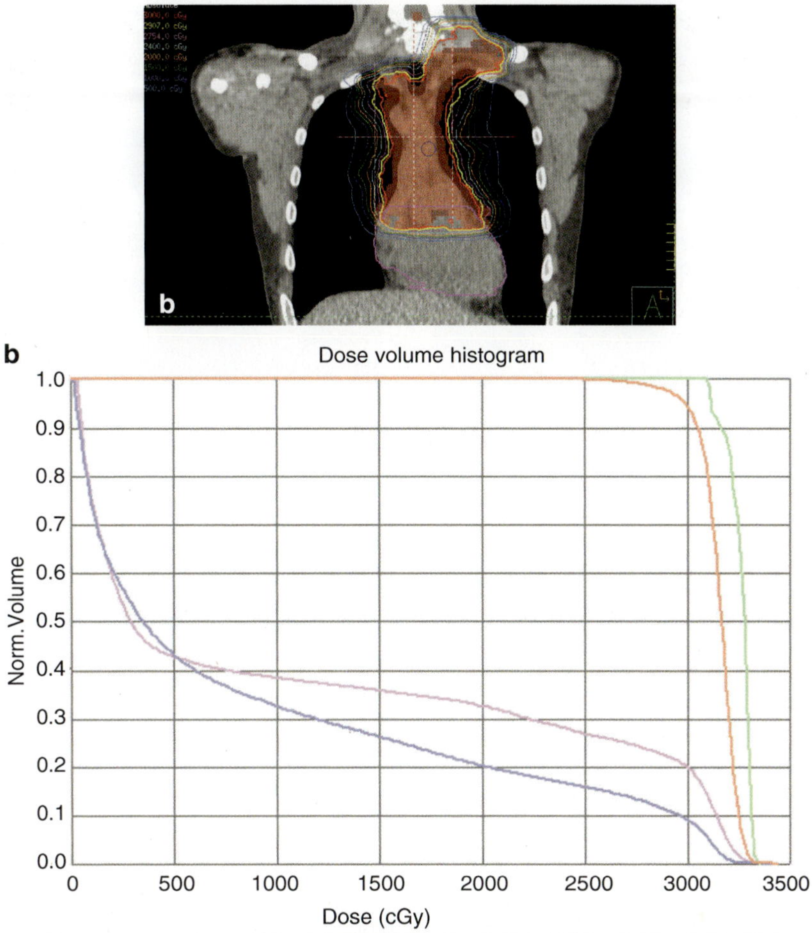

ROI Statistics

Line Type	ROI	Trial or Record	Min.	Max.	Mean	Std. Dev.
(pink line)	Heart	Aprvd BSD	30.9	3432.3	1151.9	1281.6
(green line)	LT Main coronary	Aprvd BSD	3094.5	3351.5	3258.4	58.1
(blue line)	Total Lung	Aprvd BSD	8.2	3369.2	914.8	1067.3
(orange line)	pPTV 30.6	Aprvd BSD	1535.8	3432.3	3148.6	105.5

Fig. 7.9 (continued)

they suggested that in certain patients intensification of therapy including chemotherapy and radiation by increasing the dose from 24 to 36 Gy to the mediastinum. One could also argue that may be 24 Gy is not enough to control the mediastinum, as discussed below. Radiation to a dose ≥30 Gy proved to improve both local control and disease-free survival. In spite of that, omitting radiation especially in intensified regimens that included high-dose therapy was tried by GOELAMS. The authors compared re-induction chemotherapy against intensified conditioning followed by stem cell transplantation; they reported 7-year OS and DFS of 64 % and 65 % with little information on the local control [12]. In the recently published GRAALL-LYSA LL03 study, 148 patients (90 % with T-cell LBL) were prospectively treated with a pediatric-like leukemia protocol, with CNS prophylaxis and 2 years of maintenance therapy. There were 34 relapses,

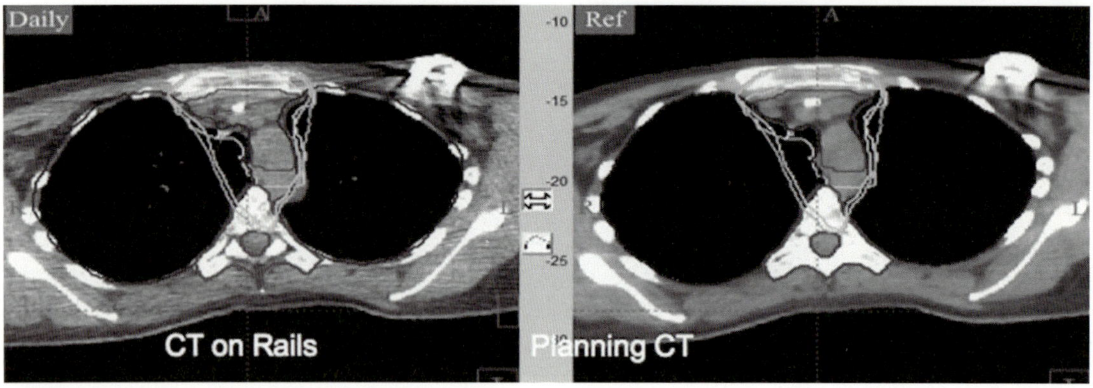

Fig. 7.10 CT on rail done for verification

yielding a 3-year event-free survival of 63 % and overall survival of 74 %. No mediastinal radiation was given. Of the 131 patients with T-LBL, 30 relapsed and went on to be salvaged. At the last follow-up, 82 of the assessed patients were still in CR. However, there was no information on patterns of relapse and the risk of mediastinal failure.

Our institution has reported different outcomes, and we have highlighted in multiple publications the importance of radiation in local control and disease-free survival.

In a study by Thomas et al., 33 patients with LBL were treated with hyper-CVAD. Seventeen of the 23 patients with mediastinal disease received mediastinal radiation, and only 1 of the 17 relapsed in the mediastinum [13]. In a subsequent publication [14] on 47 patients with T-LBL, none of the 19 patients who received mediastinal radiation had mediastinal relapse, as compared to 8 patients with mediastinal relapse among the 24 patients who did not receive radiation. We updated our experience recently with a more modernly treated cohort. Mediastinal radiation was given to 50 of 77 patients. Mediastinal relapse occurred in 3 of 50 (6 %) patients who received radiation, as opposed to in 7 of 27 (27 %) relapses among those who did not receive radiation. These results translated into an improvement in disease-free survival [15].

The discrepancy in treatment is mainly derived from the fear of toxicity that could be seen with radiation even decades later, especially that these patients who have received intensive chemotherapy. Radiation oncologists should be aware of the treatment-related toxicity as well as of the expectations when treating this disease. The role of radiation is purely to address the mediastinal disease and not to chase after small disease or involvement that might compromise the critical organs, in this case the heart and lung. There have been major technological advances that made it possible for us to target the area of interest while keeping the critical organs at risk safe from radiation [10]. There have been recent data suggesting that lower-dose threshold for critical organs should be used in radiation therapy for hematological malignancies as compared to the ones accepted for solid tumors [16]. Additionally, refining and perfecting planning using modern techniques such as IMRT [9] have made it possible to reduce the volume exposed to the prescription dose. However, robust immobilization and control of internal organ motion such as use of DIBH technique are critical.

The patient in case 1 completed his radiation and went on to receive his 2-year maintenance. Today he is 3 years out and he is still in complete remission.

Role of Craniospinal Radiation in Leukemia

Case 2: A 39-year-old man presented with left lower leg pain. Ultrasound was notable for a deep venous thrombus. He was initiated on rivaroxaban for treatment of DVT and had an IVC filter placed. At the same time, he was noted to have abnormal blood counts and therefore had a workup, which included a bone marrow biopsy that showed B-lineage acute lymphoblastic leukemia. Bone marrow obtained had 94 % blasts with immunophenotyping positive for CD20, CD19, and HLA-DRTdT cytogenetics with 47 xy plus x, white blood cell count reportedly 120,000 per microliter. CSF obtained through a spinal tap showed no involvement. The patient was initiated on induction chemotherapy with rituximab and hyper-CVAD. Day 28 bone marrow showed a complete morphologic remission but with persistent minimal residual disease. He received a total of 7 intrathecal therapies, all with cytarabine. Completed 8 cycles of chemotherapy and went on to start maintenance therapy.

Clinical Presentation and Treatment of Leukemias

Leukemias are typically classified according to the cell of origin and into acute and chronic. Myeloid neoplasms arise from bone marrow progenitor cells that develop into granulocytes, erythrocytes, monocytes, or megakaryocytes. Lymphoid neoplasms arise from cells that normally develop into B or T lymphocytes. Further, chronic are mature cells, while acute are immature cells; it is also possible for transformation of a chronic leukemia into a more acute.

The leukemias of lymphoid origin include precursor B- and T-cell lymphoblastic leukemia (i.e., acute lymphoblastic leukemia, ALL), chronic lymphocytic leukemia/small lymphocytic lymphoma (CLL/SLL), and B- and T-cell prolymphocytic leukemia. Leukemias of myeloid origin include acute myelogenous leukemia (AML) and chronic myelogenous leukemia (CML).

In addition to morphology, examined by an experienced hematopathologist, the classification of leukemia also relies on immunophenotyping and cytogenetics. The impact of the current advancement in diagnosis is major since it can not only determine the prognosis, and the risk of developing CNS disease or extramedullary disease, but also guides decision on chemotherapy regimens, the need for maintenance chemotherapy, the use of high-dose autologous or allogeneic transplant, and the type of central nervous system prophylaxis to be applied. Some examples to highlight the aforementioned are high-dose Ara-C in AML especially in the presence of inversion 16 (t16;16)(p13;q22), which has a more favorable prognosis [17, 18]; hyper-CVAD/high-dose MTX and Ara-C for ALL [6]; the need for high-dose chemotherapy and transplant in Philadelphia-positive (t(9;22) BCR-ABL) translocation ALL which affect 20–30 % of adult ALL; the addition of a tyrosine kinase inhibitor like imatinib or dasatinib [19, 20] in those with a higher risk for CNS relapse [21], such as in AML patients with inversion 16 and complex cytogenetic; and the use of targeted therapy with tyrosine kinase inhibitors in chronic myelogenous leukemia [18], arsenic trioxide in AML M3 t(15:17) [22].

For the patient in case 2, at 12 months from the initiation of his maintenance therapy, he presented with low counts, headache, and loss of vision in the left eye. A repeat bone marrow biopsy showed a hypocellular marrow with 30 % blasts and recurrence of the plus X and an additional 17p, consistent with B-lineage ALL. Immunophenotyping was positive for CD34, CD10, CD22, cytoplasmic CD79A, and CRLF2. No translocations were noted on translocation panel. Cytogenetics showed a 47 xy plus x inversion 17 in three metaphases and a 47–48 xy idem in 5 metaphases. Repeat CSF evaluation showed abundant blasts. MRI of the brain and spine were both normal. He was started on moxetumomab (an anti-CD22 mouse monoclonal antibody) on clinical protocol, as well as intrathecal chemotherapy. After 4 cycles, his bone marrow showed near-complete response with minimal residual disease. Unfortunately, his CSF continued to show blasts, and additionally he presented with decreased vision in his left eye, which on exam showed a sharply demarcated white discoloration in his cornea (Fig. 7.11).

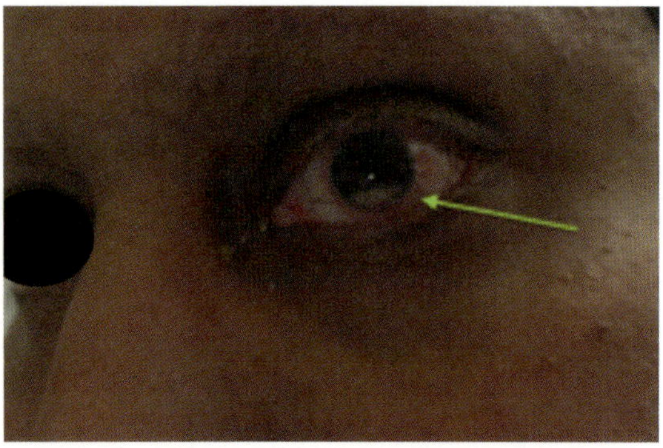

Fig. 7.11 A sharply demarcated white discoloration in the patient's cornea

Patients with ALL are at risk for CNS disease [23], with risk ranging from 20 to 50 %, while it is less common in patients with AML [24]. The observed toxicity of cranial radiation has deterred medical oncologist from using it. Alternatively high-dose and intensive chemotherapy regimens that can cross the blood-brain barrier as well as direct intrathecal therapy are used. Nevertheless, the survival of leukemia in general has improved substantially [25, 26] with the availability of multiple targeted therapies that addresses the systemic disease, which might leave the sanctuary sites only partially addressed. This is applicable also in the case of high-dose chemotherapy even in the setting of allogeneic transplant. Therefore, radiation has recently emerged as an attractive approach specifically to patients that have proved that they are sensitive to the systemic therapy but with persistent disease in the CNS. In our institution, it became the standard of care to deliver craniospinal irradiation (CSI) prior to transplant. In cases where total body irradiation, typically of 12 Gy, is planned as part of the conditioning, we give a CSI dose of 12 Gy in 6 treatments, then we immediately proceed with the TBI on days –4 to –6, and then we transplant cell infusion on day 0. It is important that CSI is delivered prior to the transplant. This is because if CNS relapse occurs in the setting of bone marrow remission in an engrafted patient, CSI can compromise the graft. Additionally, the CNS disease can potentially reseed back into the blood/bone marrow. In a recent study from MD Anderson, the role of CSI in 163 adults with leukemia was addressed and compared to those who received more limited radiation. The 1-year CNS progression-free survival was 77 % for those who received CSI or whole brain irradiation, compared to 51 % for those who received base of skull irradiation only. Furthermore, comprehensive radiation with CSI mostly benefited patients with negative marrow in the pretransplant setting [27].

Patient in case 2 underwent a sibling matched donor allogeneic stem cell transplant, and as part of the conditioning regimen, CSI was delivered to a total dose of 24 Gy using proton therapy in an effort to decrease the exit dose through the anterior critical organs including the thyroid, lung, heart, gastrointestinal, and pelvic structures (Fig. 7.12a, b).

Commonly, CSI is delivered using photon which should be an acceptable alternative in places where proton therapy is not available. Photon in a prone position provides the ability to visually check the matching gaps between fields, thus a safer delivery of this technically challenging treatment. Photon CSI can also be delivered in a supine position where the gaps are managed with IMRT. When using proton CSI, it is important for the team involved to be well versed in the proton delivery, specifically to pay attention to the distal beam edge which carries a higher RBE at the end tail. Ideally, in the case where CSI is not part of a myeloablative regimen including TBI, proton CSI can spare the vertebral bodies (which forms 50 % of the marrow). When using proton in this setting, attention should be directed to the higher RBE that can reach up to 1.6 at the distal beam edge [28, 29]. For that reason, the beam edge should be placed anteriorly to encompass 1/3 or more of the vertebral bodies to avoid the high RBE at the beam tail from falling into the cord. However, in cases where the CSI is delivered prior to a myeloablative conditioning regimen, this is less of an issue, and the field can encompass the majority of the vertebral bodies.

When treating the brain either as part of a CSI or whole brain irradiation, both eyes have to be included in the field, one because they are considered part of the meninges/CNS and second because of the high risk of eye involvement with

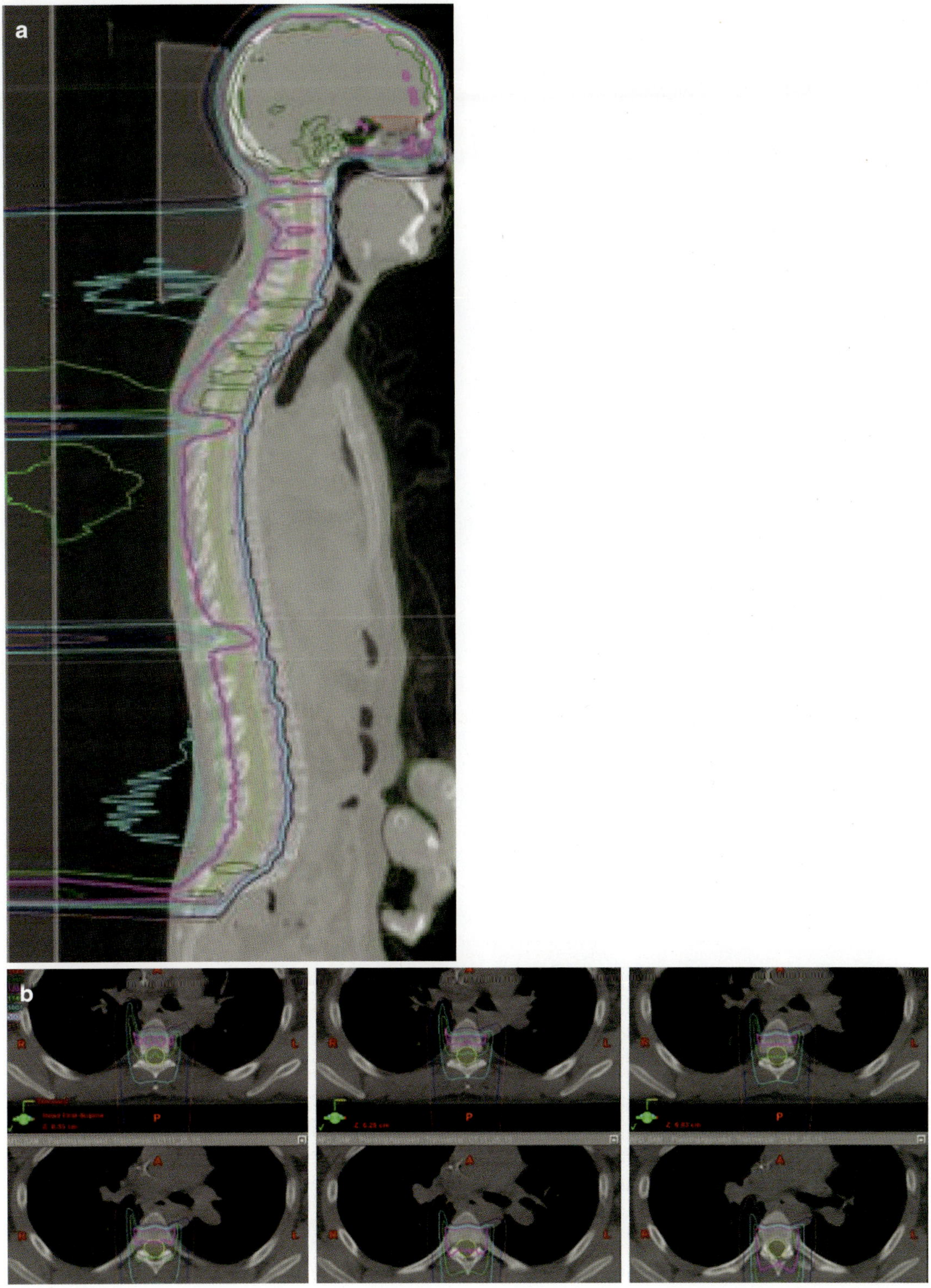

Fig. 7.12 (**a**) Proton, edge of the beam is mid-vertebral body to avoid the high RBE at the distal beam edge from falling into the cord. (**b**) Cross-sectional view of the proton isodose lines, sparing some of the vertebral bodies, and overshooting where the tissue density is lower (lung)

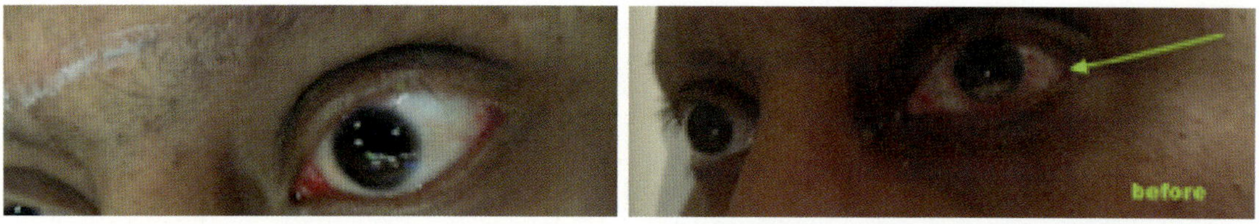

Fig. 7.13 The patient regained full vision in his left eye

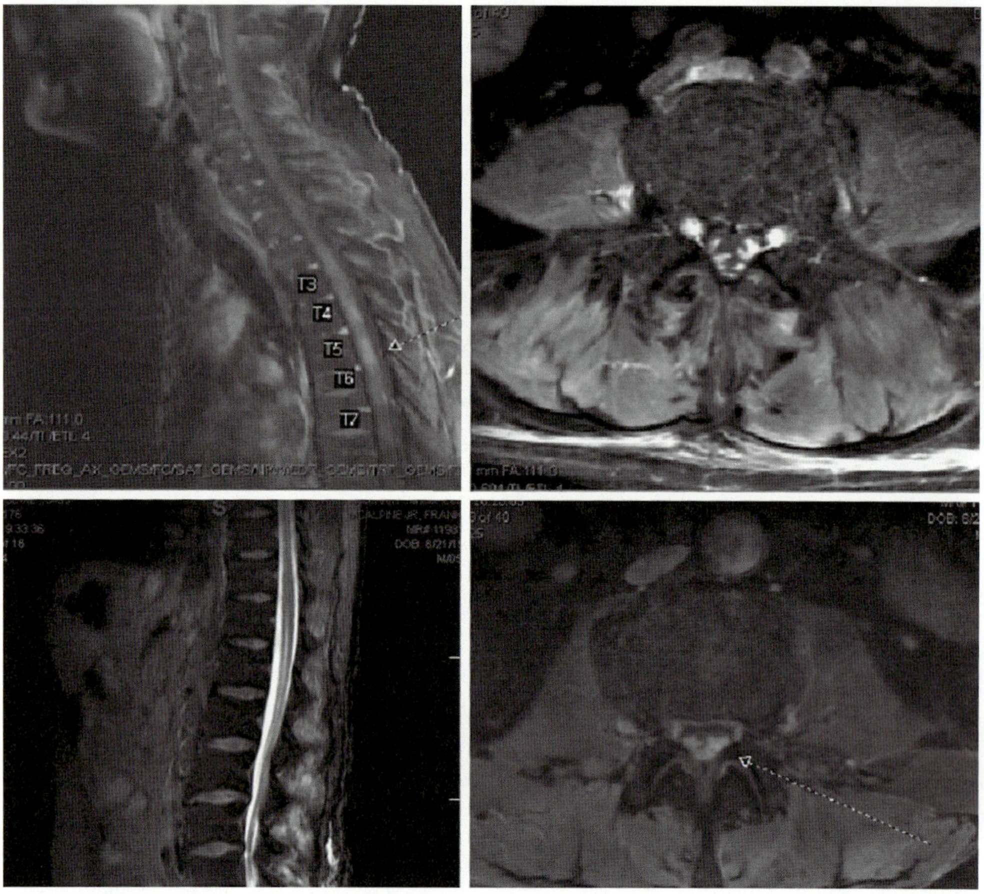

Fig. 7.14 Spine MRI showing leptomeningeal disease

leukemia. In the case presented here, the field extended anteriorly to flash the anterior chamber. However, it is acceptable in general to omit the anterior chamber because of the rarity of the occurrence of disease there [30]. In the case of cornea/iris involvement, it is believed that the risk increases with disease relapse, and it is thought to result from disruption of the epithelial cells secondary to chemotherapy [31].

The patient went on to receive his allogeneic transplant after minimal residual disease in his marrow was confirmed. He did well with no major side effects. At day 100 evaluation, he was found to have a molecular relapse, but his CSF continued to remain negative, and he regained full vision in his left eye (Fig. 7.13).

At that time he was started on blinatumomab, a monoclonal antibody and *a bispecific T-cell engager. At the last follow-up 7 months posttransplant, the patient is still in remission, by morphology, cytogenetics, and FISH analysis of the bone marrow. His last CSF study was also negative.*

Radiation oncologist often faced with the situation where the patient presents with spinal disease

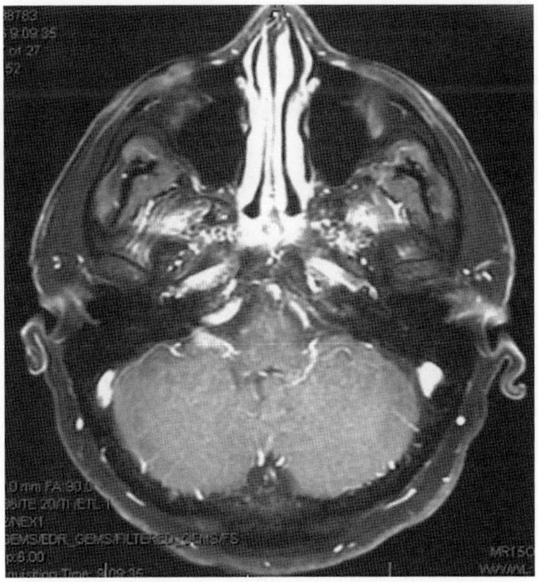

Fig. 7.15 Planning of case 3 using 3 D beams

but negative MRI. Often these patients are heavily treated including numerous intrathecal therapy, multiple systemic therapies, and or allogeneic transplant. In these cases it is advisable to give a comprehensive therapy based on the fact that the brain and spine are in a continuum as part of the CNS, and it is a matter of time before the brain will show disease too. Arguably the same logic applies to when the brain has disease while the spine is negative by imaging but with positive CSF.

Here I describe a 37-year-old man with ALL heavily pretreated who presented with lower extremity weakness and bowel incontinence to the emergency room. MRI of the spine (Fig. 7.14) *showed thick leptomeningeal disease coating the thoracolumbar spine as well as the sacrum, CSF packed with blasts. Although the radiation oncologist recommended to treat comprehensively the brain and spine, the medical oncology team decided against it. The patient was initiated on spinal irradiation omitting the brain and upper cervical spine. The patient improved, and he was able to walk 2 weeks after initiation of therapy. Unfortunately 5 weeks later, he presented with facial palsy, decreased hearing, and frank involvement of the cranial nerves* (Fig. 7.15). *The patient had to be treated with brain radiation including the cervical spine, which was challenging to match with the previous field.*

Finally, the radiation oncologist has to be alert that sometimes chemotherapy or intrathecal chemotherapy toxicity can present with similar symptoms and signs to leukemia involvement. In this case CSF fails to show blasts, brain MRI is negative, and spine MRI T2-weighted images show abnormality in the dorsal columns of the spinal cord. In a recently published data from MD Anderson, seven patients were described to have this devastating myelopathy associated with intrathecal chemotherapy and described to be idiosyncratic side effects [32].

Treatment of Chloroma and Role of Radiation

A 59-year-man presented with easy bruisability, fatigue, and recurrent infection. His white blood cell count was 1500 per microliter, and platelet count was 25,000 per microliter at presentation. Bone marrow biopsy showed 80 % blasts leading to the diagnosis of acute myeloid leukemia (AML). Cytogenetic studies showed a complex karyotype, FLT3 positive. He was started on 3 + 7 regimen at an outside hospital. His day 28 bone marrow showed persistent disease. He was transferred to our institution where he was initiated on high-dose Ara-C and mitoxantrone. A repeat bone marrow biopsy showed residual 18 % blasts. He then was started on decitabine. In the meantime, he developed pain in the sinus area and a headache. An MRI of the brain (Fig. 7.16) *showed an extensive lesion in the nasoethmoid region, extending to the right orbit, nasal cavity through the cribriform plate, and into the subfrontal epidural space. His CSF was positive for blasts suggesting CNS disease although no other lesions were seen on the MRI of the brain or spine.*

Because of the urgent symptoms, the patient was started on radiation. The dose planned was 20 Gy in 10 fractions. The question at that time was whether to address only the area in the nasoethmoid region or to think ahead that he might eventually achieve a remission and will need whole brain irradiation or CSI prior to an allotransplant. The case was discussed with the referring physicians, and it was decided to treat the area causing the problem but include the eyes to make it easier to match to a future whole

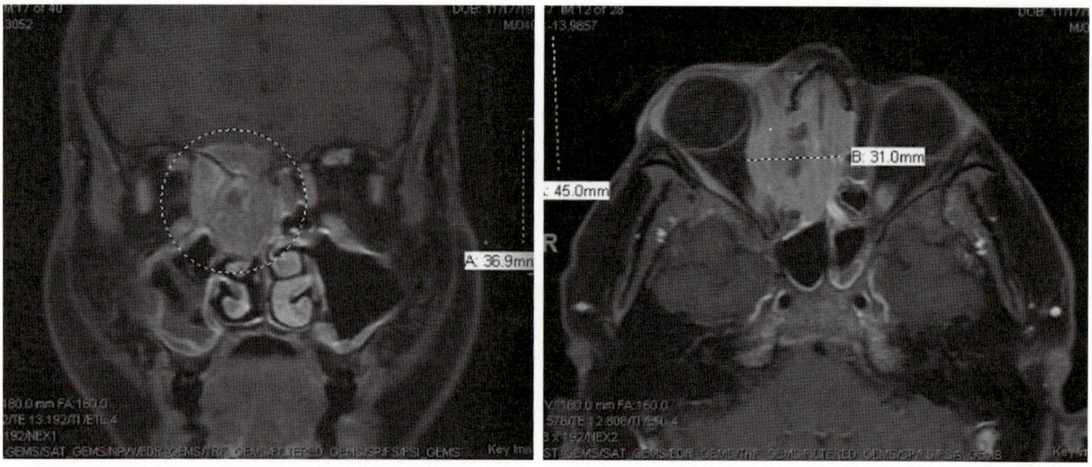

Fig. 7.16 MRI of the brain showing an extensive lesion in the nasoethmoid region, extending to the right orbit, nasal cavity through the cribriform plate, and into the subfrontal epidural space

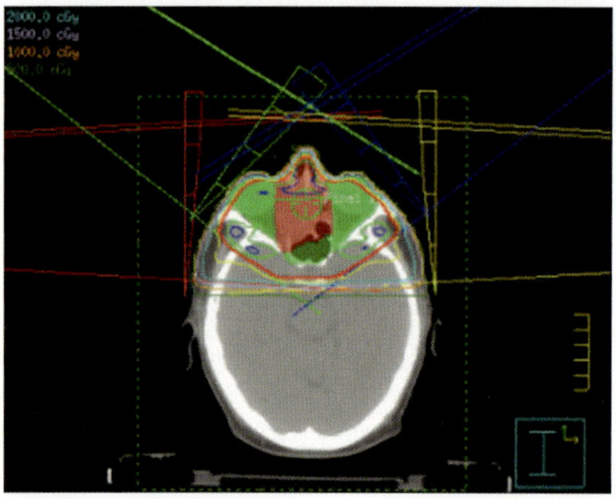

Fig. 7.17 Planning of case 3 using 3 D beams

brain field (Fig. 7.17). *The patient's symptoms improved quickly after only 6 Gy. After completion of the radiation therapy, he went on to receive further systemic therapy in an attempt to put him in remission in preparation for an allogeneic transplant. As for his CSF disease, it was managed with intrathecal chemotherapy.*

Chloroma (known in the past as granulocytic sarcoma) occurs mostly in the setting of AML but can also occur with CML. The use of radiation has been very effective in taking care of the disease even with doses that are as low as 20 Gy. Memorial Sloan Kettering published a retrospective [33] review of 38 patients treated for chloroma, showing that radiation therapy provided excellent local control (97 %) and symptom relief in 95 % of cases. Median dose ranged from 6 to 36 Gy. The fact that the local control was 97 % suggests that lower doses of radiation are as effective and should be used.

Conclusions

Radiation therapy still plays a role in the treatment of leukemias. The key is to understand that leukemias are very sensitive to radiation, to doses as low as 20 Gy. Since it is a systemic disease that can be managed effectively with chemotherapy, radiation fields have to be limited to the area at risk for local relapse (like in the case of LBL) or in treating chloromas. Radiation also can serve an important role in addressing the CNS disease by overcoming the blood-brain barrier and effectively eradicating disease in the CNS. Radiation therapy can therefore potentially contribute to improve the outcome of many patients, especially those who fall short of complete remission due to CNS involvement.

References

1. Soslow RA, Baergen RN, Warnke RA. B-lineage lymphoblastic lymphoma is a clinicopathologic entity distinct from other histologically similar aggressive lymphomas with blastic morphology. Cancer. 1999;85(12):2648–54.

2. Campo E, Swerdlow SH, Harris NL, Pileri S, Stein H, Jaffe ES. The 2008 WHO classification of lymphoid neoplasms and beyond: evolving concepts and practical applications. Blood. 2011;117(19):5019–32.
3. Kobayashi R, Takimoto T, Nakazawa A, Fujita N, Akazai A, Yamato K, et al. Inferior outcomes of stage III T lymphoblastic lymphoma relative to stage IV lymphoma and T-acute lymphoblastic leukemia: long-term comparison of outcomes in the JACLS NHL T-98 and ALL T-97 protocols. Int J Hematol. 2014;99(6):743–9.
4. Jain N, Lamb AV, O'Brien S, Ravandi F, Konopleva M, Jabbour E, et al. Early T-cell precursor acute lymphoblastic leukemia/lymphoma (ETP-ALL/LBL) in adolescents and adults: a high-risk subtype. Blood. 2016;127(15):1863–9.
5. Reiter A, Schrappe M, Ludwig WD, Tiemann M, Parwaresch R, Zimmermann M, et al. Intensive ALL-type therapy without local radiotherapy provides a 90% event-free survival for children with T-cell lymphoblastic lymphoma: a BFM group report. Blood. 2000;95(2):416–21.
6. Kantarjian HM, O'Brien S, Smith TL, Cortes J, Giles FJ, Beran M, et al. Results of treatment with hyper-CVAD, a dose-intensive regimen, in adult acute lymphocytic leukemia. J Clin Oncol Off J Am Soc Clin Oncol. 2000;18(3):547–61.
7. Le Gouill S, Lepretre S, Briere J, Morel P, Bouabdallah R, Raffoux E, et al. Adult lymphoblastic lymphoma: a retrospective analysis of 92 patients under 61 years included in the LNH87/93 trials. Leukemia. 2003;17(11):2220–4.
8. Dabaja BS, Rebueno NC, Mazloom A, Thorne S, Perrin KJ, Tolani N, et al. Radiation for Hodgkin's lymphoma in young female patients: a new technique to avoid the breasts and decrease the dose to the heart. Int J Radiat Oncol Biol Phys. 2011;79(2):503–7.
9. Voong KR, McSpadden K, Pinnix CC, Shihadeh F, Reed V, Salehpour MR, et al. Dosimetric advantages of a "butterfly" technique for intensity-modulated radiation therapy for young female patients with mediastinal Hodgkin's lymphoma. Radiat Oncol. 2014;9:94.
10. Specht L, Dabaja BS, Illidge T, Wilson LD, Hoppe RT, International Lymphoma Radiation Oncology G. Modern radiation therapy for primary cutaneous lymphomas: field and dose guidelines from the International Lymphoma Radiation Oncology Group. Int J Radiat Oncol Biol Phys. 2015;92(1):32–9.
11. Hoelzer D, Gokbuget N, Digel W, Faak T, Kneba M, Reutzel R, et al. Outcome of adult patients with T-lymphoblastic lymphoma treated according to protocols for acute lymphoblastic leukemia. Blood. 2002;99(12):4379–85.
12. Hunault M, Truchan-Graczyk M, Caillot D, Harousseau JL, Bologna S, Himberlin C, et al. Outcome of adult T-lymphoblastic lymphoma after acute lymphoblastic leukemia-type treatment: a GOELAMS trial. Haematologica. 2007;92(12):1623–30.
13. Thomas DA, O'Brien S, Cortes J, Giles FJ, Faderl S, Verstovsek S, et al. Outcome with the hyper-CVAD regimens in lymphoblastic lymphoma. Blood. 2004;104(6):1624–30.
14. Dabaja BS, Ha CS, Thomas DA, Wilder RB, Gopal R, Cortes J, et al. The role of local radiation therapy for mediastinal disease in adults with T-cell lymphoblastic lymphoma. Cancer. 2002;94(10):2738–44.
15. Abstract selected for presentation in an ePoster Discussion session at ASTRO's 2016 Annual Meeting. 25–28 Sept. Boston, MA.
16. Pinnix CC, Smith GL, Milgrom S, Osborne EM, Reddy JP, Akhtari M, et al. Predictors of radiation pneumonitis in patients receiving intensity modulated radiation therapy for Hodgkin and non-Hodgkin lymphoma. Int J Radiat Oncol Biol Phys. 2015;92(1):175–82.
17. Byrd JC, Ruppert AS, Mrozek K, Carroll AJ, Edwards CG, Arthur DC, et al. Repetitive cycles of high-dose cytarabine benefit patients with acute myeloid leukemia and inv(16)(p13q22) or t(16;16)(p13;q22): results from CALGB 8461. J Clin Oncol Off J Am Soc Clin Oncol. 2004;22(6):1087–94.
18. Druker BJ, Guilhot F, O'Brien SG, Gathmann I, Kantarjian H, Gattermann N, et al. Five-year follow-up of patients receiving imatinib for chronic myeloid leukemia. N Engl J Med. 2006;355(23):2408–17.
19. Ottmann OG, Hoelzer D. The ABL tyrosine kinase inhibitor STI571 (Glivec) in Philadelphia positive acute lymphoblastic leukemia – promises, pitfalls and possibilities. Hematol J Off J Eur Haematol Assoc/EHA. 2002;3(1):2–6.
20. Ottmann OG, Wassmann B, Hoelzer D. Therapy of Philadelphia chromosome positive acute lymphatic leukemia (Ph + ALL) with an inhibitor of abl-tyrosine kinase (Glivec). Med Klin. 2002;97 Suppl 1:16–21.
21. Schrappe M, Reiter A, Ludwig WD, Harbott J, Zimmermann M, Hiddemann W, et al. Improved outcome in childhood acute lymphoblastic leukemia despite reduced use of anthracyclines and cranial radiotherapy: results of trial ALL-BFM 90. German-Austrian-Swiss ALL-BFM Study Group. Blood. 2000;95(11):3310–22.
22. Daver N, Cortes J, Ravandi F, Patel KP, Burger JA, Konopleva M, et al. Secondary mutations as mediators of resistance to targeted therapy in leukemia. Blood. 2015;125(21):3236–45.
23. Gustafsson G, Schmiegelow K, Forestier E, Clausen N, Glomstein A, Jonmundsson G, et al. Improving outcome through two decades in childhood ALL in the Nordic countries: the impact of high-dose methotrexate in the reduction of CNS irradiation. Nordic Society of Pediatric Haematology and Oncology (NOPHO). Leukemia. 2000;14(12):2267–75.
24. Shihadeh F, Reed V, Faderl S, Medeiros LJ, Mazloom A, Hadziahmetovic M, et al. Cytogenetic profile of patients with acute myeloid leukemia and central nervous system disease. Cancer. 2012;118(1):112–7.

25. Kantarjian HM, Thomas D, Ravandi F, Faderl S, Jabbour E, Garcia-Manero G, et al. Defining the course and prognosis of adults with acute lymphocytic leukemia in first salvage after induction failure or short first remission duration. Cancer. 2010;116(24):5568–74.
26. Pui CH, Howard SC. Current management and challenges of malignant disease in the CNS in paediatric leukaemia. Lancet Oncol. 2008;9(3):257–68.
27. Walker GV, Shihadeh F, Kantarjian H, Allen P, Rondon G, Kebriaei P, et al. Comprehensive craniospinal radiation for controlling central nervous system leukemia. Int J Radiat Oncol Biol Phys. 2014;90(5):1119–25.
28. Chaudhary P, Marshall TI, Perozziello FM, Manti L, Currell FJ, Hanton F, et al. Relative biological effectiveness variation along monoenergetic and modulated Bragg peaks of a 62-MeV therapeutic proton beam: a preclinical assessment. Int J Radiat Oncol Biol Phys. 2014;90(1):27–35.
29. Paganetti H. Relating proton treatments to photon treatments via the relative biological effectiveness-should we revise current clinical practice? Int J Radiat Oncol Biol Phys. 2015;91(5):892–4.
30. Allen RA, Straatsma BR. Ocular involvement in leukemia and allied disorders. Arch Ophthalmol. 1961;66:490–508.
31. Bhadresa GN. Changes in the anterior segment as a presenting feature in leukaemia. Br J Ophthalmol. 1971;55(2):133–5.
32. Cachia D, Kamiya-Matsuoka C, Pinnix CC, Chi L, Kantarjian HM, Cortes JE, et al. Myelopathy following intrathecal chemotherapy in adults: a single institution experience. J Neurooncol. 2015;122(2):391–8.
33. Bakst R, Wolden S, Yahalom J. Radiation therapy for chloroma (granulocytic sarcoma). Int J Radiat Oncol Biol Phys. 2012;82(5):1816–22.

Primary CNS Lymphoma

8

Chelsea Pinnix

Abstract

Primary central nervous system lymphoma (PCNSL) is an uncommon extranodal form of non-Hodgkin lymphoma affecting the brain, leptomeninges, eyes, or the spinal cord, in the absence of systemic involvement. The predominant risk factor for disease development is immunodeficiency. PCNSL is an acquired immune deficiency syndrome (AIDS) defining malignancy; however, the incidence in this patient population is decreasing due to advancements in antiretroviral treatment. On the other hand, among immunocompetent individuals, the incidence of PCNSL has increased over the past few decades, representing 3–4% of all primary brain tumors (Eby et al. Cancer 62(11):2461–2465, 1988). The explanation for the growing incidence is not clear. PCNSL has a predilection for the elderly population with a median age of diagnosis of 55 years and peak incidence in the sixth and seventh decades of life (Hochberg and Miller, J Neurosurg 68(6):835–853, 1988; Fine and Mayer, Ann Intern Med 119(11):1093–1104, 1993).

The cornerstone of therapy is a systemic treatment with intravenous high-dose methotrexate (Mtx). There is an ongoing controversy regarding the role of consolidative therapies, including radiation therapy (RT) and autologous stem cell transplantation (ASCT). In this review, we will explore diagnostic considerations, prognosis, as well as primary and salvage therapy for PCNSL. We will highlight the data supporting various therapeutic strategies, with an emphasis on the role of RT in this rare hematologic malignancy.

Introduction

Primary central nervous system lymphoma (PCNSL) is an uncommon extranodal form of non-Hodgkin lymphoma affecting the brain, leptomeninges, eyes, or the spinal cord, in the

C. Pinnix, MD, PhD
Department of Radiation Oncology,
MD Anderson Cancer Center,
1515 Holcombe Blvd, Unit #97,
Houston, TX 77030, USA
e-mail: ccpinnix@mdanderson.org

B.S. Dabaja, A.K. Ng (eds.), *Radiation Therapy in Hematologic Malignancies*,
DOI 10.1007/978-3-319-42615-0_8

absence of systemic involvement. The predominant risk factor for disease development is immunodeficiency. PCNSL is an acquired immune deficiency syndrome (AIDS) defining malignancy; however, the incidence in this patient population is decreasing due to advancements in antiretroviral treatment. On the other hand, among immunocompetent individuals, the incidence of PCNSL has increased over the past few decades, representing 3–4 % of all primary brain tumors [1]. The explanation for the growing incidence is not clear. PCNSL has a predilection for the elderly population with a median age of diagnosis of 55 years and peak incidence in the sixth and seventh decades of life [2, 3].

The cornerstone of therapy is a systemic treatment with intravenous high-dose methotrexate (Mtx). There is an ongoing controversy regarding the role of consolidative therapies, including radiation therapy (RT) and autologous stem cell transplantation (ASCT). In this review, we will explore diagnostic considerations, prognosis, as well as primary and salvage therapy for PCNSL. We will highlight the data supporting various therapeutic strategies, with an emphasis on the role of RT in this rare hematologic malignancy.

Case 1

A 71-year-old woman presented with a 3-week history of worsening memory deficits. Computed tomography (CT) imaging of the head without contrast revealed a large hyperdense mass within the left frontal lobe with vasogenic edema and mass effect on the left lateral ventricle (Fig. 8.1a). *Follow-up magnetic resonance imaging (MRI) confirmed the presence of a large heterogeneous enhancing mass measuring 5.1 × 3.4 × 2.6 cm in the left frontal lobe* (Fig. 8.1b). *There were small satellite lesions present as well as a second enhancing lesion within the right ventricle. There was surrounding T2-fluid-attenuated inversion recovery (FLAIR) hyperintense signal in the white matter of the frontal lobe* (Fig. 8.1c). *Stereotactic biopsy revealed CD20-positive (CD20+) diffuse large B-cell lymphoma (DLBCL) with high-grade features and an activated B-cell (ABC)-like immunophenotype. The Ki-67 was 90–95 %. Fluorescent in situ hybridization (FISH) studies for BCL-2 and Myc gene rearrangements were negative. Positron emission tomography (PET)-CT imaging was negative for extracranial disease. Bone marrow biopsy was negative for lymphoma involvement. Ophthalmologic evaluation did not reveal evidence of ocular disease.*

Clinical Presentation

Patients with PCNSL often have presenting symptoms that reflect the periventricular location of the lymphoma. In a retrospective review of 248 cases of intracerebral PCNSL, 70 % of patients presented with a focal neurologic deficit, 43 % had neuropsychiatric symptoms, and 33 % had signs of increased intracranial pressure [4]. Given that most tumors are located deep in the white matter, seizures are not as common as in other cases of primary brain neoplasms, with only 14 % of patients presenting with seizures in this series.

The eye, specifically the vitreous and/or the retina, is a common site of initial disease and a potential location for relapse in PCNSL. Roughly 20–25 % of patients with PCNSL will have ocular involvement at diagnosis [5]. Primary intraocular lymphoma (PIOL) affects the vitreous or retina in the absence of the brain, leptomeninges, spinal cord, or systemic disease. For patients with PIOL, brain relapse is the rule, as 50–80 % of patients will have cerebral lymphomatous involvement, often within 2 years of PIOL diagnosis [6]. Patients often present with floaters, blurry vision, or painless decrease in visual acuity [7, 8]. Bilateral ocular involvement is common [5].

Histopathology

Greater than 95 % of PCNSL tumors are CD20+ DLBCL; however other histologic lymphoma variants can affect the CNS, including T-cell lymphoma, Burkitt's lymphoma, and indolent B-cell lymphomas (most notably marginal zone lymphoma of mucosa-associated lymphoid tissue, MALT) [9–11]. Indeed,

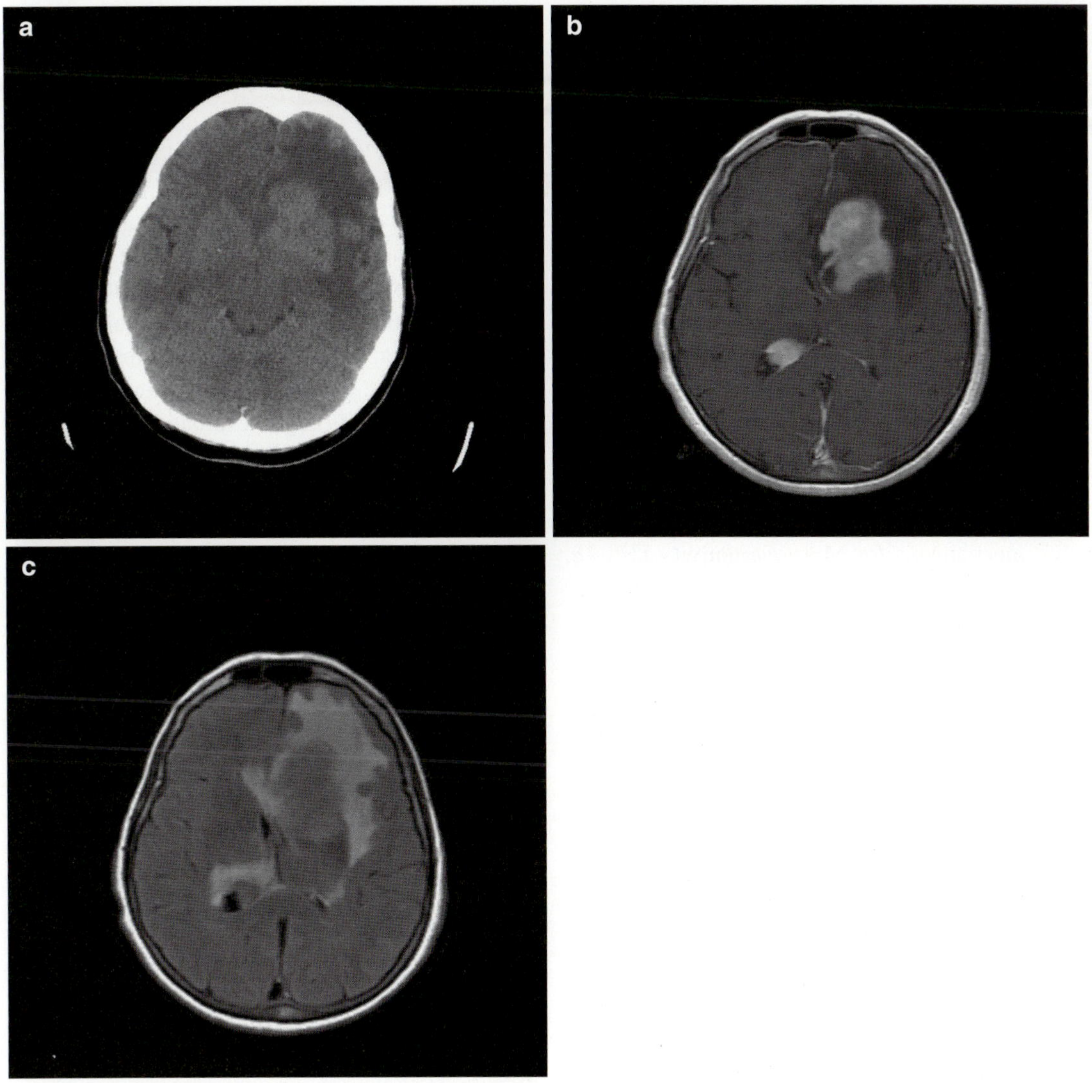

Fig. 8.1 Brain imaging in a 71-year-old woman with PCNSL. (**a**) Axial CT without contrast reveals a dominant mass in the left frontal lobe. (**b**) Axial T1 post-contrast image demonstrates the heterogeneously enhancing large left frontal mass as well as an enhancing lesion in the right ventricle. (**c**) Corresponding T2-FLAIR axial image illustrating vasogenic edema with mass effect on the left lateral ventricle

according to the *WHO Classification of Tumours of Haematopoietic and Lymphoid Tissue*, the term PCNSL refers only to DLBCL affecting the CNS in immunocompetent patients with exclusion of other histologies [12].

The DLBCL cells in PCNSL express typical B-cell markers, including CD19, CD20, and CD79a. MUM1 expression is present in greater than 90 % of cases, and BCL6 expression is also common [13]. In nodal DLBCL, gene expression profiling has identified two distinct cell of origin (COO) phenotypes, the "activated B-cell" (ABC) and "germinal center B-cell" (GCB) types that are predictive of disease aggression and outcome [14, 15]. The immunohistochemical Hans classifier, based on CD10, BCL6, and MUM1 expression, is routinely used as gene expression profiling surrogates to distinguish the two subgroups in the setting of systemic DLBCL [16]. While recent data does suggest a predominance of the non-GCB phenotype among PCNSL cells, this classification is of limited clinical utility, as no association of COO subtype with clinical outcome has been demonstrated among patients with PCNSL [17, 18].

Myc expression has also been evaluated in PCNSL tumor cells given the poor prognosis of PCNSL compared to systemic DLBCL. Myc rearrangements, as detected by fluorescent in situ hybridization (FISH), occur in roughly 10–15 % of DLBCLs and confer poor clinical outcome, especially when paired with rearrangements of the BCL-2 gene (i.e., “double-hit lymphomas”) [19, 20]. In PCNSL, despite the low frequency of Myc rearrangements (3–9 %), Myc protein overexpression is common (73–92 %) suggesting other mechanisms for Myc overactivity [17, 18, 21]. However, in the limited data available, Myc overexpression did not correlate with adverse clinical outcome. Taken together, this suggests that prognostic markers used in nodal DLBCL are of limited utility in PCNSL. This is likely due to differences in disease biology.

Diagnosis and Work-Up

When there is suspicion for PCNSL, the initial radiographic study of choice is a contrast-enhanced cranial MRI. Despite the absence of a pathognomonic MRI characteristic, there are several radiographic findings suggestive of PCNSL [22]. Lesions are typically solitary (in 2/3 of cases) involving the supratentorial brain with ventricular or meningeal surface contact. Edema is prominent; however it is less than observed in malignant gliomas or metastatic lesions. Given the hypercellularity and high nuclear to cytoplasmic ratio of PCNSL tumor cells, the predominant mass is usually isointense on T1 and T2 sequences and exhibits restricted diffusion on diffusion-weighted imaging. Diffuse and homogeneous contrast enhancement is the rule. In cases of immunosuppressed patients with PCNSL, ring enhancement is frequent. Necrosis, hemorrhage, and calcifications are rare.

Stereotactic-guided biopsy is the method of choice for obtaining tissue for definitive diagnosis. If possible, it is highly recommended that glucocorticoid administration be avoided prior to biopsy, as there is a potential for dramatic steroid-induced tumor regression that will result in a nondiagnostic biopsy [23]. In the absence of a contraindication to lumbar puncture, a cerebrospinal fluid (CSF) sample should be obtained. CSF studies include cytology, flow cytometric analysis, cell count, and protein and glucose levels. Concurrent systemic involvement should be excluded with bone marrow biopsy and positron emission tomography-computed tomography (PET-CT) imaging with or without contrasted CT imaging of the chest, abdomen, and pelvis. A detailed ophthalmologic evaluation with a slit lamp examination should be performed to screen for intraocular involvement that often manifests as a cellular infiltration of the vitreous and subretinal tumor cell deposits. Serum studies including HIV, blood urea nitrogen (BUN), creatinine, lactate dehydrogenase (LDH), and hepatitis B and C serologies are also part of baseline work-up evaluation. Ultrasound of the testis should be considered in elderly men who present with DLBCL involving the CNS.

Case 1

The patient initiated a systemic therapy with rituximab, methotrexate, procarbazine, and vincristine (R-MPV). Restaging MRI after 2 cycles of therapy demonstrated improvement (Fig. 8.2a). *She completed a total of five cycles of therapy. Repeat MRI revealed a complete regression of the known lymphoma involvement within the left frontal lobe and right ventricle* (Fig. 8.2b). *She was then referred for consolidative low-dose whole brain radiation therapy (WBRT).*

Treatment

Surgery

It has been widely accepted that aggressive surgical resection has little role in the management of PCNSL given a potential increased risk of permanent neurologic deficit coupled with no evidence of improvement in overall survival [4, 24]. However, this standard has been recently challenged by a retrospective analysis of a large phase

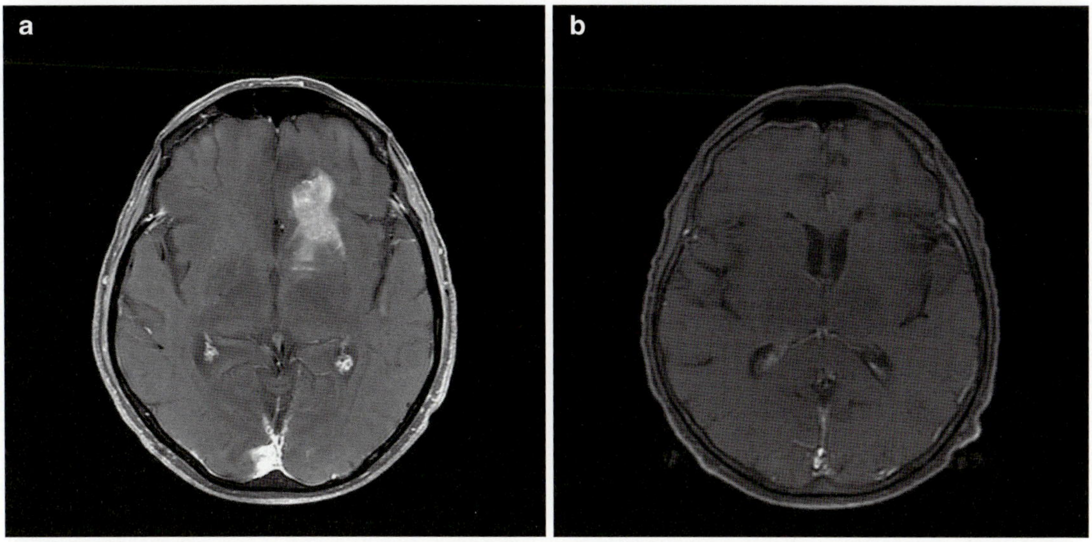

Fig. 8.2 MRI after methotrexate-based chemotherapy. T1 post-contrast axial image demonstrates a partial response after 2 cycles of R-MPV (rituximab, methotrexate, procarbazine, and vincristine) (**a**) and a complete response after 5 cycles (**b**)

III randomized trial, the German PCNSL Study Group-1 (GPSG-1) trial. In this analysis of several hundred patients, compete resection was associated with an increase in progression-free survival (PFS) [25]. In light of this observation, many centers will consider a complete surgical resection of well-circumscribed single lesions in non-eloquent areas. Otherwise, stereotactic-guided biopsy should be considered standard of care, given the lower risk of postoperative morbidity.

Radiation Therapy Alone

Historically RT has been the cornerstone of therapy for PCNSL, a highly radiosensitive tumor. Responses to whole brain RT (WBRT) are rapid and robust with an overall response rate (ORR) of greater than 90 %. Unfortunately however these responses are short lived. The Radiation Therapy Oncology Group (RTOG) conducted a phase II prospective trial between 1983 and 1987 of WBRT alone for patients with PCNSL (RTOG 83–15) [26]. Forty-one patients were enrolled and received RT to the whole brain to a dose of 40 Gy followed by a 20 Gy boost to gross disease. The results were disappointing with a median overall survival (OS) of only 11.6 months. The dominant pattern of failure was local, with 61 % failure rate within the radiated brain field in contrast to 7 % distant failure rate. One- and two-year OS rates were 48 % and 28 %, respectively. Of the 25 documented local recurrences, 22 (88 %) were within the 60 Gy region. Given the inability to further dose escalate without excessive severe toxicity such as brain necrosis, these data highlighted the need for therapy beyond RT alone to improve outcomes among patients with newly diagnosed PCNSL.

Combined Modality Therapy

Given the disappointing results of the RTOG 83–15 trial, subsequent studies focused on the potential of combined modality therapy (CMT) to improve outcomes. In RTOG 88–06, cyclophosphamide, doxorubicin, vincristine, and dexamethasone (CHOD) were administered prior to 41.4 Gy in 1.8 Gy fractions to the whole brain followed by a boost of 18 Gy, for a cumulative tumor bed boost of 59.4 Gy [27]. Unfortunately results from this prospective study were on par with outcomes obtained with RT alone. The median OS was 16.1 months with a 2-year OS rate of 42 %. It is hypothesized that the ineffectiveness of CHOP like regimens relates to the poor penetration of these agents across the blood-brain barrier (BBB).

The dilemma of inadequate BBB penetration of systemically administered chemotherapeutic agents has been addressed with the implementation of high-dose Mtx-based regimens. Rapid infusion of greater than 3 g/m^2 Mtx intravenously (IV) results in consistent CSF concentrations that have antitumor activity in the CNS [28, 29]. Leucovorin must be administered to prevent bone marrow and end organ damage (especially kidneys), while lymphoma cells in the CNS are offered little rescue given the poor BBB penetration of leucovorin. In one of the first studies to evaluate high-dose Mtx-based regimens in patients with PCNSL, DeAngelis and colleagues at the Memorial Sloan Kettering Cancer Center (MSKCC) evaluated pre-RT IV and intra-Ommaya Mtx followed by cranial RT (40 Gy to the whole brain followed by 14.4 Gy boost) and consolidative high-dose Ara-C among 31 patients with PCNSL [30]. In a nonrandomized fashion, outcomes were compared with 16 patients treated with RT alone. Median OS was improved among patients treated with combined modality therapy (42.5 months) versus RT alone (21.7 months). The median time to recurrence was also improved (41 months versus 10 months). These improvements in OS were reproducible in other studies, with a median OS of 32–36 months reported when patients were treated with combined modality therapy [31–33].

The improvement in clinical outcome with Mtx-based CMT did not come without a cost. With longer follow-up, profound neurotoxicity was appreciated, with patients older than 60 being at the highest risk. In long-term follow-up of the 31 patients treated with CMT at MSKCC, delayed neurotoxicity was reported in 10 patients (32 %) [34]. At 48-month follow-up, 100 % of patients 60 years or older developed neurotoxicity compared with 35 % of patients less than 60. For patients greater than 60 years of age, symptoms began at a median of 13.2 months (range 6–52 months) and consisted of dementia, urinary incontinence, and gait ataxia often requiring custodial care. The neurotoxicity was fatal in three patients. MRI findings consisted of atrophy and diffuse white matter changes in the absence of disease recurrence. Given the high incidence of long-term neurotoxicity after Mtx and high-dose whole brain RT (40 Gy with 14.4 Gy boost), the focus of subsequent studies shifted to the omission or delay of WBRT.

Omission of WBRT

In the largest randomized trial conducted in PCNSL, the G-PCNSL-SG-1 trial sought to evaluate whether high-dose Mtx-based chemotherapy alone was not inferior to the same chemotherapy regimen followed by whole brain RT to 45 Gy in 30 fractions of 1.5 Gy daily without a boost. 551 patients were enrolled at 74 German centers, but only 318 patients were treated according to protocol. Among these 318 patients, the median OS was 32.4 months among patients that received WBRT, and 37.1 months in patients treated with chemotherapy alone ($p=0.71$). Median progression-free survival (PFS) was improved among patients treated with WBRT but was not statistically significant (18.3 months versus 11.9 months, $p=0.14$). Treatment-related neurotoxicity was lower among patients who had RT omitted (49 % versus 26 %). The authors concluded that the PFS benefit of WBRT must be weighed against the increased risk of neurotoxicity, given the lack of demonstrable OS benefit. Many in the medical oncology community regarded the results of the trial as a justification for permanent omission of WBRT as part of upfront therapy for patients with PCNSL. However this trial is fraught with many limitations that restrict the ability to make definitive conclusions regarding the role of consolidative WBRT. The trial was drastically underpowered (~60 %) to address the primary hypothesis, and therefore unplanned subset analyses were even further underpowered. Poor protocol adherence was common with major violations noted in 30 % of patients. For instance, 29 % of patients who did not achieve complete response (CR) in the no RT arm actually received WBRT, while 24 % of patients assigned to receive cranial RT did not receive it. Additional limitations of the trial included suboptimal chemotherapy use, the absence of quality assurance, and insufficient neurotoxicity evaluation. Finally only 58 % of the original cohort was included in the analysis which undoubtedly undermines the results of the study. It has also been suggested that the unbalanced effect from salvage therapy between the arms that favored the experimental no radiation cohort also undermines conclusions drawn from this trial [35].

Reduced Dose WBRT

In an effort to maintain the potential benefit of consolidative WBRT in improving PFS while limiting risk of long-term neurotoxicity, the group at MSCKK pioneered a reduced dose WBRT (rdWBRT) approach after high-dose Mtx-based polychemotherapy. In the multicenter phase II trial of 52 patients with median age of 60 years (range 30–79) patients were treated with 5–7 cycles of rituximab, Mtx (3.5 g/m^2), procarbazine, and vincristine (R-MPV) followed by rdWBRT to 23.4 Gy in 1.8 Gy fractions and 2 cycles of consolidative high-dose Ara-C if CR was achieved. 31 patients achieved CR and received rdWBRT after R-MPV. For this group of patients, the median PFS was 7.7 years, and the median OS was not reached at a median follow-up of 5.9 years. 2-year PFS was 77 % and 3-year OS was 87 %. Rigorous neurocognitive testing was a component of the trial, and no severe long-term neurotoxicity was demonstrated. Disease progression occurred in 35 % of patients treated with rdWBRT ($n = 11$); two patients developed ocular relapse and nine patients had parenchymal brain relapse. Given these impressive results with minimal neurotoxicity, the role of rdWBRT is being evaluated in a randomized fashion by the RTOG (RTOG 1114).

Autologous Stem Cell Transplant

Efforts to identify strategies to augment therapy in the absence of WBRT continue at many centers. Recently the interest in consolidative high-dose chemotherapy and autologous stem cell transplant (ASCT) has increased. Theoretically the high concentration of chemotherapy drugs given IV will allow for concentrations in the CSF adequate to provide cytotoxic effects. Initial studies using a common regimen in systemic DLBCL, BEAM (BCNU, etoposide, Ara-C, melphalan), have been disappointing with 3-year event-free survival (EFS) of 25 % and 3-year OS of 60 % [36]. When conditioning regimens containing agents known to penetrate the CNS are utilized (such as thiotepa), the outcomes improve. In a single publication reporting on the outcome of two prospective single arm studies that treated patients with Mtx-based chemotherapy followed by high-dose carmustine and thiotepa and ASCT with or without WBRT, the median OS was 104 months with 5-year OS of 70 %[37]. The group at MSKCC recently published their results with R-MPV followed by high-dose chemotherapy and ASCT with TBC (thiotepa, busulfan, and cyclophosphamide) [38]. Among 32 patients, 81 % proceeded to frontline ASCT. With a median follow-up of 45 months, median PFS and OS were not reached, and 2-year PFS and OS were 79 % and 81 %, respectively. To date there is no evidence of neurotoxicity although follow-up time is limited. WBRT was omitted among patients who received ASCT. The results of R-MPV followed by rdWBRT compare favorably with this trial; however it should be noted that in the ASCT study, there were three transplant-related deaths, while the rdWBRT phase II study was without mortality related to consolidative WBRT. Two ongoing randomized trials being conducted by the International Extranodal Lymphoma Study Group and ANOCEF/GOELAMS will provide key data regarding the clinical benefit and toxicity associated with consolidative WBRT versus ASCT after Mtx-based polychemotherapy. (NCT01011920 and NCT00863460).

Intensive Polychemotherapy Alone

Another approach being utilized in patients with newly diagnosed PCNSL is highly intensive polychemotherapy alone without consolidative ASCT or WBRT. In a CALGB multicenter study, Alliance 50202, 44 patients were treated with an aggressive induction regimen of rituximab, Mtx (8 g/m^2), and temozolomide (MT-R) for 4 cycles followed by consolidative etoposide and high-dose Ara-C (EA) for patients that achieved a CR [39]. At a median follow-up of 4.9 years, the

2-year PFS was 57 % and median OS was not reached. There was no reported neurotoxicity; however formal neurocognitive testing was not a component of the trial. This regimen of MT-R is now being evaluated in a subsequent randomized trial (CALGB 51101) comparing consolidative dose intensive EA to high-dose chemotherapy with carmustine and thiotepa followed by ASCT.

Salvage Therapy

Given the growing trend to omit cranial RT from the upfront management of PCNSL, RT is often used as salvage therapy in the setting of relapsed or refractory disease. In a retrospective study of salvage WBRT for recurrent or refractory PCNSL in 48 patients, the ORR was 79 % with 58 % patients achieving CR after WBRT to a median dose of 40 Gy (range 21.6–50.4 Gy) [40]. The 1-year OS after RT was 54 % with 16-month median OS. Treatment-related neurotoxicity occurred in 22 % of patients with those greater than age of 60 and a history of Mtx within 6 months of RT at the greatest risk. In another retrospective study of 27 patients given WBRT to a median dose of 36 Gy as salvage after Mtx failure, the ORR was 74 % (37 % CR) [41]. The median OS from the time of RT was 10.9 months. Neurotoxicity occurred in 15 % of patients and was associated with RT dose of greater than 36 Gy. Taken together these studies support a valid role for WBRT as salvage after Mtx failure with ORR of greater than 70 % and modest rates of late neurotoxicity. To date there are no salvage chemotherapy regimens that result in such high ORR rates.

Case 1

The patient was treated to the whole brain and the posterior aspect of the bilateral orbits via opposed lateral fields with 6-MV photons to a total dose of 23.4 Gy at 1.8 Gy per fraction (Fig. 8.3). *Step and shoot technique was used to reduce hot spots to less than 107 %. Upon completion of WBRT, she received 2 cycles of high-dose Ara-C according to the Memorial Sloan Kettering Cancer Center regimen. Eighteen months posttreatment, the patient is doing well without evidence of disease and no neurocognitive toxicity recorded on neurocognitive testing.*

Case 2

A 54-year-old male presented with weakness and numbness of his left arm followed by difficulty with ambulation. He went to his local emergency room where MRI revealed an intensely enhancing mass with restricted diffusion in the right posterior frontal lobe measuring 3.5 × 2.5 × 3.2 cm with diffuse edema and compression of the adjacent body of the right lateral ventricle (Fig. 8.4a–f). *He was administered steroids and scheduled for stereotactic biopsy. The biopsy was subsequently postponed due to significant regression of the lesion. Ultimately the lesion regrew, and biopsy revealed diffuse large B-cell lymphoma with a Ki-67 of 80–90 %. PET-CT revealed no evidence of disease outside of the brain. Ultrasound of the testicles was normal. Bone marrow biopsy was negative. Ophthalmologic examination was normal. After 5 cycles of R-MPV, he still had radiographic evidence of persistent enhancing tumor in the right frontal lobe. An additional 2 cycles were given and the tumor persisted. Radiation therapy was considered at that time, but ultimately he was referred for autologous stem cell transplantation out of concern for radiation toxicity. He underwent autologous transplant with BCNU, thiotepa, and rituximab. Unfortunately he had residual frontal lobe enhancement and surrounding T2 hyperintensity consistent with persistent disease. He was then referred for radiation therapy. He was treated to the whole brain to 23.4 Gy followed by a 16.2 Gy boost to the right frontal region with intensity-modulated radiation therapy (IMRT) for a cumulative dose of 39.6 Gy to the persistent disease* (Fig. 8.5). *Postradiation therapy MRI revealed resolution of the enhancement within the right frontal lobe.*

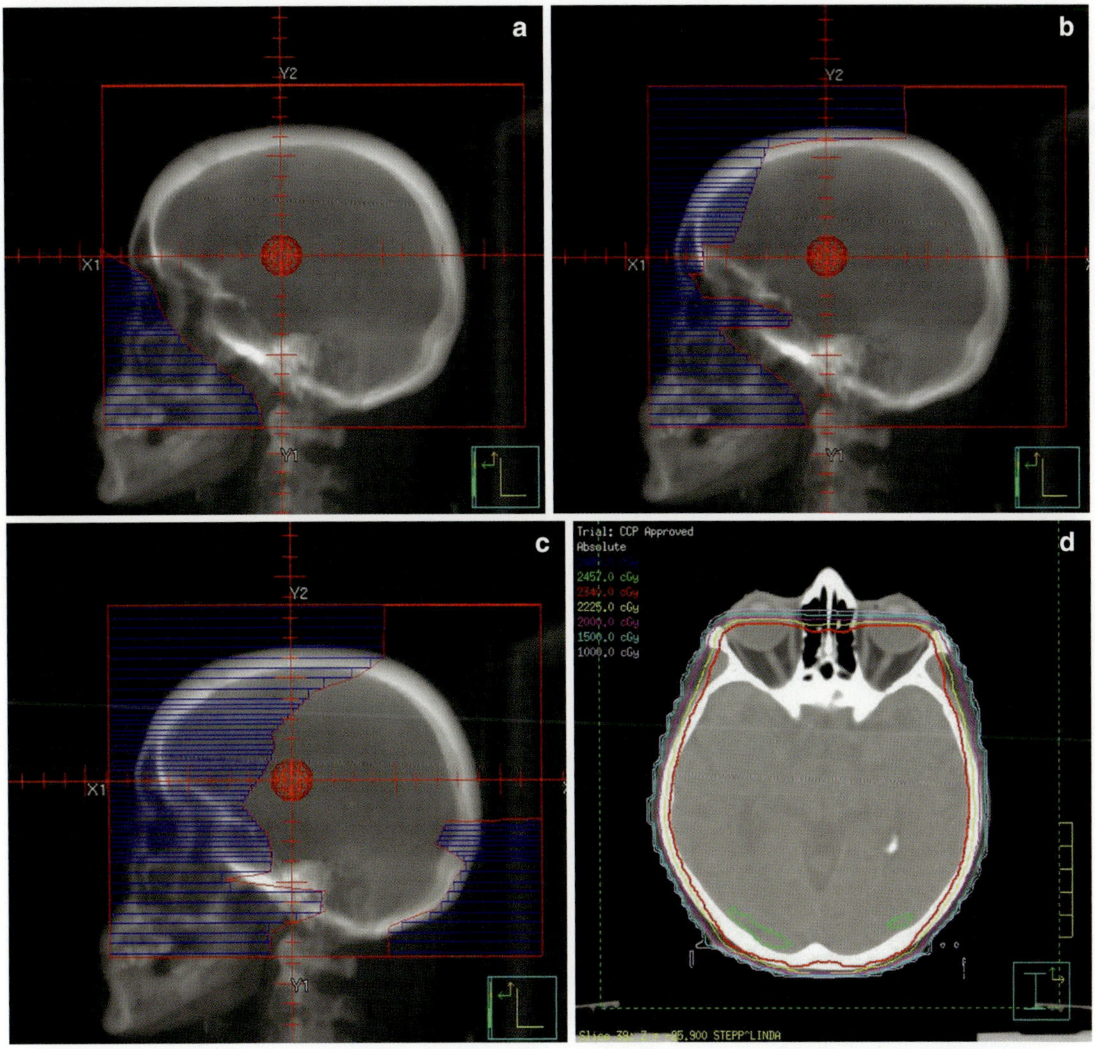

Fig. 8.3 Low-dose whole brain radiation therapy to 23.4 Gy in a patient with a complete radiographic response to 5 cycles of R-MPV. (**a**) Opposed lateral 6-MV photon fields targeting the whole brain and the posterior aspect of the bilateral orbits. (**b**, **c**) Step and shoot fields aimed at reducing hot spots to less than 107 %. (**d**) Axial CT image depicting isodose lines with prescription dose of 23.4 Gy

Radiation Technique

Radiation fields should target the whole brain with equally weighted opposed lateral photon beams with energy of 4–10 MV. CT-based planning is utilized to ensure adequate coverage of the frontal lobes at the cribriform plate and the posterior two-thirds of the globes bilaterally. The inferior border can be placed either at the bottom of C1 or C2. In patients with confirmed ocular involvement, the field should include the entire eye without lens sparing.

After a CR to upfront Mtx chemotherapy, we advocate rdWBRT to 23.4 Gy in 1.8 Gy fractions. MRI should be used to define disease response; however the clinician should recognize that small residual MRI abnormalities may not represent active gross disease and should not prohibit a patient from receiving rdWBRT [36]. For patients

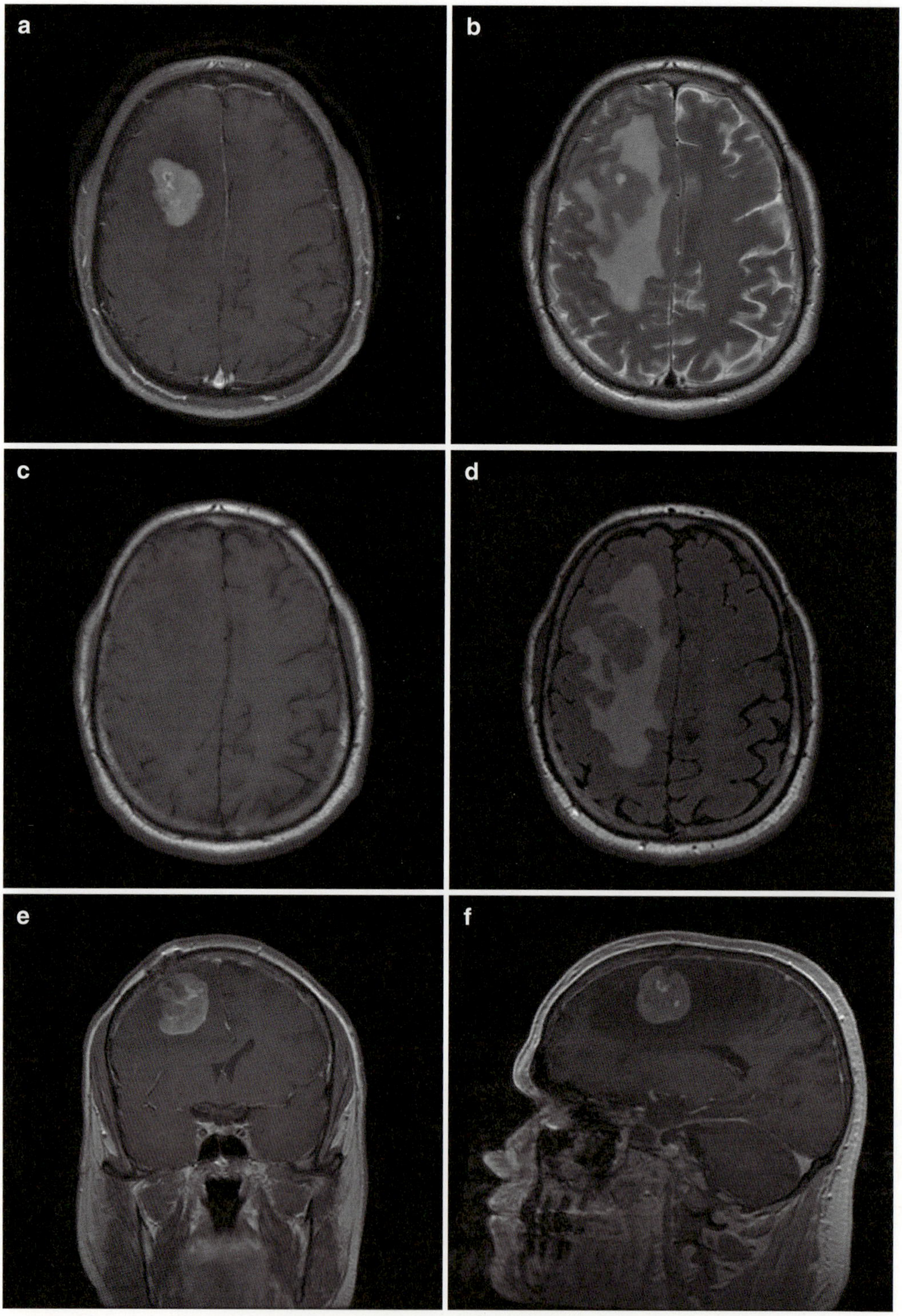

Fig. 8.4 MRI in a 55-year-old male patient with PCNSL. (**a**) T1 post-contrast axial image demonstrates an intensely enhancing tumor in the right posterior frontal lobe high convexity region. (**b**) T2-FLAIR axial image showing extensive edema. (**c**) T1-weighted axial image reveals the frontal mass is isointense relative to gray matter. (**d**) T2-weighted image demonstrates the frontal lobe mass that is isointense to mildly hypointense with surrounding edema. (**e**, **f**) Coronal and sagittal post-contrast images illustrating the solidly enhancing right frontal mass with compression of the anterior portion of the body of the right lateral ventricle

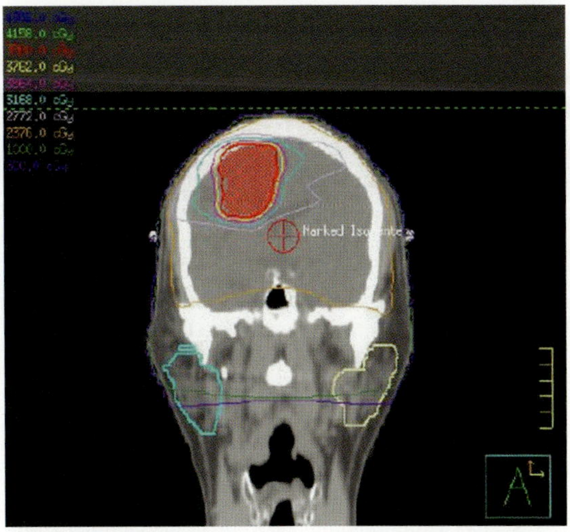

Fig. 8.5 Whole brain radiation to 23.4 Gy followed by a right frontal boost with IMRT to 39.6 Gy

being treated solely with WBRT who are not candidates for systemic therapy, doses of 40–45 Gy should be used. In the salvage setting, 36–45 Gy is appropriate.

The clinical value of partial-brain radiation was explored in a retrospective study of 43 patients with PCNSL, of whom 74 % had unifocal disease, and 60 % received systemic therapy [42]. Partial brain RT was administered to a median dose of 50 Gy with median margin size of 4 cm. At 5 years the infield brain recurrence rate was 57 %, and out of field brain recurrence rate was 49 %. The authors concluded that focal RT with margins less than 4 cm were associated with high rates of out of field recurrences. Given these observations, consolidative radiation fields should contain the whole brain out of concern for out of field parenchymal brain recurrences. Partial brain radiation has also been explored in the salvage setting. Gamma knife radiotherapy was evaluated in the setting of relapsed primary and secondary CNS lymphoma in a small retrospective study of six patients [43]. All patients experienced improvement in neurologic symptoms without neurotoxicity; however disease progression occurred 3–13 months after the first gamma knife procedure. Taken together these data suggest a limited role for partial brain radiation outside of a protocol setting.

While limited data suggests a minimal role for partial brain radiation, it is unclear if there is value to a tumor boost, particularly in cases of persistent disease. In the ongoing HOVON, 105 trial patients that achieve only a partial response (PR) to induction chemotherapy are treated with simultaneous integrated boost technique. The whole brain is to receive 30 Gy in 20 fractions of 1.5 Gy, with the residual disease receiving 40 Gy in 2.0 Gy fractions. In an effort to minimize toxicity associated with higher whole brain doses, in our clinical practice, we often utilize simultaneous integrated boost or sequential boost technique to treat patients with persistent gross disease with the goal of achieving doses of greater than or equal to 40 Gy in fraction sizes of 2 Gy or less.

Integrated IMRT to address the local disease is an appealing approach especially when the failure is in multiple areas. When patients receive multiple therapies and show multiple progressions in different areas, the integrated IMRT should include all areas seen on the different MRI corresponding to each progression. Physicians can fuse all the MRI available and contour abnormalities seen on different dates. An illustration with a patient who progressed after four different chemotherapy regimens before presenting for a definitive dose of radiation is provided. We illustrated the whole brain treatment to 30 Gy while boosting daily the areas of disease progression from his different MRI to a dose of 45 Gy using IMRT. This is to illustrate the use of IMRT as an integrated boost as practiced currently.

Conclusion

The prognosis of PCNSL has improved over the last few decades; however the optimal therapy remains to be established. With high-dose Mtx as the backbone of therapy, high-dose WBRT to doses greater than 45 Gy, while associated with improved PFS, is limited by severe long-term neurotoxicity, especially in the older patient population. Newer strategies, especially rdWBRT to 23.4 Gy, demonstrate promising results in long-term follow-up of a single institutional phase II trial without neurotoxicity. Other considerations for consolidative therapy include intensive chemotherapy as well as ASCT. Future clinical trials should help to better define the optimal consolidative approach.

References

1. Eby NL, et al. Increasing incidence of primary brain lymphoma in the US. Cancer. 1988;62(11):2461–5.
2. Hochberg FH, Miller DC. Primary central nervous system lymphoma. J Neurosurg. 1988;68(6):835–53.
3. Fine HA, Mayer RJ. Primary central nervous system lymphoma. Ann Intern Med. 1993;119(11):1093–104.
4. Bataille B, et al. Primary intracerebral malignant lymphoma: report of 248 cases. J Neurosurg. 2000;92(2):261–6.
5. Peterson K, et al. The clinical spectrum of ocular lymphoma. Cancer. 1993;72(3):843–9.
6. Ursea R, et al. Ophthalmic, ultrasonographic findings in primary central nervous system lymphoma with ocular involvement. Retina. 1997;17(2):118–23.
7. Grimm SA, et al. Primary intraocular lymphoma: an International Primary Central Nervous System Lymphoma Collaborative Group Report. Ann Oncol. 2007;18(11):1851–5.
8. Char DH, et al. Primary intraocular lymphoma (ocular reticulum cell sarcoma) diagnosis and management. Ophthalmology. 1988;95(5):625–30.
9. Shenkier TN, et al. Primary CNS lymphoma of T-cell origin: a descriptive analysis from the international primary CNS lymphoma collaborative group. J Clin Oncol. 2005;23(10):2233–9.
10. Monabati A, et al. Primary burkitt lymphoma of the brain in an immunocompetent patient. Case report. J Neurosurg. 2002;96(6):1127–9.
11. Tu PH, et al. Clinicopathologic and genetic profile of intracranial marginal zone lymphoma: a primary low-grade CNS lymphoma that mimics meningioma. J Clin Oncol. 2005;23(24):5718–27.
12. Kluin PM, Deckert M, Ferry JA. Primary diffuse large B cell lymphoma of the CNS., in WHO classification of tumours of haematopoietic and lymphoid tissue (IARC WHO Classification of tumours). Lyon: IARC; 2008. p. 240–1.
13. Giannini C, Dogan A, Salomao DR. CNS lymphoma: a practical diagnostic approach. J Neuropathol Exp Neurol. 2014;73(6):478–94.
14. Alizadeh AA, et al. Distinct types of diffuse large B-cell lymphoma identified by gene expression profiling. Nature. 2000;403(6769):503–11.
15. Bea S, et al. Diffuse large B-cell lymphoma subgroups have distinct genetic profiles that influence tumor biology and improve gene-expression-based survival prediction. Blood. 2005;106(9):3183–90.
16. Hans CP, et al. Confirmation of the molecular classification of diffuse large B-cell lymphoma by immunohistochemistry using a tissue microarray. Blood. 2004;103(1):275–82.
17. Brunn A, et al. Frequent triple-hit expression of MYC, BCL2, and BCL6 in primary lymphoma of the central nervous system and absence of a favorable MYC(low) BCL2 (low) subgroup may underlie the inferior prognosis as compared to systemic diffuse large B-cell lymphomas. Acta Neuropathol. 2013;126(4):603–5.
18. Gill KZ, et al. MYC protein expression in primary diffuse large B-cell lymphoma of the central nervous system. PLoS One. 2014;9(12):e114398.
19. Klapper W, et al. Structural aberrations affecting the MYC locus indicate a poor prognosis independent of clinical risk factors in diffuse large B-cell lymphomas treated within randomized trials of the German High-Grade Non-Hodgkin's Lymphoma Study Group (DSHNHL). Leukemia. 2008;22(12):2226–9.
20. Akyurek N, et al. Prognostic significance of MYC, BCL2, and BCL6 rearrangements in patients with diffuse large B-cell lymphoma treated with cyclophosphamide, doxorubicin, vincristine, and prednisone plus rituximab. Cancer. 2012;118(17):4173–83.
21. Cady FM, et al. Del(6)(q22) and BCL6 rearrangements in primary CNS lymphoma are indicators of an aggressive clinical course. J Clin Oncol. 2008;26(29):4814–9.
22. Mansour A, et al. MR imaging features of intracranial primary CNS lymphoma in immune competent patients. Cancer Imaging. 2014;14(1):22.
23. Porter AB, et al. Primary central nervous system lymphoma can be histologically diagnosed after previous corticosteroid use: a pilot study to determine whether corticosteroids prevent the diagnosis of primary central nervous system lymphoma. Ann Neurol. 2008;63(5):662–7.
24. DeAngelis LM, et al. Primary CNS lymphoma: combined treatment with chemotherapy and radiotherapy. Neurology. 1990;40(1):80–6.
25. Weller M, et al. Surgery for primary CNS lymphoma? Challenging a paradigm. Neuro Oncol. 2012;14(12):1481–4.
26. Nelson DF, et al. Non-Hodgkin's lymphoma of the brain: can high dose, large volume radiation therapy improve survival? Report on a prospective trial by the Radiation Therapy Oncology Group (RTOG): RTOG 8315. Int J Radiat Oncol Biol Phys. 1992;23(1):9–17.
27. Schultz C, et al. Preirradiation chemotherapy with cyclophosphamide, doxorubicin, vincristine, and dexamethasone for primary CNS lymphomas: initial report of radiation therapy oncology group protocol 88–06. J Clin Oncol. 1996;14(2):556–64.
28. Borsi JD, Moe PJ. A comparative study on the pharmacokinetics of methotrexate in a dose range of 0.5 g

to 33.6 g/m2 in children with acute lymphoblastic leukemia. Cancer. 1987;60(1):5–13.

29. Shapiro WR, Young DF, Mehta BM. Methotrexate: distribution in cerebrospinal fluid after intravenous, ventricular and lumbar injections. N Engl J Med. 1975;293(4):161–6.
30. DeAngelis LM, et al. Combined modality therapy for primary CNS lymphoma. J Clin Oncol. 1992;10(4):635–43.
31. Ferreri AJ, et al. High-dose cytarabine plus high-dose methotrexate versus high-dose methotrexate alone in patients with primary CNS lymphoma: a randomised phase 2 trial. Lancet. 2009;374(9700):1512–20.
32. Glass J, et al. Preirradiation methotrexate chemotherapy of primary central nervous system lymphoma: long-term outcome. J Neurosurg. 1994;81(2): 188–95.
33. O'Brien PC, et al. Combined-modality therapy for primary central nervous system lymphoma: long-term data from a Phase II multicenter study (Trans-Tasman Radiation Oncology Group). Int J Radiat Oncol Biol Phys. 2006;64(2):408–13.
34. Abrey LE, DeAngelis LM, Yahalom J. Long-term survival in primary CNS lymphoma. J Clin Oncol. 1998;16(3):859–63.
35. Citterio G, Ferreri AJ, Reni M. Current uses of radiation therapy in patients with primary CNS lymphoma. Expert Rev Anticancer Ther. 2013;13(11):1327–37.
36. Abrey LE, et al. Report of an international workshop to standardize baseline evaluation and response criteria for primary CNS lymphoma. J Clin Oncol. 2005;23(22):5034–43.
37. Kasenda B, et al. Prognosis after high-dose chemotherapy followed by autologous stem-cell transplantation as first-line treatment in primary CNS lymphoma--a long-term follow-up study. Ann Oncol. 2012;23(10):2670–5.
38. Omuro A, et al. R-MPV followed by high-dose chemotherapy with TBC and autologous stem-cell transplant for newly diagnosed primary CNS lymphoma. Blood. 2015;125:1403–10.
39. Rubenstein JL, et al. Intensive chemotherapy and immunotherapy in patients with newly diagnosed primary CNS lymphoma: CALGB 50202 (Alliance 50202). J Clin Oncol. 2013;31(25):3061–8.
40. Hottinger AF, et al. Salvage whole brain radiotherapy for recurrent or refractory primary CNS lymphoma. Neurology. 2007;69(11):1178–82.
41. Nguyen PL, et al. Results of whole-brain radiation as salvage of methotrexate failure for immunocompetent patients with primary CNS lymphoma. J Clin Oncol. 2005;23(7):1507–13.
42. Shibamoto Y, et al. Is whole-brain irradiation necessary for primary central nervous system lymphoma? Patterns of recurrence after partial-brain irradiation. Cancer. 2003;97(1):128–33.
43. Matsumoto Y, et al. Effectiveness and limitation of gamma knife radiosurgery for relapsed central nervous system lymphoma: a retrospective analysis in one institution. Int J Hematol. 2007;85(4):333–7.

Primary Testicular Lymphoma

9

Andrew Wirth and Chan Yoon Cheah

Abstract

Adjuvant testicular irradiation is a component of standard care for patients with stage I–II primary testicular lymphomas following anthracycline-based chemotherapy and improves both local disease control and overall outcome in appropriately selected patients. It can also be considered in advanced stage III/IV patients on a case-by-case basis.

Introduction and Clinical Case

Primary testicular lymphoma (PTL) is a rare, clinically aggressive form of extra-nodal lymphoma, with an estimated annual incidence of 0.09–0.26 per 100,000. It accounts for <5 % of testicular malignancies and 1–2 % of NHL [1, 2]. Patients typically present in their mid- to late 60s [3–6]. PTL is the commonest testicular malignancy in men aged >60 years and the most common bilateral testicular neoplasm [7]. Patients typically present with a firm, painless testicular mass that is associated with a hydrocele in approximately 40 % of cases [3, 8]. Synchronous bilateral involvement occurs in up to 10 % of cases and constitutional symptoms may occur in 20–30 % [2, 9]. PTL has a propensity to relapse in extra-nodal sites including the CNS, skin, contralateral testis and pleura [4, 6, 10–12]. HIV infection is a known risk factor for aggressive NHL, and HIV-positive patients with PTL are younger, often with highly aggressive histology and a very poor prognosis prior to the introduction of combined antiretroviral therapy [13, 14]. The current standard of care for PTL consists of rituximab, cyclophosphamide, doxorubicin, vincristine and prednisone (R-CHOP) chemoimmunotherapy, central nervous system (CNS) prophylaxis and loco-regional radiotherapy. In this chapter an illustrative case of PTL is presented followed by a discussion of the appropriate evaluation and management, with a focus on the role of radiotherapy.

A. Wirth (✉)
Division of Radiation Oncology and Cancer Imaging, Peter MacCallum cancer Centre, East Melbourne, VIC, Australia
e-mail: andrew.wirth@petermac.org

C.Y. Cheah
Department of Lymphoma/Myeloma, UT MD Anderson Cancer Center, 1515 Holcombe Blvd, Houston, TX 77030, USA
e-mail: ccheah@mdanderson.org

B.S. Dabaja, A.K. Ng (eds.), *Radiation Therapy in Hematologic Malignancies*,
DOI 10.1007/978-3-319-42615-0_9

Case Presentation and Initial Evaluation

A 49-year-old male in good previous health presented to his local doctor with a 2-month history of a right scrotal mass, which was uncomfortable but not painful. He denied weight loss, fevers or night sweats. On examination his local doctor found a solid, non-tender 3 cm mass inseparable from the testis. Blood biochemistry revealed a normal β-HCG, AFP, LDH and liver and renal function and a FBE was normal. A scrotal ultrasound demonstrated a solid 2.5 cm testicular mass. The patient was referred to a urologist. The urologist ordered a computerised tomographic (CT) scan that demonstrated no abnormality beyond the testis, and the patient underwent an inguinal orchiectomy. The pathology demonstrated DLBCL involving the rete testis without invasion of the epididymis or tunica albuginea.

The patient was then referred to a haematologist. Physical examination was again unremarkable, and in particular there was no lymphadenopathy or hepatosplenomegaly, and a thorough examination of the skin revealed no suspicious lesions. The staging was completed with bone marrow aspiration and trephine, positron emission tomography (PET) scan, magnetic resonance imaging (MRI) of the brain and cerebrospinal fluid (CSF) examination for cytology and flow cytometry. These examinations were all normal. HIV serology was negative. The patient therefore had stage I disease.

Systemic Therapy Given Following Orchiectomy

The patient was informed of the planned management programme and its acute and late toxicities including infertility and hypogonadism. The patient declined sperm collection. The patient commenced a course of R-CHOP chemotherapy and completed 6 cycles at 3 weekly intervals. Intrathecal ara-c was administered during the R-CHOP, and two cycles of high-dose methotrexate were delivered following completion of R-CHOP. Treatment was delivered on time with no major toxicities.

Testicular Irradiation

The patient underwent a course of testicular radiation of 30.6 Gy in 17 fractions. The patient was simulated in a supine position with legs slightly apart and the penis displaced and immobilised superiorly (Figs. 9.1 and 9.2). The irradiated field was marked clinically using anatomical landmarks and was intended to encompass the entire scrotal sac/contents. The upper border of the clinically marked field was 1.5 cm above the superior aspect of the palpated testis/scrotal sac. Mapping can be also done using the CT simulation images that will also help to determine the electron energy needed (Fig. 9.3a–c). The patient was treated with a direct anterior 16 MeV electron beam. Verification was performed daily by palpation to confirm clinical landmarks so as to ensure the entire scrotum was encompassed throughout the course of treatment. Skin collimation was made to block the excess dose to the rectum (Fig. 9.4). No bolus was used in this case since the skin dose is already high when using 16 MeV, obviously, and when using lower energies, bolus might be needed to ensure a good skin dose especially if the skin is involved. During the treatment

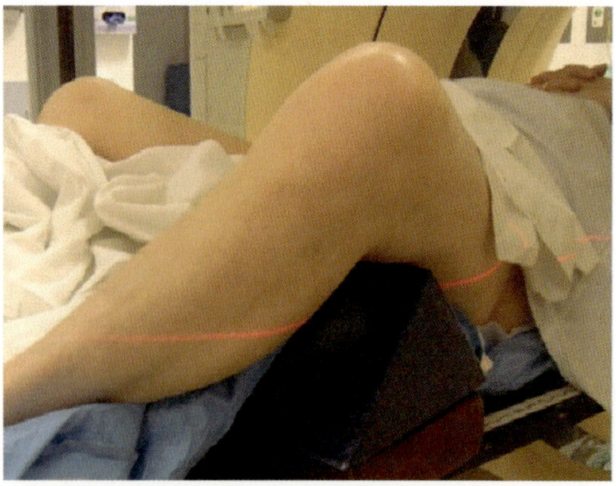

Fig. 9.1 Patient setup in a frog leg for scrotal irradiation

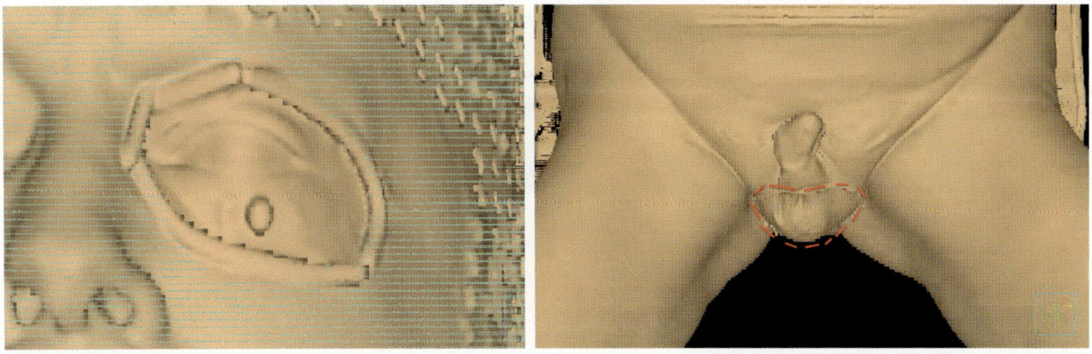

Fig. 9.2 Patient setup, skin rendering showing the in tomato colour the edge of the field, the position of the penis in a frog leg position for scrotal irradiation

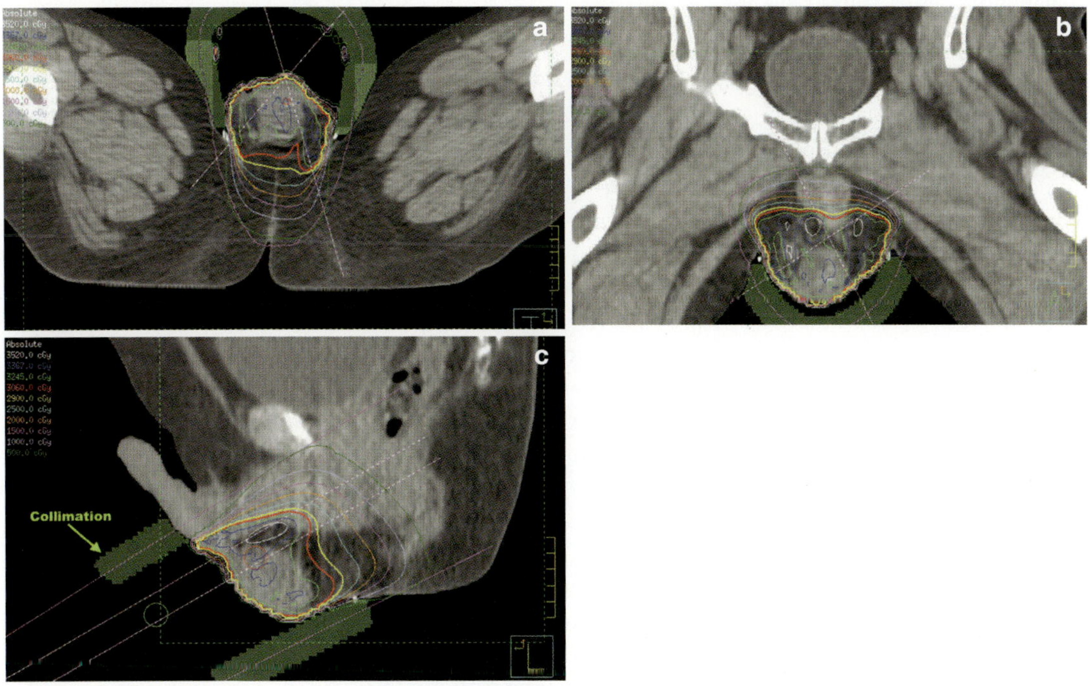

Fig. 9.3 CT planning showing the 100 % isodone line in *red* in (**a**) axial, (**b**) coronal, (**c**) sagittal views

patients should be kept warm and relaxed; otherwise the scrotum might retract and the field might not cover it well. Regional nodal irradiation was not given in this patient with stage I disease.

Supportive Care and Follow-Up

The patient was seen weekly during radiotherapy, with particular attention to scrotal and perineal skin care. Patients invariably end up with grade 2/3 dermatitis, especially at the end of the radiation course or the week following; skin care with sitz baths and local moisturisers is quite often needed. A follow-up plan is to include regular clinical assessment looking for evidence of tumour recurrence or late toxicity including features of hypogonadism. Periodic measurements of serum testosterone and gonadotropins will be performed and replacement therapy instituted if clinically appropriate with appropriate endocrinology consultation.

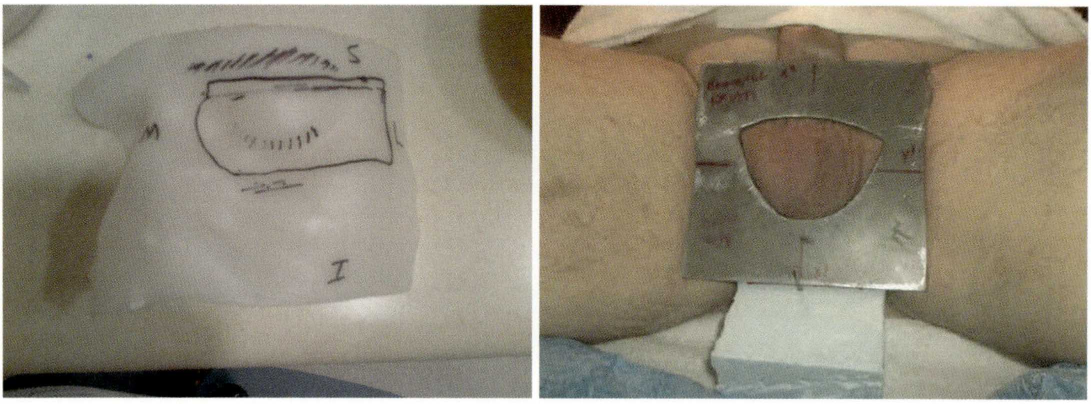

Fig. 9.4 Treatment set using the skin collimation while making sure that the whole scrotum is exposed out of the skin collimation during the daily treatment

Discussion and Rationale

Pathology

The majority of PT-DLBCL cases are of activated B-cell type [5, 15–20]. This predominance of ABC type may partially account for the historically poor outcomes from PTL [21, 22]. Although co-expression of MYC and Bcl-2 protein may contribute to the inferior survival of ABC-type nodal DLBCL, cytogenetic "double-hit" cases with concurrent rearrangements of *MYC* and *BCL2* and/or *BCL6* in PTL are infrequent [23–25]. MYD88 mutations are also more frequent in PTL than nodal DLBCL [26, 27]. Other histologies that present as PTL include mantle cell lymphoma, extra-nodal NK-cell lymphoma, peripheral T-cell lymphoma, extra-nodal marginal zone lymphoma, ALK1-negative anaplastic large cell lymphoma and paediatric follicular lymphoma [18, 28–39]. The biological basis for the propensity of PTL for extra-nodal relapse is unknown, but may include the development of an immune escape phenotype origin in an immune privileged site behind the blood-testis barrier and overexpression of the chemokine receptor CXCR4 [40–47]. Chapuy et al.'s recent observed copy gains in 9p24.1/CD274 (PD-L1) were present in >40 % of a cohort of 43 PTL cases and were associated with overexpression of PD1 ligands [48].

Rationale for the Initial Evaluation, Staging and Prognosis

Initial imaging of a scrotal swelling should include ultrasonography, which may demonstrate focal or diffuse areas of hypo-echogenicity with hypervascularity in an enlarged testis [49, 50]. Magnetic resonance imaging (MRI) allows simultaneous evaluation of the testis, para-testicular spaces and spermatic cord. Findings in testicular lymphoma include T2 hypointensity and strong heterogeneous gadolinium enhancement [51]. Inguinal orchiectomy is mandatory for the diagnosis as well as for optimal local disease control. Expert hemato-pathological review is essential with the performance of appropriate immunohistochemistry, as distinguishing some cases of PTL from seminoma can be difficult [52].

Recommended staging includes positron emission tomography (PET)-CT and bone marrow biopsy. It is essential to perform baseline MRI of the brain and lumbar puncture for CSF analysis by both cytology and flow cytometry, given the propensity of PTL to disseminate to the CNS [53]. The skin should be thoroughly examined as it is a common site of extra-nodal recurrence and cutaneous "DLBCL, leg type" has been concurrently reported with PTL [54]. HIV serology should be performed.

Staging is based on the Ann Arbor system [55]; 60–70 % of patients have stage I–II at presentation [2, 4, 12, 56]. Patients with isolated bilateral involvement of the testes have similar prognosis to stage I/II disease, and it is reasonable to consider such cases as having stage I disease [57, 58].

For the majority of patients with PTL who present with limited stage disease, the IPI is typically <2 and therefore has limited prognostic utility [59]. A number of adverse prognostic markers have been reported including older age, advanced stage, B symptoms, poor performance status, more than one extra-nodal site of involvement, tumour size >10 cm, raised LDH or β-2 microglobulin, low albumin, left testis involvement and infiltration of adjacent tissues [1, 2, 4, 6, 11, 12, 60–65]. A Dutch series found evidence of transformed extra-nodal marginal zone lymphoma associated with smaller tumour size, less frequently elevated LDH, absence of B symptoms, more frequent stage IE disease and lower IPI than "pure" DLBCL, with a non-significant trend towards improved survival [32].

PTL is characterised by a pattern of continuing relapses for more than 10–15 years after initial treatment. Relapse typically involves sanctuary sites such as the contralateral testis and CNS, but may occur at multiple extra-nodal sites including the lung, soft tissue, adrenals, liver and bone marrow [4, 6, 11, 12].

Rationale for Systemic Therapy

The outcomes of patients treated with orchiectomy and/or radiation alone are poor [2, 3, 66]. Available data on the efficacy of systemic therapy are drawn from either non-randomised phase II studies or retrospective series and suggest an inferior prognosis to nodal DLBCL, with no plateau in PFS and OS curves in retrospective studies [5, 6, 9, 11, 12, 56, 63]. There is evidence that the prognosis of PTL has improved over time as treatment strategies have evolved [2, 11]. The SEER registry analysis reported a median OS of 1.8 years for patients diagnosed in 1980–1985 but with the median not yet reached for those diagnosed 20 years later [2]. Three-weekly CHOP was the most commonly used regimen for PTL prior to the introduction of rituximab, achieving 5-year OS of 30–52 % [11, 67]. Small series evaluating the addition of bleomycin, increasing dose density or intensified chemotherapy regimens such as hyperfractionated cyclophosphamide, doxorubicin, vincristine and dexamethasone (Hyper-CVAD) have not been shown to improve outcomes and are challenging to deliver in older patients [10, 63, 68].

A small retrospective analysis from the British Columbia Cancer Agency (BCCA) demonstrated no improvement in 5-year rates of progression or OS with the addition of rituximab; however the use of rituximab was associated with improvements in both time to progression ($p=0.006$) and overall survival (OS) ($p=0.009$) on multivariate analysis [64].

The reported results of limited systemic therapy have been mixed. Connors et al. reported excellent results with three cycles of CHOP or a 6-week regimen termed ACOB (cyclophosphamide, doxorubicin, vincristine, bleomycin and prednisolone) [68]. However, other series including a large IELSG analysis and a single-centre study from Australia suggest that patients who receive <6 cycles of chemotherapy have a poorer outcome; therefore limited chemotherapy is not recommended for PTL [6, 12].

Few prospective clinical trials in PTL have been conducted. The GOELAMS protocol was based on three cycles of VCAP (vindesine, cyclophosphamide, doxorubicin and prednisolone) and IT chemotherapy (vindesine, cyclophosphamide, epirubicin, prednisolone and bleomycin for patients aged over 60). Radiotherapy was given to regional lymph nodes as well as to whole brain [69]. With a median follow-up of 73.5 months, the DFS and OS were 70 % and 65 %, respectively, with one CNS relapse.

Aviles et al. reported a single-arm study using 6 cycles of R-CEOP (rituximab, cyclophosphamide 1500 mg/m^2, epirubicin 120 mg/m^2, vincristine and prednisolone) dosed at 14-day intervals. Scrotal/contralateral testis irradiation (30 Gy) was given to patients achieving CR to chemotherapy. CNS prophylaxis comprised 4 cycles of high-dose intravenous methotrexate (6 g/m^2) with leucovorin rescue [70]. Of the 38 patients enrolled, 86 % achieved CR and the actuarial 5-year EFS and OS were 70 % and 66 %, respectively. No CNS relapses were reported in this study.

Finally, the International Extranodal Lymphoma Study Group (IELSG) has reported a phase II multicentre study of 53 patients with stage I/II DLBCL-type PTL. Treatment was 3-weekly R-CHOP with IT methotrexate, followed by loco-regional irradiation [59]. Ninety-eight percent achieved CR, and after a median follow-up of 65 months, the 5-year PFS and OS were 74 % and 85 %, respectively. The 5-year actuarial incidence of CNS relapse was 6 %. The excellent results in this study established R-CHOP Q21 with IT methotrexate and loco-regional radiation as the reference treatment for patients with limited stage PTL, including those with bilateral testicular involvement.

Novel therapeutic strategies for DLBCL may have applicability to PTL. The addition of lenalidomide [71] or the tyrosine kinase inhibitor ibrutinib [72] to R-CHOP [73–76] appears to be well tolerated and effective. Lenalidomide has been detected in the semen of male patients and has been reported as having efficacy for myeloma invading the testis [77, 78]. Pomalidomide, another immunomodulatory drug, appears to be synergistic with rituximab [79] and has excellent CNS penetration [80]. Other agents of interest for DLBCL include the CXCR4 inhibitor plerixafor and small molecule inhibitors of the NF-kB, STAT3 and NF-kB signalling pathways [81]. The recent finding of PD1 overexpression in many cases of PTL makes this an appealing therapeutic target [48]. Currently, 3-weekly R-CHOP (or an equivalent anthracycline-based regimen) with intrathecal methotrexate and loco-regional RT is the international standard of care for stage I–II PTL.

CNS Prophylaxis

The reported incidence of CNS involvement in PTL varies widely but has been as high as 44 % [4, 6, 11, 56, 82]. The IELSG retrospective study reported a 10-year actuarial risk of CNS involvement of 34 % that appears to be substantially greater than nodal DLBCL [12, 83]. The addition of rituximab to anthracycline-based chemotherapy has not had an appreciable impact on the rate of CNS relapse risk [83, 84].

IT chemotherapy has been used in many retrospective series; however methodological limitations make it difficult to draw firm conclusions about its efficacy [4–6, 11]. In two prospective clinical trials that used IT chemotherapy alone, the reported CNS relapse rate was 6 %, whereas a study that used both IT and systemic methotrexate reported no CNS relapses among 38 patients [59, 69, 70]. In all three studies, the crude incidence of CNS relapse was significantly less than for historic controls. Parenchymal CNS relapse is more common than isolated leptomeningeal relapse [12, 85]. As the penetration of IT methotrexate into brain parenchyma is limited, there is conceptual appeal to the use of high-dose systemic methotrexate for CNS prophylaxis, as it achieves higher drug levels in brain parenchyma [86, 87]. This concept is supported both by the results of the Aviles study noted above and the apparent benefit of high-dose systemic methotrexate as CNS prophylaxis for nodal DLBCL [88–91]. The merits of this approach are reflected in treatment guidelines, and the ongoing IELSG-30 prospective protocol incorporates IV methotrexate (1.5 g/m^2) in addition to IT liposomal cytarabine (ClinicalTrials.gov identifier: NCT00945724) [92]. Although prophylactic cranial irradiation (PCI) has been used to reduce the incidence of CNS relapse (as in the GOELAMS study), and may be effective, the use of PCI is not routinely recommended due to the risks of late neurocognitive toxicity [93].

Discussion of Prophylactic Testicular Irradiation

Rationale

It is recognised that patients treated by orchidectomy and anthracycline-based chemotherapy have an appreciable risk of relapse in the contralateral testis [1, 3, 4, 9, 12, 57, 59, 65, 67, 69, 94, 95]. This presumably reflects poor penetration of commonly used chemotherapy agents into the intact testis. There are no randomised trial data regarding the use of prophylactic testicular irradiation, nor regarding the optimal dose or technique. Available data are derived from retrospective studies and a small number of non-randomised prospective trials. Mazloom et al. reported the MD Anderson Cancer Center experience and found that 3/35 (9 %) patients who did not receive testicular irradiation relapsed in the contralateral testis, compared to 4 % in patients who receive a median testicular radiation dose of 30.6 Gy [11]. Individual series have reported rates of contralateral testicular relapse ranging from 0 to 35 % [96]. In the largest retrospective multicentre series, reported by the IELSG, testicular relapse was a component of 43 of 195 treatment failures, with a 15-year actuarial incidence of contralateral testicular relapse of 42 % in the absence of scrotal irradiation [12]. A number of individual studies have reported a low incidence of testicular relapse following prophylactic scrotal irradiation, typically ranging from 0 to 10 %, though reportedly as high as 20 % in one series, which may reflect uncertainty about the quality of radiotherapy delivery in older series [96, 97]. Prophylactic scrotal radiation in the IELSG retrospective study was associated with a statistically significantly lower incidence of testicular relapse from 42 % to fewer than 10 % ($p=0.011$). Importantly, this local control advantage was associated with an improvement in both 5-year PFS (70 % v 36 %, $p=0.00001$) and OS (66 % v 38 %, $p=0.00001$), which remained statistically significant on multivariate analysis [12]. Other studies have also suggested an association between the use of adjuvant RT and improved survival, although it is uncertain to what extent this reflects patient selection for adjuvant irradiation [2, 98].

Prophylactic testicular irradiation was used in three of the four reported prospective studies of PTL. In two phase II studies reported by Aviles et al., all patients received prophylactic testicular irradiation and no testicular relapses were reported [10, 70]. Similarly in the more recently reported IELSG-10 prospective study, adjuvant testicular radiation (median dose 30 Gy, range 24–40 Gy) was used routinely with no testicular relapses observed [59]. Based on the preponderance of data from both retrospective and prospective trials, prophylactic testicular irradiation is considered standard of care for patients with stage I–II PTL.

Adjuvant scrotal radiation may have a greater impact in patients with limited stage disease, as the competing risks of systemic relapse appear to increase with advancing initial stage. In the IELSG retrospective series, contralateral testicular relapse as a component of the first site of failure occurred in 28 %, 14 % and 16 % of patients with stages I, II and III–IV, respectively. Corresponding figures for sole initial site of failure were 10 %, 2 % and 2 %, respectively [12]. Although the absolute benefit from prophylactic testicular irradiation may be smaller for more advanced stage disease, given the relatively low morbidity of this treatment, it is reasonable to consider it for all patients having potentially curative chemotherapy. Despite the demonstrated efficacy of scrotal irradiation, these findings have not yet been fully translated into routine practice, as the SEER data suggest that only 30–40 % of patients appear to receive RT, without an apparent increase in utilisation over time [2].

Testicular Radiotherapy Volume

The entire testis, tunica albuginea, epididymis and spermatic cord are often reported to be involved in pathological studies of PTL and constitute the CTV for testicular irradiation [62, 96]. In rare cases of overt skin involvement, the skin also forms part of the CTV.

Testicular Radiotherapy Dose

Scrotal irradiation doses reported in the literature have ranged from 18 Gy to over 50 Gy, but are most commonly reported in the range of 25–30 Gy [96]. The prospective studies reported by Aviles and the more recent publication of the IELSG prospective intergroup study both used testicular doses in the range of 25–30 with a high degree of efficacy [10, 59, 70]. As there is some evidence from the IELSG retrospective analysis that doses less than 30 Gy were associated with a lower survival rate, 30 Gy may be considered a reasonable standard of care [12]. Radiotherapy should be fully fractionated to minimise acute scrotal skin morbidity.

Radiotherapy Technique

Several radiotherapy techniques have been described for irradiation of the scrotum, and as with other aspects of radiotherapy for PTL, they have not been compared in prospective clinical trials. In fact, many reported series either do not describe the techniques used or provide inadequate information on techniques used both for testicular and nodal irradiation. Some older series describe techniques that may have provided inadequate or marginal coverage of the testis [96]. A group of Dutch investigators have reported an extensive review of radiotherapy techniques for PTL, including a survey of techniques used in Dutch centres and a phantom study to compare PTV and critical organ dosimetry using various techniques. The three techniques compared were a direct anterior electron beam, a direct anterior photon beam and a wedge pair photon beam [96]. They found that the most commonly used technique in Holland was an anterior electron beam used in 10 of 16 eligible centres surveyed. The most homogeneous dosimetric coverage of the PTV was achieved using either of the photon techniques, but this came at the cost of higher doses to normal tissues such as anus and rectum. Although the doses to normal tissues were within conventional tolerances, it can be argued, particularly in younger patients, that photon techniques are best avoided to minimise exposure of pelvic and perineal structures in order to minimise the risk of second malignancies. A key message is that the method used in any centre needs to be evaluated carefully from a physics and dosimetric perspective to ensure adequate coverage.

The use of bolus over the scrotal surface is not always clearly described in reports of testicular irradiation for PTL. It should certainly be included in rare cases of overt scrotal skin infiltration to avoid underdosing potentially involved skin. It has been reported that invasion of the tunica albuginea is observed in approximately half of cases of PTL at pathological examination [62, 96]. Given that the skin is only a few mm thick, techniques that spare skin may also lead to underdosing of the tunica and potentially increase the risk of in-field failure.

Patient setup will depend on the technique used. Most surveyed Dutch centres used clinical palpation both to define the CTV and for verification during treatment [96]. Given the variation in scrotal anatomy due to fluctuation in temperature or patient anxiety, clinical localisation may in fact be superior to imaging-based localisation, although CT planning and CBCT verification have been used in some centres and potentially offer better documentation of dosimetry and selection of electron energy [96].

Considerations for the Use of Nodal Irradiation

For patients with stage I PTL, radiation is generally confined to the scrotum, and there is no clear role for adjuvant irradiation to apparently uninvolved para-aortic-pelvic nodes. In studies in which scrotal RT only was used for stage I disease, the reported incidence of isolated nodal relapse is low [99].

It is not possible to draw firm conclusions regarding the role of RT to involved regional lymph nodes in patients treated with R-CHOP for stage II disease, because of small numbers of patients reported in the literature with stage II disease treated with or without nodal radiation. Even in the IELSG retrospective study with over 300 cases, it was not possible to make meaningful observations on the role of nodal irradiation in stage II disease [12]. In the IELSG-10 study, of 13 stage II patients, nine received nodal RT, and the single relapse occurred in one of these patients, within the radiotherapy field [59]. The four patients not treated with RT were all in remission at the time of reporting.

The broader literature on the role of adjuvant radiotherapy for DLBCL suggests a benefit for patients with localised and/or bulky disease even in the era of R-CHOP [100–103]. It is uncertain whether the principles of consolidative nodal radiotherapy derived from more common presentations of DLBCL can be translated to the setting of testicular lymphoma, as the pattern of recurrence in PTL is unusual and is dominated by widespread extra-nodal relapse. Despite these caveats, for patients with stage II disease who present with involvement of the pelvic and para-aortic lymph nodes, it is common for adjuvant RT to be delivered to initially involved nodes following chemotherapy, and this may be considered a reasonable standard of care [59]. For patients who present with stage III to IV, the benefit of regional nodal irradiation is even less certain, and radiotherapy would not be used routinely. A possible exception would be cases where there is a dominant sight of nodal disease that is bulky (>7 or 10 cm) or responds slowly or incompletely to initial chemotherapy, particularly in the elderly patient who is unsuitable for aggressive salvage therapy.

Nodal Radiotherapy Dose and Volume

When regional nodal radiation is given for patients in a complete remission documented on PET, radiotherapy should be directed to the initial sites of involvement or the initial site of bulky disease – involved node or involved site technique [104] – to avoid unnecessary exposure of normal tissues [105]. The GTV consists of residual post-chemotherapy lymph node enlargement, and the CTV represents the pre-chemotherapy tumour volume adjusted for concentric reduction in the transverse tumour dimensions following chemotherapy. A dose of 30 Gy in 15–20 fractions is appropriate for patients achieving a complete response to chemotherapy.

Discussion of Supportive Care and Follow-Up

Testicular irradiation is associated with acute cutaneous toxicity, and in some cases, this may lead to a period of discomfort lasting several weeks. The acute toxicities of abdominal and pelvic irradiation include lethargy, mild nausea and a possible short-term disturbance of bowel function. In addition, in some patients for whom a large part of the pelvic marrow is irradiated may develop cytopenias, which can sometimes be long lasting.

The major long-term toxicity of scrotal irradiation to a dose of 30 Gy is infertility. In addition, patients undergoing testicular irradiation to a dose of 14–20 Gy or more experience progressive decline in testosterone production and need to be aware of the possible need for hormone replacement in the future [106–109]. Patients having abdominal pelvic radiation may be at increased risk of secondary malignancies 10 years or more after radiation.

Conclusion

Adjuvant testicular irradiation is a component of standard care for patients with stage I–II primary testicular lymphomas following anthracycline-based chemotherapy and improves both local disease control and overall outcome in appropriately selected patients [2, 12, 98]. Nodal irradiation for stage II disease is widely used and should be considered on a case-by-case basis, as should testicular irradiation for patients with stage III–IV disease.

References

1. Moller MB, d'Amore F, Christensen BE. Testicular lymphoma: a population-based study of incidence, clinicopathological correlations and prognosis. The Danish Lymphoma Study Group, LYFO. Eur J Cancer. 1994;30A(12):1760–4.
2. Gundrum JD, et al. Primary testicular diffuse large B-cell lymphoma: a population-based study on the incidence, natural history, and survival comparison with primary nodal counterpart before and after the introduction of rituximab. J Clin Oncol. 2009;27(31):5227–32.
3. Shahab N, Doll DC. Testicular lymphoma. Semin Oncol. 1999;26(3):259–69.
4. Fonseca R, et al. Testicular lymphoma is associated with a high incidence of extranodal recurrence. Cancer. 2000;88(1):154–61.
5. Hasselblom S, et al. Testicular lymphoma--a retrospective, population-based, clinical and immunohistochemical study. Acta Oncol. 2004;43(8):758–65.
6. Seymour JF, et al. Primary large-cell non-Hodgkin's lymphoma of the testis: a retrospective analysis of patterns of failure and prognostic factors. Clin Lymphoma. 2001;2(2):109–15.
7. Vitolo U, Ferreri AJ, Zucca E. Primary testicular lymphoma. Crit Rev Oncol Hematol. 2008;65(2):183–9.

8. Horne MJ, Adeniran AJ. Primary diffuse large B-cell lymphoma of the testis. Arch Pathol Lab Med. 2011;135(10):1363–7.
9. Crellin AM, et al. Non-Hodgkin's lymphoma of the testis. Radiother Oncol. 1993;27(2):99–106.
10. Aviles A, et al. Testicular lymphoma: organ-specific treatment did not improve outcome. Oncology. 2004;67(3–4):211–4.
11. Mazloom A, et al. Outcome of patients with diffuse large B-cell lymphoma of the testis by era of treatment: the M. D. Anderson Cancer Center experience. Leuk Lymphoma. 2010;51(7):1217–24.
12. Zucca E, et al. Patterns of outcome and prognostic factors in primary large-cell lymphoma of the testis in a survey by the International Extranodal Lymphoma Study Group. J Clin Oncol. 2003;21(1):20–7.
13. Verma N, et al. Primary testicular lymphoma and AIDS. Ann Clin Lab Sci. 2010;40(1):75–9.
14. Barta SK, et al. Treatment factors affecting outcomes in HIV-associated non-Hodgkin lymphomas: a pooled analysis of 1546 patients. Blood. 2013;122(19):3251–62.
15. Booman M, et al. Primary testicular diffuse large B-cell lymphomas have activated B-cell-like subtype characteristics. J Pathol. 2006;210(2):163–71.
16. Li D, Xie P, Mi C. Primary testicular diffuse large B-cell lymphoma shows an activated B-cell-like phenotype. Pathol Res Pract. 2010;206(9):611–5.
17. Al-Abbadi MA, et al. Primary testicular diffuse large B-cell lymphoma belongs to the nongerminal center B-cell-like subgroup: a study of 18 cases. Mod Pathol. 2006;19(12):1521–7.
18. Kemmerling R, et al. Primary testicular lymphoma: a strictly homogeneous hematological disease? Oncol Rep. 2010;23(5):1261–7.
19. Hans CP, et al. Confirmation of the molecular classification of diffuse large B-cell lymphoma by immunohistochemistry using a tissue microarray. Blood. 2004;103(1):275–82.
20. Colomo L, et al. Clinical impact of the differentiation profile assessed by immunophenotyping in patients with diffuse large B-cell lymphoma. Blood. 2003;101(1):78–84.
21. Alizadeh AA, et al. Distinct types of diffuse large B-cell lymphoma identified by gene expression profiling. Nature. 2000;403(6769):503–11.
22. Davis RE, et al. Chronic active B-cell-receptor signalling in diffuse large B-cell lymphoma. Nature. 2010;463(7277):88–92.
23. Hu S, et al. MYC/BCL2 protein coexpression contributes to the inferior survival of activated B-cell subtype of diffuse large B-cell lymphoma and demonstrates high-risk gene expression signatures: a report from The International DLBCL Rituximab-CHOP Consortium Program. Blood. 2013;121(20):4021–31; quiz 4250.
24. Bernasconi B, et al. Gene translocations in testicular lymphomas. Leuk Lymphoma. 2014;55:1410–2.
25. Menter T, et al. Phenotype profiling of primary testicular diffuse large B-cell lymphomas. Hematol Oncol. 2014;32(2):72–81.
26. Ngo VN, et al. Oncogenically active MYD88 mutations in human lymphoma. Nature. 2011;470(7332):115–9.
27. Kraan W, et al. High prevalence of oncogenic MYD88 and CD79B mutations in diffuse large B-cell lymphomas presenting at immune-privileged sites. Blood Cancer J. 2013;3:e139.
28. Epstein AS, et al. Testis-isolated mantle cell lymphoma: a unique case. Clin Lymphoma Myeloma Leuk. 2011;11(5):439–41.
29. Licci S, Morelli L, Covello R. Primary mantle cell lymphoma of the testis. Ann Hematol. 2011;90(4):483–4.
30. Liang DN, et al. Extranodal nasal type natural killer/T-cell lymphoma of testis: report of seven cases with review of literature. Leuk Lymphoma. 2012;53(6):1117–23.
31. Jun HJ, et al. Orbital infiltration as the first site of relapse of primary testicular T-cell lymphoma. Cancer Res Treat. 2007;39(1):40–3.
32. Kuper-Hommel MJ, et al. Clinical and pathological features of testicular diffuse large B-cell lymphoma: a heterogeneous disease. Leuk Lymphoma. 2012;53(2):242–6.
33. Lagmay J, et al. Primary testicular presentation of ALK-1-negative anaplastic large cell lymphoma in a pediatric patient. J Pediatr Hematol Oncol. 2009;31(5):330–2.
34. Bacon CM, et al. Primary follicular lymphoma of the testis and epididymis in adults. Am J Surg Pathol. 2007;31(7):1050–8.
35. Finn LS, et al. Primary follicular lymphoma of the testis in childhood. Cancer. 1999;85(7):1626–35.
36. Pakzad K, et al. Follicular large cell lymphoma localized to the testis in children. J Urol. 2002;168(1):225–8.
37. Pileri SA, et al. Primary follicular lymphoma of the testis in childhood: an entity with peculiar clinical and molecular characteristics. J Clin Pathol. 2002;55(9):684–8.
38. Liu Q, et al. Follicular lymphomas in children and young adults: a comparison of the pediatric variant with usual follicular lymphoma. Am J Surg Pathol. 2013;37(3):333–43.
39. Heller KN, et al. Primary follicular lymphoma of the testis: excellent outcome following surgical resection without adjuvant chemotherapy. J Pediatr Hematol Oncol. 2004;26(2):104–7.
40. Dunn GP, et al. Cancer immunoediting: from immunosurveillance to tumor escape. Nat Immunol. 2002;3(11):991–8.
41. Thompsett AR, et al. V(H) gene sequences from primary central nervous system lymphomas indicate derivation from highly mutated germinal center B cells with ongoing mutational activity. Blood. 1999;94(5):1738–46.

42. Booman M, et al. Mechanisms and effects of loss of human leukocyte antigen class II expression in immune-privileged site-associated B-cell lymphoma. Clin Cancer Res. 2006;12(9):2698–705.
43. Riemersma SA, et al. Extensive genetic alterations of the HLA region, including homozygous deletions of HLA class II genes in B-cell lymphomas arising in immune-privileged sites. Blood. 2000;96(10): 3569–77.
44. Bart J, et al. An oncological view on the blood-testis barrier. Lancet Oncol. 2002;3(6):357–63.
45. Mital P, Hinton BT, Dufour JM. The blood-testis and blood-epididymis barriers are more than just their tight junctions. Biol Reprod. 2011;84(5):851–8.
46. Fijak M, Bhushan S, Meinhardt A. Immunoprivileged sites: the testis. Methods Mol Biol. 2011;677: 459–70.
47. Domanska UM, et al. A review on CXCR4/CXCL12 axis in oncology: no place to hide. Eur J Cancer. 2013;49(1):219–30.
48. Chapuy B, et al. Actionable genetic features of primary testicular and primary central nervous system lymphomas in ASH Annual Meeting Abstracts. 2014.
49. Moorjani V, et al. Sonographic appearance of primary testicular lymphoma. AJR Am J Roentgenol. 1991;157(6):1225–6.
50. Srisuwan T, et al. Clinics in diagnostic imaging (134). Testicular lymphoma. Singapore Med J. 2011;52(3): 204–8.
51. Tsili AC, et al. Primary diffuse large B-cell testicular lymphoma: magnetic resonance imaging findings. Andrologia. 2012;44 Suppl 1:845–7.
52. Ponti G, et al. The impact of histopathologic diagnosis on the proper management of testis neoplasms. Nat Clin Pract Oncol. 2008;5(10):619–22.
53. Benevolo G, et al. Final results of a multicenter trial addressing role of CSF flow cytometric analysis in NHL patients at high risk for CNS dissemination. Blood. 2012;120(16):3222–8.
54. Muniesa C, et al. Primary cutaneous diffuse large B-cell lymphoma, leg type and secondary cutaneous involvement by testicular B-cell lymphoma share identical clinicopathological and immunophenotypical features. J Am Acad Dermatol. 2012;66(4): 650–4.
55. Rosenberg SA. Validity of the Ann Arbor staging classification for the non-Hodgkin's lymphomas. Cancer Treat Rep. 1977;61(6):1023–7.
56. Lagrange JL, et al. Non-Hodgkin's lymphoma of the testis: a retrospective study of 84 patients treated in the French anticancer centres. Ann Oncol. 2001;12(9):1313–9.
57. Go RS, Gundrum JD. Uncertainty and discordance in the staging and prognosis of diffuse large B-cell lymphoma with isolated bilateral testicular involvement. Am J Hematol. 2009;84(11):762–3.
58. Wittekind C, et al. UICC-TNM Supplement. A commentary on uniform use (second edition). 2nd ed. New York: Wiley-Liss Publishers; 2001.
59. Vitolo U, et al. First-line treatment for primary testicular diffuse large B-cell lymphoma with rituximab-CHOP, CNS prophylaxis, and contralateral testis irradiation: final results of an international phase II trial. J Clin Oncol. 2011;29(20):2766–72.
60. Wang Y, et al. Three prognostic factors influence clinical outcomes of primary testicular lymphoma. Tumour Biol. 2013;34(1):55–63.
61. Cao B, et al. A clinical analysis of primary testicular diffuse large B-cell lymphoma in China. Hematology. 2011;16(5):291–7.
62. Ferry JA, et al. Malignant lymphoma of the testis, epididymis, and spermatic cord. A clinicopathologic study of 69 cases with immunophenotypic analysis. Am J Surg Pathol. 1994;18(4):376–90.
63. Park B-B, et al. Consideration of aggressive therapeutic strategies for primary testicular lymphoma. Am J Hematol. 2007;82(9):840–5.
64. Telio D, et al. Diffuse large B-cell lymphoma with testicular involvement: outcome and risk of CNS relapse in the rituximab era. ASH Annu Meet Abstr. 2011;118(21):780.
65. Touroutoglou N, et al. Testicular lymphoma: late relapses and poor outcome despite doxorubicin-based therapy. J Clin Oncol. 1995;13(6):1361–7.
66. Buskirk SJ, et al. Primary lymphoma of the testis. Int J Radiat Oncol Biol Phys. 1982;8(10):1699–703.
67. Tondini C, et al. Diffuse large-cell lymphoma of the testis. J Clin Oncol. 1999;17(9):2854–8.
68. Connors JM, et al. Testicular lymphoma: improved outcome with early brief chemotherapy. J Clin Oncol. 1988;6(5):776–81.
69. Linassier C, et al. Stage I-IIE primary non-Hodgkin's lymphoma of the testis: results of a prospective trial by the GOELAMS Study Group. Clin Lymphoma. 2002;3(3):167–72.
70. Aviles A, et al. Rituximab and dose-dense chemotherapy in primary testicular lymphoma. Clin Lymphoma Myeloma. 2009;9(5):386–9.
71. Zhang LH, et al. Lenalidomide efficacy in activated B-cell-like subtype diffuse large B-cell lymphoma is dependent upon IRF4 and cereblon expression. Br J Haematol. 2013;160(4):487–502.
72. Wilson WH, et al. The Bruton's Tyrosine Kinase (BTK) inhibitor, ibrutinib (PCI-32765), has preferential activity in the ABC subtype of relapsed/refractory De Novo Diffuse Large B-Cell Lymphoma (DLBCL): interim results of a multicenter, open-label, phase 2 study. ASH Annu Meet Abstr. 2012;120(21):686.
73. Nowakowski GS, et al. Lenalidomide can be safely combined with R-CHOP (R2CHOP) in the initial chemotherapy for aggressive B-cell lymphomas: phase I study. Leukemia. 2011;25(12):1877–81.
74. Chiappella A, et al. Lenalidomide plus cyclophosphamide, doxorubicin, vincristine, prednisone and rituximab is safe and effective in untreated elderly diffuse large B-cell lymphoma patients: phase I study by the Fondazione Italiana Linfomi. Haematologica. 2013;98(11):1732–8.

75. Tilly H, et al. Phase 1b study of lenalidomide in combination with rituximab-CHOP (R2-CHOP) in patients with B-cell lymphoma. Leukemia. 2013;27(1):252–5.
76. Wang M, et al. Oral lenalidomide with rituximab in relapsed or refractory diffuse large cell, follicular and transformed lymphoma: a phase II clinical trial. Leukemia. 2013;27:1902–9.
77. Chen N, et al. Distribution of lenalidomide into semen of healthy men after multiple oral doses. J Clin Pharmacol. 2010;50(7):767–74.
78. Miyao K, et al. Testicular invading refractory multiple myeloma during bortezomib treatment successfully treated with lenalidomide: a case report. Ann Hematol. 2014;93(3):529–30.
79. Hernandez-Ilizaliturri FJ, et al. Immunomodulatory drug CC-5013 or CC-4047 and rituximab enhance antitumor activity in a severe combined immunodeficient mouse lymphoma model. Clin Cancer Res. 2005;11(16):5984–92.
80. Li Z, et al. Pomalidomide shows significant therapeutic activity against CNS lymphoma with a major impact on the tumor microenvironment in murine models. PLoS One. 2013;8(8):e71754.
81. Lam LT, et al. Cooperative signaling through the signal transducer and activator of transcription 3 and nuclear factor-{kappa}B pathways in subtypes of diffuse large B-cell lymphoma. Blood. 2008;111(7): 3701–13.
82. Lote K, Holte H, Kvaloy S. Testicular lymphoma is associated with a high risk of extranodal recurrence. Cancer. 2000;89(3):713–4.
83. Zhang J, Chen B, Xu X. Impact of rituximab on incidence of and risk factors for central nervous system relapse in patients with diffuse large B-cell lymphoma: a systematic review and meta-analysis. Leuk Lymphoma. 2013;0(ja):1–16.
84. Rubenstein JL, et al. Phase I study of intraventricular administration of rituximab in patients with recurrent CNS and intraocular lymphoma. J Clin Oncol. 2007;25(11):1350–6.
85. Siegal T, Goldschmidt N. CNS prophylaxis in diffuse large B-cell lymphoma: if, when, how and for whom? Blood Rev. 2012;26(3):97–106.
86. Balis FM, et al. Methotrexate distribution within the subarachnoid space after intraventricular and intravenous administration. Cancer Chemother Pharmacol. 2000;45(3):259–64.
87. Zylber-Katz E, et al. Pharmacokinetics of methotrexate in cerebrospinal fluid and serum after osmotic blood–brain barrier disruption in patients with brain lymphoma. Clin Pharmacol Ther. 2000;67(6):631–41.
88. Tilly H, et al. Intensive conventional chemotherapy (ACVBP regimen) compared with standard CHOP for poor-prognosis aggressive non-Hodgkin lymphoma. Blood. 2003;102(13):4284–9.
89. Holte H, et al. Dose-densified chemoimmunotherapy followed by systemic central nervous system prophylaxis for younger high-risk diffuse large B-cell/follicular grade 3 lymphoma patients: results of a phase II Nordic Lymphoma Group study. Ann Oncol. 2013;24(5):1385–92.
90. Abramson JS, et al. Intravenous methotrexate as central nervous system (CNS) prophylaxis is associated with a low risk of CNS recurrence in high-risk patients with diffuse large B-cell lymphoma. Cancer. 2010;116(18):4283–90.
91. Cheah CY, et al. A multicentre retrospective comparison of central nervous system prophylaxis strategies among patients with high-risk diffuse large B-cell lymphoma. Br J Cancer. 2014;111(6): 1072–9.
92. McMillan A, et al. Guideline on the prevention of secondary central nervous system lymphoma: British Committee for Standards in Haematology. Br J Haematol. 2013;163(2):168–81.
93. Greene-Schloesser D, et al. Radiation-induced brain injury: a review. Front Oncol. 2012;2:73.
94. Sussman EB, et al. Malignant lymphoma of the testis: a clinicopathologic study of 37 cases. J Urol. 1977;118(6):1004–7.
95. Connors JM. Problems in lymphoma management: special sites of presentation. Oncology (Williston Park). 1998;12(2):185–91; discussion 192–5.
96. Brouwer CL, et al. Scrotal irradiation in primary testicular lymphoma: review of the literature and in silico planning comparative study. Int J Radiat Oncol Biol Phys. 2013;85(2):298–308.
97. Conrad AL, Go RS. Contralateral testicular relapse after prophylactic radiation in a patient with primary testicular diffuse large B-cell lymphoma. Eur J Haematol. 2009;83(6):603–5.
98. Visco C, et al. Non-Hodgkin's lymphoma affecting the testis: is it curable with doxorubicin-based therapy? Clin Lymphoma. 2001;2(1):40–6.
99. Zietman AL, et al. The management and outcome of stage IAE non Hodgkin's lymphoma of the testis. J Urol. 1996;155(3):943–6.
100. Wirth A. The rationale and role of radiation therapy in the treatment of patients with diffuse large B-cell lymphoma in the Rituximab era. Leuk Lymphoma. 2007;48(11):2121–36.
101. Phan J, et al. Benefit of consolidative radiation therapy in patients with diffuse large B-cell lymphoma treated with R-CHOP chemotherapy. J Clin Oncol. 2010;28(27):4170–6.
102. Martelli M, et al. Diffuse large B-cell lymphoma. Crit Rev Oncol Hematol. 2013;87(2):146–71.
103. Held G, et al. Role of radiotherapy to bulky disease in elderly patients with aggressive B-cell lymphoma. J Clin Oncol. 2014;32(11):1112–8.
104. Illidge T, Specht L, Yahalom J, et al. Modern radiation therapy for nodal non-Hodgkin lymphoma-target definition and dose guidelines from the International Lymphoma Radiation Oncology Group. Int J Radiat Oncol Biol Phys. 2014;89(1):49–58.
105. Hoskin PJ, et al. Recommendations for the use of radiotherapy in nodal lymphoma. Clin Oncol (R Coll Radiol). 2013;25(1):49–58.

106. Shapiro E, et al. Effects of fractionated irradiation of endocrine aspects of testicular function. J Clin Oncol. 1985;3(9):1232–9.
107. Lowry L, et al. Reduced dose radiotherapy for local control in non-Hodgkin lymphoma: a randomised phase III trial. Radiother Oncol. 2011;100(1):86–92.
108. Shalet SM, et al. Vulnerability of the human Leydig cell to radiation damage is dependent upon age. J Endocrinol. 1989;120(1):161–5.
109. Petersen PM, et al. Effect of graded testicular doses of radiotherapy in patients treated for carcinoma-in-situ in the testis. J Clin Oncol. 2002;20(6):1537–43.

10 Radiation Therapy in the Management of Mantle Cell Lymphoma

Sarah A. Milgrom

Abstract

Mantle cell lymphoma (MCL) comprises 3–6 % of non-Hodgkin lymphoma cases, with an annual incidence of 0.5 per 100,000 in Western countries. It is an aggressive malignancy that is usually disseminated at diagnosis; therefore, chemotherapy is typically the backbone of treatment. However, MCL is exquisitely radiosensitive, and radiation therapy (RT) can be an important modality that contributes to cure in early-stage disease and provides durable palliation in advanced cases. In this chapter, patients with early- and advanced-stage MCL will be discussed, with a focus on the role of RT in management.

Background

Mantle cell lymphoma (MCL) comprises 3–6 % of non-Hodgkin lymphoma cases, with an annual incidence of 0.5 per 100,000 in Western countries [1]. It is an aggressive malignancy that is usually disseminated at diagnosis; therefore, chemotherapy is typically the backbone of treatment. However, MCL is exquisitely radiosensitive, and radiation therapy (RT) can be an important modality that contributes to cure in early-stage disease and provides durable palliation in advanced cases. In this chapter, patients with early- and advanced-stage MCL will be discussed, with a focus on the role of RT in management.

Early-Stage Mantle Cell Lymphoma

Clinical Presentation, Early-Stage Case

A healthy 69-year-old man was noted on a routine eye examination to have a pink growth extending along the inferior bulbar conjunctiva of the left eye (Fig. 10.1). The remaining ophthalmologic examination was normal. A biopsy of the conjunctival mass revealed a diagnosis of MCL. This patient is typical, with respect to demographics: the median age at diagnosis of MCL is 68 years, and the male-to-female ratio is 3:1 [1].

S.A. Milgrom, MD
Department of Radiation Oncology,
MD Anderson Cancer Center, 1515 Holcombe Blvd,
Houston, TX 77030, USA
e-mail: samilgrom@mdanderson.org

B.S. Dabaja, A.K. Ng (eds.), *Radiation Therapy in Hematologic Malignancies*,
DOI 10.1007/978-3-319-42615-0_10

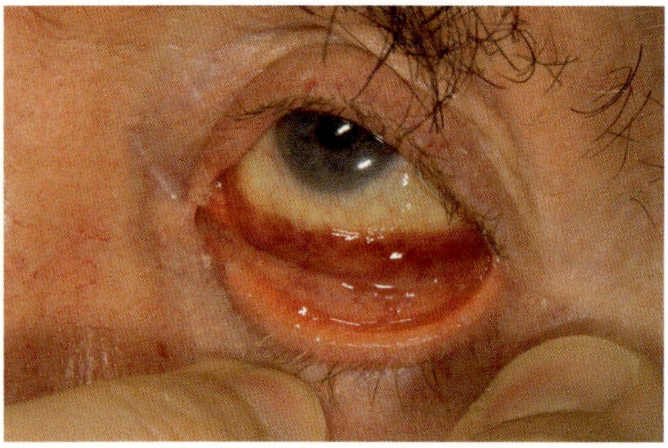

Fig. 10.1 MCL involving the inferior bulbar conjunctiva of the left eye

A careful history and physical examination was performed. The patient had an excellent performance status. He had no symptoms attributable to the eye. He denied constitutional symptoms of fever, night sweats, and weight loss. The conjunctival lesion was the only abnormality appreciated on physical examination. Special attention was paid to the nodal basins, liver, and spleen, all of which were unremarkable.

Pathology, Early-Stage Case

An incisional biopsy of the conjunctival mass was performed. It should be noted that a fine-needle aspiration is typically insufficient to make the diagnosis of MCL. The biopsy revealed a glandular epithelium, largely replaced by lymphocytes with features typical of MCL, which arises from immature B-cells. The neoplastic cells tend to be small to medium sized, with irregular nuclear contours, inconspicuous nucleoli, and scant cytoplasm.

This patient's neoplasm was noted to have a diffuse pattern of growth. Three histological patterns (mantle zone, nodular, and diffuse) and three cytological variants (classical, blastoid, and pleomorphic) have been described. Data suggest that these pathological differences correlate with clinical behavior, for example, pleomorphic and blastoid variants demonstrate a particularly aggressive course [1, 2].

The immunohistochemistry results for this case were typical for MCL. The cells were positive for B-cell markers (including CD19, CD20, and PAX5), CD5, CD43, and cyclin D1; they were negative for CD10 and CD23. The translocation t(11;14) was detected by fluorescent in situ hybridization (FISH). This genetic anomaly is regarded as the primary genetic event in MCL. It places the cyclin D1 gene downstream of the IgH promoter, resulting in the overexpression of cyclin D1 and consequent accelerated passage through the cell cycle [1]. It should be noted, however, that a small subset of MCL cases is negative for the t(11;14) translocation and for cyclin D1 overexpression [3, 4]. A proportion of these cases bear translocations involving cyclin D2 and cyclin D3 [5, 6]. SOX11 expression may be useful for the identification of the cyclin D1-negative subtype [7].

Staging and Prognostic Factors, Early-Stage Case

A complete staging evaluation was performed. Bloodwork, including a complete blood count (CBC) with differential, comprehensive metabolic panel (CMP), β_2-microglobulin, and lactate dehydrogenase (LDH), was within normal limits. A contrast-enhanced PET-CT scan revealed no other sites of disease. A bone marrow biopsy, which must be performed in all cases, was negative for lymphoma by histology and flow cytometry. An esophagogastroduodenoscopy and colonoscopy with random biopsies showed no evidence of lymphoma. Evaluation of the gastrointestinal tract is critical to establish the diagnosis of limited stage disease, as occult involvement by MCL is detected in the majority of patients [8]. CNS involvement is exceedingly rare; therefore, CSF analysis and neuroimaging should be reserved for patients with neurological symptoms, blastoid histology, or Ki-67 > 30% [9, 10]. Thus, in this patient, a complete staging evaluation, including bloodwork, PET-CT scan, bone marrow biopsy, and gastrointestinal endoscopy, confirmed that his disease was limited to the left conjunctiva.

Only 10 % of MCL cases are early stage at diagnosis [11]. Anytime the diagnosis of localized MCL is suspected, a thorough evaluation must be performed to exclude the presence of occult systemic disease. The proportion of patients diagnosed with limited stage disease has been decreasing over time, likely due to more sensitive assays of the bone marrow and more frequent evaluation of the gastrointestinal tract, both of which are commonly involved by disease [11, 12].

As observed in this case, extranodal disease is common in MCL. The most frequently involved sites are the gastrointestinal tract, head and neck, and reticuloendothelial system. Less commonly involved extranodal sites include the lung, skin, musculoskeletal system, and breast. Data suggest that the primary site of disease involvement is a predictor of survival. For example, patients with primary disease of the head and neck have superior survival, compared to those with primary nodal disease ($P<0.001$) [13].

Treatment and Management, Early-Stage Case

For his stage IAE MCL of the left conjunctiva, this patient was treated with three cycles of R-CHOP (rituximab, cyclophosphamide, doxorubicin, vincristine, and prednisone). He had a complete clinical and radiographic response to chemotherapy. Then, he received consolidative RT to the initially involved site.

Because early-stage MCL is rare, data regarding its management and outcomes are limited. A large series, reported by the International Lymphoma Radiation Oncology Group (ILROG), consists of 160 stage I–II MCL patients treated at 13 institutions. The majority of patients (59 %) received chemotherapy followed by consolidative RT. The remaining patients were treated with chemotherapy alone (23 %) or definitive RT alone (18 %). The most common chemotherapy regimen was R-CHOP or R-CHOP-like, and RT was to a median dose of 35 Gy (range 12–45 Gy). The authors reported favorable outcomes for the cohort, irrespective of the modality of treatment given, with disease-free and overall survival rates of 65 and 76 % at 5 years and of 44 % and 63 % at 10 years, respectively [14]. These findings demonstrate that patients with limited stage MCL can achieve long-term disease control even with radiation therapy alone and de-escalation of therapy should be considered in early-stage presentation.

A smaller series from the British Columbia Cancer Agency suggests an important role of RT in the management of limited stage MCL. The authors reported on 26 patients with non-bulky-stage IA–IIA MCL. They observed superior progression-free survival in patients whose initial therapy consisted of RT ± chemotherapy, when compared to those who did not receive RT (68 % vs. 11 % at 5 years, $P=0.002$). Furthermore, there was a trend toward improved overall survival (71 % vs. 25 % at 6 years, $P=0.13$). All patients with PFS beyond 6 years had received RT as a part of their upfront management [15]. ILROG trial.

Researchers from Princess Margaret Hospital reported on 21 patients with stage I–II MCL who were managed with curative intent. Among the 17 patients treated with a combination of chemotherapy (typically CHOP or R-CHOP) and RT (median 35 Gy), the overall response rate was 100 % (15 complete response, 1 unconfirmed complete response, 1 partial response). For five patients, a partial or unconfirmed complete response after chemotherapy was transformed to a complete response after RT. Local control was maintained in all but one patient, whose disease relapsed both locally and distantly. Distant relapse was common. The 5-year progression-free survival rate was 43.8 %, with a median time to event of 3.2 years. The median overall survival time was 6.4 years [16]. It is worth to mention that these patients were subsequently included in the aforementioned ILROG study.

Lastly, an analysis using the National Cancer Database (NCDB) assessed outcomes of early-stage MCL. The authors identified 2539 patients with stage I–II MCL. Of these, 70 % were treated with chemotherapy alone, 11 % with RT alone, and 19 % with a combination of chemotherapy and RT. Patients who received combined modality therapy experienced significantly better overall survival than patients treated with either chemotherapy or RT alone (3-year overall survival 79.8 % for chemotherapy + RT, 67.8 % for chemotherapy alone, 72.4 % for RT alone, $P<0.001$). After correction for indication bias through inverse probability treatment weighting, combined modality therapy was found to reduce the risk of overall mortality compared with monotherapy (hazard ratio 0.65, $P=0.029$) [17].

Taken together, these studies suggest that the incorporation of RT into management is associated with improved outcomes in limited stage MCL. Patients who are fit should receive chemoimmunotherapy followed by consolidative RT. RT alone is appropriate in patients considered unsuitable for systemic therapy [1].

Radiation Field, Dose, and Technique, Early-Stage Case

In this case, consolidative RT targeted the entire left conjunctiva. Technique varies between institutions, some uses electron, and others use photon with intensity-modulated radiation therapy (IMRT). In case 1, treatment was delivered using a single appositional 16-MeV electron beam. The total dose of 24 Gy was given at 2 Gy per fraction (Fig. 10.2a). Custom skin collimation was used to sharpen the penumbra and protect adjacent structures; in this case since we used 16 MeV, the eyelid served as a bolus, and patient was treated with closed eyes. It should be looked at on a case-by-case basis to make sure that the target is well covered. It is also felt that when the conjunctiva is involved, the whole orbit has to be treated as opposed to when the lacrimal gland is involved, only targeting the lacrimal gland is acceptable.

The step of planning starts with the simulation where the physician outlines the tentative area of interest using CT wires; this area can be later easily identified by the planning team as the presumed edge of the skin collimation. CT simulation scan will be obtained, the eye will be contoured as the CTV, and plan will be generated taking into consideration that a skin collimation will be used. At the same time, the skin collimation making will start as follows: an aquaplast material is used to template the face and the eye during the simulation (Fig. 10.2b) and will be used as the negative to produce a clay material (Fig. 10.2c 1, 2, 3), the skin collimation will be drawn on the clay by the physician, and the shape of the skin collimation will be copied from the skin rendering from the treatment planning system (Fig. 10.2d). The skin collimation thickness will be produced according to the electron energy used. It is advisable on day one to verify with the area treated by applying the skin collimation and generating the field using CT wires and rerun the plan on the new scan to make sure we are not missing the target (Fig. 10.2e).

The ILROG RT guidelines for nodal and extranodal non-Hodgkin lymphomas are a valuable reference for the radiation oncologist treating MCL [18, 19]. As described in the guidelines, an involved site RT (ISRT) approach should be used, in which the gross tumor volume (GTV) equates to the clinically and radiographically evident tumor, the clinical target volume (CTV) encompasses the GTV as well as potential sites of microscopic disease, the internal target volume (ITV) considers uncertainties in position of the CTV within the patient, and the planning target volume (PTV) accounts for differences in patient positioning with each treatment. In patients treated with consolidative RT after a complete response to chemotherapy, RT should target the pre-chemotherapy site of disease, taking into consideration changes in anatomy following disease response. In patients who are not candidates for or decline chemotherapy, RT may be used as a single modality; in this setting, a more generous area may be irradiated to account for adjacent microscopic disease.

MCL responds to low RT doses. M'kacher et al. demonstrated the exquisite radiosensitivity of MCL cells in vitro [20]. These findings have been supported by clinical experience. When RT is used with curative intent, a dose of 24–30 Gy is recommended in most cases; however, as described below, lower doses may be preferable in certain settings [18].

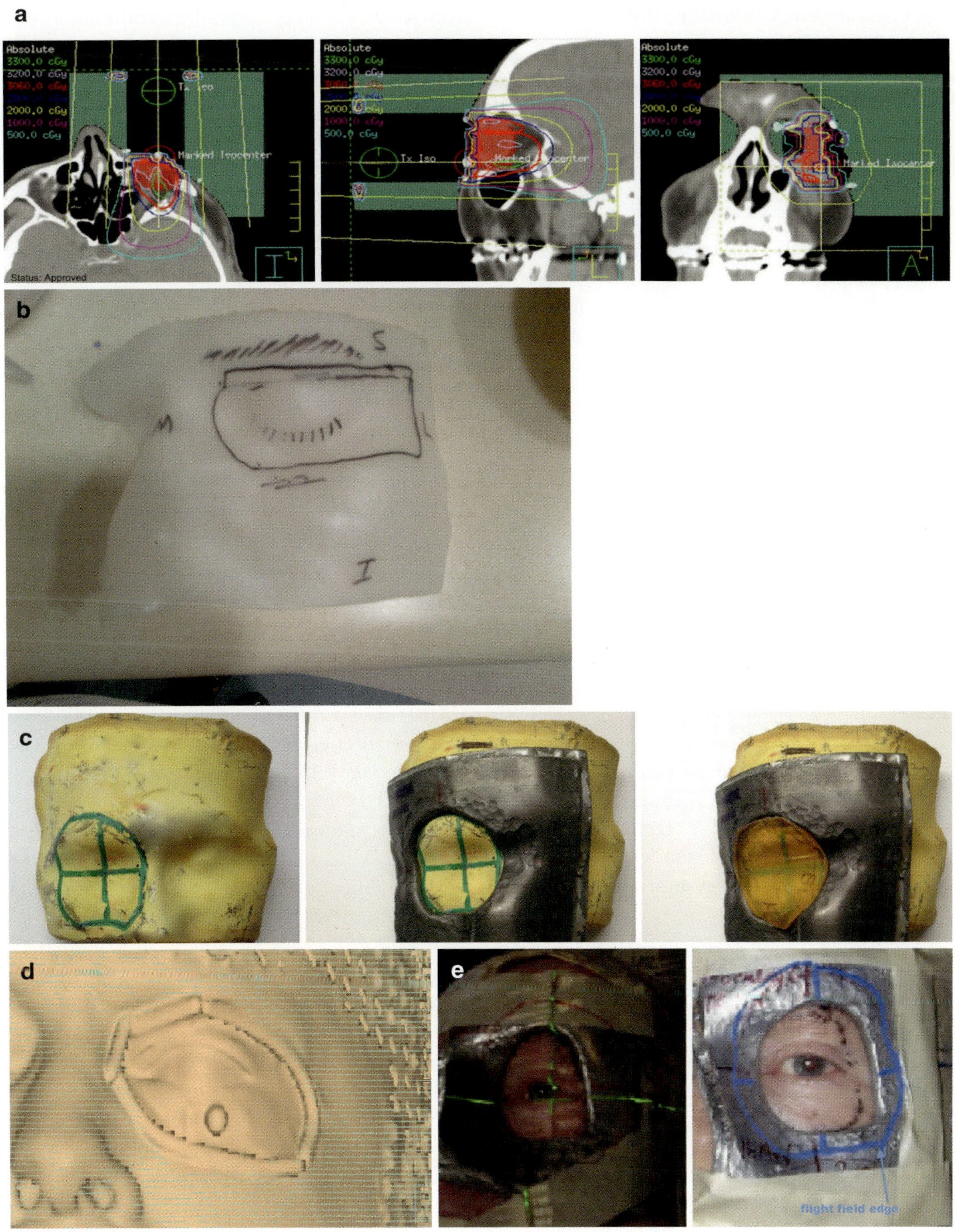

Fig. 10.2 (**a**) Axial, sagittal, and coronal slices from an RT plan that targeted the left conjunctiva, using a single appositional 16-MeV electron beam. The total dose of 24 Gy was given at 2 Gy per fraction. Custom skin collimation was used to reduce penumbra and protect adjacent structures. (**b**) Aquaplast mold used to template the face. (**c**) Clay mold showing how to mark for the skin collimation (1), the skin collimation (2), and (3) the bolus added to bring the dose superficially. (**d**) Skin rendering used to mark the skin collimation on the clay mold. (**e**) Patient daily setup

Posttreatment Considerations, Early-Stage Case

This patient developed dryness and irritation of the eye near the end of RT. His symptoms responded well to lubricating eye drops and had improved significantly by 1 month after treatment.

After the completion of therapy, he was seen in routine follow-up every 3–6 months for 5 years, and annually thereafter. Each follow-up visit included a history and physical examination, bloodwork (including a CBC, CMP, and LDH), and a contrast-enhanced CT scan of the neck, chest, abdomen, and pelvis. Six years after the completion of treatment, this patient remained clinically and radiographically without evidence of disease.

Advanced-Stage Mantle Cell Lymphoma

Clinical Presentation, Advanced-Stage Case 1

A 69-year-old man presented with a sore throat. He was prescribed several courses of antibiotics, which did not provide relief. Ultimately, he was referred to an otolaryngologist, who appreciated an oropharyngeal mass. A biopsy of the mass confirmed MCL.

The patient had an excellent performance status. His only symptom was throat pain. He denied fevers, night sweats, and weight loss. A physical examination was notable for lymphadenopathy of the neck, axillae, and inguinal regions. The largest node, in the left neck, measured 6 cm. No hepatosplenomegaly was appreciated.

Pathology, Advanced-Stage Case 1

This patient's oropharyngeal biopsy revealed MCL, blastoid variant. The pharyngeal mucosa was extensively replaced by lymphoma. The neoplastic cells were positive for CD5, CD20, PAX5, and cyclin D1; they were negative for CD10. The anti-Ki-67 antibody showed a proliferation rate of 90%. Translocation t(11;14) was detected by FISH.

Blastoid or blastic variant MCL describes cases with a homogeneous population of cells displaying lymphoblastic morphology. It represents 10–15% of MCL cases. Patients with blastoid variant MCL experience particularly short durations of response after chemotherapy and poor overall survival [2].

Staging and Prognostic Factors, Advanced-Stage Case 1

A complete staging evaluation was remarkable for an elevated white blood cell count (WBC, 19,000/μL) and LDH level (1400 IU/L). A PET scan showed a hypermetabolic mass involving the oropharynx and multi-compartmental adenopathy above and below the diaphragm. A bone marrow biopsy revealed involvement by disease, with MCL comprising 10% of the cellularity.

The MCL International Prognostic Index (MIPI) is a validated prognostic stratification tool for patients with advanced-stage MCL. The formula takes into account age, performance status, LDH level, and WBC to divide patients into low-, intermediate-, and high-risk groups, which have markedly different outcomes. In the initial publication, the median survival of the high-risk group was 29 months, of the intermediate-risk group was 51 months, and of the low-risk group had not been reached at a median follow-up of 32 months (5-year overall survival rate of the low-risk group was 60%) [21, 22]. Variations of the MIPI have been introduced. The simplified MIPI is calculable at the bedside, with similar concordance but lower discriminatory power. The biologic MIPI incorporates the Ki-67 proliferation index, which improves the discriminatory power for progression-free survival [23]. These scores may be used to develop individualized, risk-adapted treatment plans. These formulas placed this patient in the high-risk category, so his outcome was expected to be poor, and aggressive management was indicated.

Treatment and Management, Advanced-Stage Case 1

For his high-risk disease, this patient received induction treatment with four cycles of rituximab and dose intensified CHOP (maxi-CHOP) alternating with rituximab and high-dose cytarabine. His disease responded completely. Then, he underwent autologous stem cell transplantation (ASCT) with a conditioning regimen of carmustine, etoposide, cytarabine, and melphalan (BEAM). This regimen, published by the Nordic Lymphoma Group [24], is one of a variety of approaches used to intensify therapy and improve outcomes in MCL.

CHOP chemotherapy, used historically to treat MCL, was associated with poor outcomes. Early studies demonstrated that the addition of rituximab to CHOP improved the overall response rate (94 % vs. 75 %), complete response rate (34 % vs. 7 %), and median time to treatment failure (21 months vs. 14 months); however, no improvement was observed in progression-free survival (25 % at 2 years) or overall survival (76 % at 2 years) [25]. Given these poor outcomes, intensification of therapy has been studied. One approach that has demonstrated promising outcomes is first-line consolidation with high-dose chemotherapy (HDC) and ASCT. Multiple groups have reported their favorable experiences [26, 27]. As one example, the Nordic group published the regimen that was used to treat this patient. In their trial, MCL patients who responded to induction therapy with rituximab and maxi-CHOP alternating with high-dose cytarabine were subsequently consolidated with HDC/ASCT. This regimen resulted in excellent 6-year progression-free and overall survival rates of 66 % and 70 %, respectively [24]. Further follow-up showed an impressive median event-free and overall survival of 7.4 years and over 10 years, respectively [28]. An alternative approach that does not incorporate ASCT is rituximab in combination with fractionated cyclophosphamide, vincristine, doxorubicin, and dexamethasone (hyper-CVAD), alternating with high-dose methotrexate and cytarabine (R-hyper-CVAD/MA). This intensive regimen has yielded favorable outcomes. For example, in the SWOG 0213 study, R-hyper-CVAD/MA was associated with a median progression-free survival of 4.8 years and overall survival of 6.8 years; the 2-year progression-free and overall survival rates were 63 % and 76 %, respectively [29].

This patient tolerated intensified chemotherapy and ASCT well. However, 3 weeks after ASCT, he developed rapidly progressive oropharyngeal swelling. A tonsillar biopsy confirmed refractory MCL. Of note, in the Nordic Study, high MIPI score and Ki-67 expression level were independent predictors of poor outcome [28]. This patient had both of these risk factors.

He was referred to Radiation Oncology for consideration of palliative irradiation of his oropharyngeal disease. At the time of consultation, he had severe dysphagia, necessitating that he grinds his food and preventing him from swallowing pills. His voice had a muffled quality. Physical examination revealed significant tonsillar swelling and bilateral cervical adenopathy. There was no trismus or limitation of tongue mobility. Small, firm bilateral neck nodes were appreciable. No other site of adenopathy or hepatosplenomegaly was appreciated. A contrast-enhanced CT scan confirmed enlargement of the palatine and lingual tonsils, as well as bilateral neck adenopathy (Fig. 10.3a).

Radiation Field, Dose, and Technique, Advanced-Stage Case 1

RT was started urgently to address this patient's rapidly progressive oropharyngeal disease. Initially, he was treated with opposed lateral beams to a total dose of 7.5 Gy in 3 fractions (see Fig. 10.3b). After completing this initial phase of therapy, his voice had returned to normal, he was able to swallow solid foods, and a CT scan revealed a reduction in tonsillar swelling (Fig. 10.3c). Then, his treatment was continued with intensity-modulated RT (IMRT) to minimize dose to the adjacent salivary glands (Fig. 10.3d). He received an additional 16 Gy in 8 fractions, using IMRT. Thus, the oropharynx was treated to a total dose of 23.5 Gy. At the

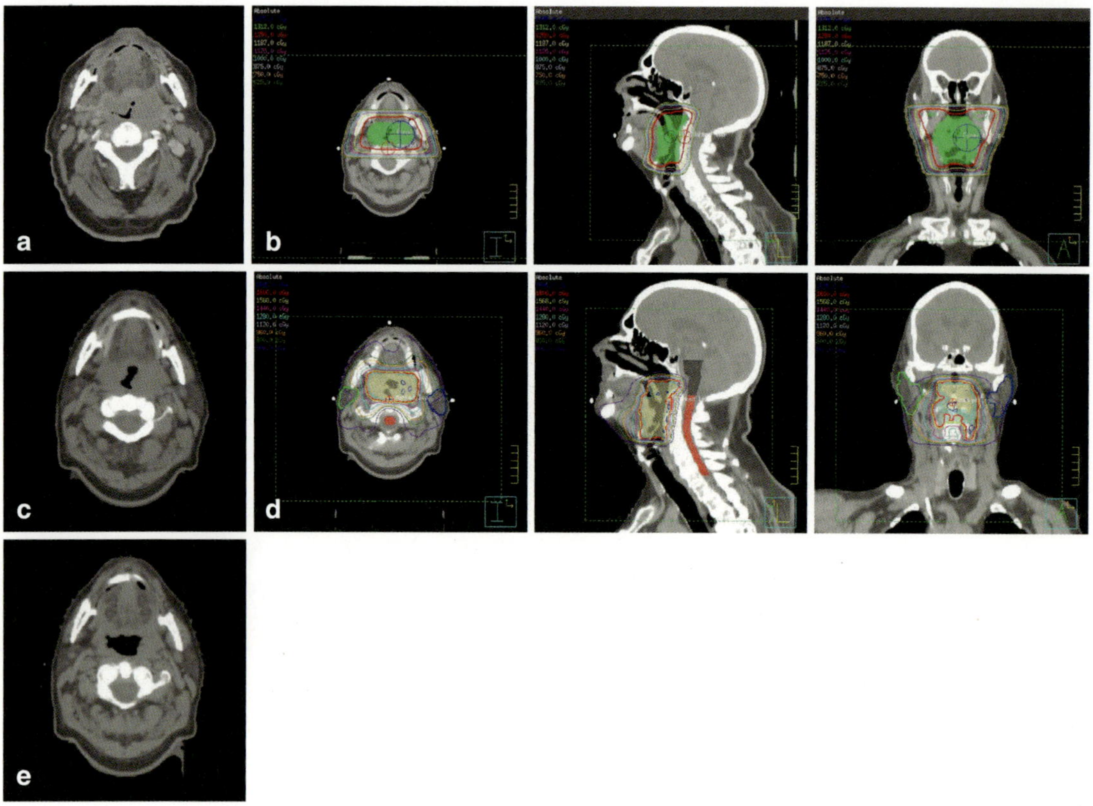

Fig. 10.3 (**a**) A contrast-enhanced CT scan demonstrating the enlargement of the palatine and lingual tonsils and bilateral neck adenopathy. A tonsillar biopsy confirmed MCL. (**b**) Axial, sagittal, and coronal slices from an opposed lateral beam RT plan. Treatment with this plan was initiated urgently to deliver a total dose of 7.5 Gy, at 2.5 Gy per fraction, for this patient's rapidly progressive oropharyngeal disease. (**c**) A non-contrast CT scan performed after the initial phase of RT (7.5 Gy) demonstrated a therapeutic response. (**d**) Axial, sagittal, and coronal slices from an intensity-modulated RT (IMRT) plan that was used to deliver an additional 16 Gy in 8 fractions. IMRT was used to minimize dose to the adjacent salivary glands. (**e**) A non-contrast CT scan performed after the completion of RT (23.5 Gy) demonstrated an excellent therapeutic response

completion of therapy, his symptoms had resolved completely. A CT scan revealed an excellent therapeutic response (Fig. 10.3e).

RT provides effective disease control in MCL, with relatively low doses. One group reported on 38 sites in 21 consecutive patients that were treated with RT to a mean dose of 30 Gy (range 10.5–45 Gy). The overall local response rate was 100 %, with a complete response obtained in 64 % of sites and partial response in 36 %. The average time to response was 20 days, with 78 % of sites demonstrating a response before RT was complete. Of the 16 sites that were initially symptomatic, 94 % exhibited palliation, most (87 %) before the completion of RT [30].

Another group confirmed these findings with a report of 68 sites in 39 patients that were treated with RT to a median dose of 30.6 Gy (range 18–40 Gy). The overall local response rate was 94 %. The response was complete in 69 % of sites and partial in 25 %. The majority of patients were treated with palliative intent, and 95 % of patients in this subgroup experienced symptomatic relief from RT. The authors emphasize that patients were heavily pretreated with chemotherapy, so RT provides benefit even in patients with chemorefractory disease. In this series, nine sites (13 %) exhibited local relapse in the previously irradiated area at a median of 7 months (range 2–21 months) after RT. The only factor that was associated with increased risk of relapse was large tumor size. No correlation was found with the radiation dose, suggesting that low doses are adequate, and no benefit is obtained from dose escalation [31].

The ILROG guidelines recommend a dose of 24–30 Gy for mantle cell lymphoma [18]. This dose should be used when RT is administered with definitive intent or with palliative intent in cases for which durable disease control is of major clinical concern. However, MCL is exquisitely radiosensitive, and lower doses may be indicated in some settings, as summarized in Advanced Case 2.

Posttreatment Considerations, Advanced-Stage Case 1

This patient experienced an excellent clinical and radiographic response to RT. He did experience acute grade 2 mucositis, which was managed with sucralfate and magic mouthwash.

Despite the dramatic local response to RT, this patient's prognosis is poor. In general, patients with MCL that have relapsed after ASCT experience a median overall survival of 19 months, with significantly inferior survival ($P<0.001$) observed in those with a short (<12 months) interval between ASCT and relapse, as observed in this case [32].

For his refractory disease, this patient was started on salvage rituximab and ibrutinib. There is no standard therapy for relapsed/refractory MCL; multiple chemo-immunotherapy regimens have been explored, but durable disease control has been difficult to achieve. Ibrutinib, a small-molecule inhibitor of Bruton's tyrosine kinase (BTK), has shown a promising activity. A multicenter phase II study evaluating ibrutinib in patients with relapsed or refractory MCL reported an overall response rate of 68 %, with a complete response in 21 % of patients. The median duration of response was 17.5 months, median progression-free survival was 14 months, and estimated overall survival rate at 18 months was 58 % [33].

Other regimens that have been studied in the relapsed/refractory setting include rituximab, gemcitabine, and oxaliplatin [34]; rituximab, dexamethasone, cytarabine, and cisplatin (R-DHAP) [35]; R-hyper-CVAD/MA [36]; rituximab, fludarabine, cyclophosphamide, and mitoxantrone [37]; and bendamustine and rituximab (BR) [38]. These regimens typically yield an initial response but only short-term disease control, with a median progression-free survival of <2 years. Initial data suggest that the consolidation of salvage therapy with allogeneic stem cell transplantation results in the best outcomes [32].

Clinical Presentation, Advanced-Stage Case 2

A 73-year-old man presented with a progressive, firm right axillary mass. A CT scan revealed axillary, mediastinal, and retroperitoneal adenopathy. A biopsy of the axillary mass demonstrated MCL. The patient had a good performance status and denied fevers, night sweats, and weight loss. His physical examination was remarkable for multi-station adenopathy, above and below the diaphragm.

Pathology, Advanced-Stage Case 2

The pathologic findings of the axillary nodal biopsy were typical of MCL. Histological sections revealed lymphoid tissue with complete effacement of the architecture by small- to medium-sized lymphoid cells with irregular nuclear contours. By immunohistochemistry, the cells were positive for CD5, CD20, and cyclin D1. They were negative for CD10. Approximately 40 % of cells were positive for Ki-67.

Staging and Prognostic Factors, Advanced-Stage Case 2

A complete staging evaluation revealed a normal WBC (5600/μL) and LDH (613 IU/L). A PET scan showed hypermetabolic adenopathy above

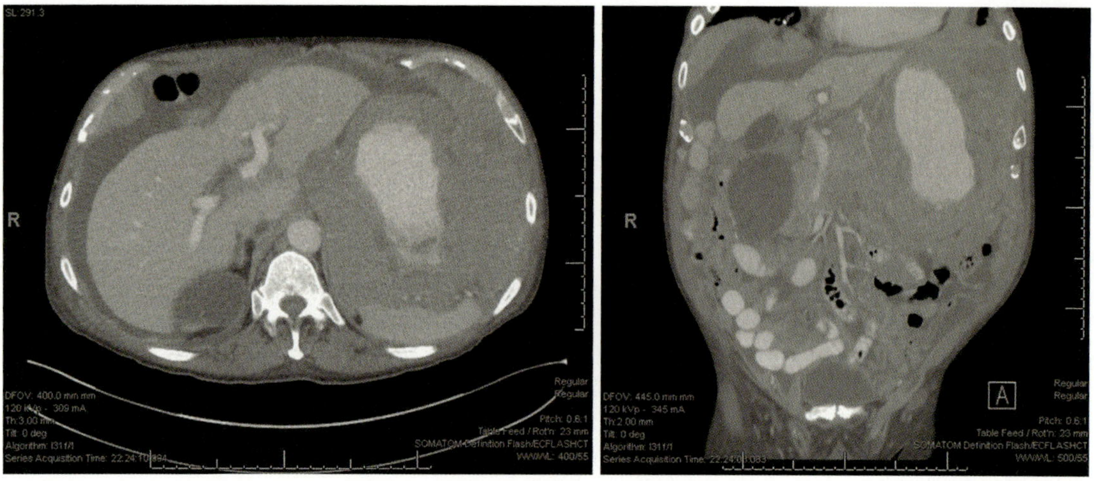

Fig. 10.4 A contrast-enhanced CT scan demonstrating extensive MCL throughout the abdomen and pelvis. Findings include gastric wall thickening, adenopathy, peritoneal implants, and ascites

and below the diaphragm. The gastric wall was diffusely thickened and hypermetabolic. FDG-avid masses were seen throughout the peritoneal cavity. A bilateral bone marrow biopsy showed no morphologic, immunohistochemical, or flow cytometric support for MCL.

This patient's biologic MIPI placed him in the high-risk group.

Treatment and Management, Advanced-Stage Case 2

For his advanced-stage MCL, this patient was treated initially with ibrutinib and rituximab, on a protocol assessing this regimen in the frontline setting. After 2 months, this therapy was discontinued, due to disease progression and side effects. Then, he was started on rituximab, bortezomib, and lenalidomide, agents that have shown activity in relapsed or refractory MCL [39–43]. His disease continued to progress rapidly, and his performance status declined. His intra-abdominal disease became quite symptomatic, causing significant distension, discomfort, and early satiety. A CT scan of the abdomen and pelvis revealed increased thickening of the diffusely infiltrated gastric wall, extensive adenopathy, increased peritoneal implants, and underlying ascites (Fig. 10.4). Paracenteses did not provide relief. Ascitic fluid contained MCL cells. The patient was referred to Radiation Oncology for consideration of palliative treatment of his abdominopelvic disease.

Radiation Field, Dose, and Technique, Advanced-Stage Case 2

The patient was treated with 4 Gy, at 2 Gy per fraction, to the abdomen and pelvis, using AP-PA 18-MV photon beams (Fig. 10.5). Similar to the indolent non-Hodgkin lymphomas, MCL is exquisitely radiosensitive. High local response rates are achieved with a dose of just 4 Gy, even in patients with chemorefractory disease [44, 45]. This treatment is well tolerated and more convenient than protracted dosing schedules. This "boom boom" RT is useful when a durable response is less critical or when normal tissue tolerance precludes the use of higher doses.

Posttreatment Considerations, Advanced-Stage Case 2

The patient tolerated RT extremely well. Within 1 week after the completion of therapy, he reported an improvement in the symptoms associated with his intra-abdominal disease. His

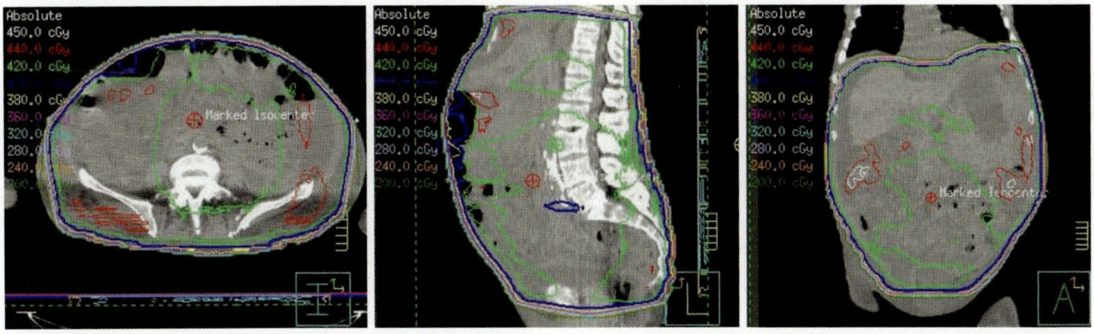

Fig. 10.5 Axial, sagittal, and coronal slices from an 18-MV photon AP-PA treatment plan that was used to deliver 4 Gy, at 2 Gy per fraction to the abdomen and pelvis

prognosis remained poor, but he achieved effective palliation.

Conclusions

Typically, MCL demonstrates aggressive clinical behavior and is disseminated at the time of diagnosis. However, the neoplastic cells are exquisitely radiosensitive, responding rapidly to low radiation doses. Therefore, RT is an important treatment modality that can contribute to cure and provide palliation. Indications for RT include consolidation therapy after initial chemotherapy in localized MCL and palliative therapy in the setting of advanced disease. The radiation oncologist should be aware of the significant benefit that MCL patients can derive from RT.

References

1. Cheah CY, Seymour JF, Wang ML. Mantle cell lymphoma. J Clin Oncol Off J Am Soc Clin Oncol. 2016; 34(11):1256–1269.
2. Bernard M, Gressin R, Lefrere F, Drenou B, Branger B, Caulet-Maugendre S, et al. Blastic variant of mantle cell lymphoma: a rare but highly aggressive subtype. Leukemia. 2001;15(11):1785–91.
3. Pileri SA, Falini B. Mantle cell lymphoma. Haematologica. 2009;94(11):1488–92.
4. de Boer CJ, van Krieken JH, Schuuring E, Kluin PM. Bcl-1/cyclin D1 in malignant lymphoma. Ann Oncol Off J Eur Soc Med Oncol/ESMO. 1997;8 Suppl 2:109–17.
5. Gesk S, Klapper W, Martin-Subero JI, Nagel I, Harder L, Fu K, et al. A chromosomal translocation in cyclin D1-negative/cyclin D2-positive mantle cell lymphoma fuses the CCND2 gene to the IGK locus. Blood. 2006;108(3):1109–10.
6. Fu K, Weisenburger DD, Greiner TC, Dave S, Wright G, Rosenwald A, et al. Cyclin D1-negative mantle cell lymphoma: a clinicopathologic study based on gene expression profiling. Blood. 2005;106(13):4315–21.
7. Mozos A, Royo C, Hartmann E, De Jong D, Baro C, Valera A, et al. SOX11 expression is highly specific for mantle cell lymphoma and identifies the cyclin D1-negative subtype. Haematologica. 2009;94(11): 1555–62.
8. Romaguera JE, Medeiros LJ, Hagemeister FB, Fayad LE, Rodriguez MA, Pro B, et al. Frequency of gastrointestinal involvement and its clinical significance in mantle cell lymphoma. Cancer. 2003;97(3):586–91.
9. Cheah CY, George A, Gine E, Chiappella A, Kluin-Nelemans HC, Jurczak W, et al. Central nervous system involvement in mantle cell lymphoma: clinical features, prognostic factors and outcomes from the European Mantle Cell Lymphoma Network. Ann Oncol Off J Eur Soc Med Oncol/ESMO. 2013;24(8):2119–23.
10. Chihara D, Asano N, Ohmachi K, Nishikori M, Okamoto M, Sawa M, et al. Ki-67 is a strong predictor of central nervous system relapse in patients with mantle cell lymphoma (MCL). Ann Oncol Off J Eur Soc Med Oncol/ESMO. 2015;26(5):966–73.
11. Chandran R, Gardiner SK, Simon M, Spurgeon SE. Survival trends in mantle cell lymphoma in the United States over 16 years 1992–2007. Leuk Lymphoma. 2012;53(8):1488–93.
12. Zhou Y, Wang H, Fang W, Romaguer JE, Zhang Y, Delasalle KB, et al. Incidence trends of mantle cell lymphoma in the United States between 1992 and 2004. Cancer. 2008;113(4):791–8.
13. Ambinder AJ, Shenoy PJ, Nastoupil LJ, Flowers CR. Using primary site as a predictor of survival in mantle cell lymphoma. Cancer. 2013;119(8):1570–7.
14. Dabaja BS, Tsang RW, Qi S, Allen P, Hodgson D, Ricardi U, et al. Favorable outcome in stage I-II mantle cell lymphoma: a report of 160 patients from the International Lymphoma Radiation Oncology Group (ILROG). Int J Radiat Oncol Biol Phys. 2014;90(1):S151–S2.

15. Leitch HA, Gascoyne RD, Chhanabhai M, Voss NJ, Klasa R, Connors JM. Limited-stage mantle-cell lymphoma. Ann Oncol Off J Eur Soc Med Oncol/ESMO. 2003;14(10):1555–61.
16. Bernard M, Tsang RW, Le LW, Hodgson DC, Sun A, Wells W, et al. Limited-stage mantle cell lymphoma: treatment outcomes at the Princess Margaret Hospital. Leuk Lymphoma. 2013;54(2):261–7.
17. Gill BS, Vargo JA, Pai SS, Balasubramani GK, Beriwal S. Management trends and outcomes for stage I to II mantle cell lymphoma using the national cancer data base: ascertaining the ideal treatment paradigm. Int J Radiat Oncol Biol Phys. 2015;93(3): 668–76.
18. Yahalom J, Illidge T, Specht L, Hoppe RT, Li YX, Tsang R, et al. Modern radiation therapy for extranodal lymphomas: field and dose guidelines from the International Lymphoma Radiation Oncology Group. Int J Radiat Oncol Biol Phys. 2015;92(1):11–31.
19. Illidge T, Specht L, Yahalom J, Aleman B, Berthelsen AK, Constine L, et al. Modern radiation therapy for nodal non-Hodgkin lymphoma-target definition and dose guidelines from the International Lymphoma Radiation Oncology Group. Int J Radiat Oncol Biol Phys. 2014;89(1):49–58.
20. M'Kacher R, Bennaceur A, Farace F, Lauge A, Plassa LF, Wittmer E, et al. Multiple molecular mechanisms contribute to radiation sensitivity in mantle cell lymphoma. Oncogene. 2003;22(39):7905–12.
21. Hoster E, Dreyling M, Klapper W, Gisselbrecht C, van Hoof A, Kluin-Nelemans HC, et al. A new prognostic index (MIPI) for patients with advanced-stage mantle cell lymphoma. Blood. 2008;111(2):558–65.
22. Hoster E, Klapper W, Hermine O, Kluin-Nelemans HC, Walewski J, van Hoof A, et al. Confirmation of the mantle-cell lymphoma international prognostic index in randomized trials of the European Mantle-Cell Lymphoma Network. J Clin Oncol Off J Am Soc Clin Oncol. 2014;32(13):1338–46.
23. Geisler CH, Kolstad A, Laurell A, Raty R, Jerkeman M, Eriksson M, et al. The Mantle Cell Lymphoma International Prognostic Index (MIPI) is superior to the International Prognostic Index (IPI) in predicting survival following intensive first-line immunochemotherapy and autologous stem cell transplantation (ASCT). Blood. 2010;115(8):1530–3.
24. Geisler CH, Kolstad A, Laurell A, Andersen NS, Pedersen LB, Jerkeman M, et al. Long-term progression-free survival of mantle cell lymphoma after intensive front-line immunochemotherapy with in vivo-purged stem cell rescue: a nonrandomized phase 2 multicenter study by the Nordic Lymphoma Group. Blood. 2008;112(7):2687–93.
25. Lenz G, Dreyling M, Hoster E, Wormann B, Duhrsen U, Metzner B, et al. Immunochemotherapy with rituximab and cyclophosphamide, doxorubicin, vincristine, and prednisone significantly improves response and time to treatment failure, but not long-term outcome in patients with previously untreated mantle cell lymphoma: results of a prospective randomized trial of the German Low Grade Lymphoma Study Group (GLSG). J Clin Oncol Off J Am Soc Clin Oncol. 2005;23(9):1984–92.
26. Khouri IF, Saliba RM, Okoroji GJ, Acholonu SA, Champlin RE. Long-term follow-up of autologous stem cell transplantation in patients with diffuse mantle cell lymphoma in first disease remission: the prognostic value of beta2-microglobulin and the tumor score. Cancer. 2003;98(12):2630–5.
27. Dreyling M, Lenz G, Hoster E, Van Hoof A, Gisselbrecht C, Schmits R, et al. Early consolidation by myeloablative radiochemotherapy followed by autologous stem cell transplantation in first remission significantly prolongs progression-free survival in mantle-cell lymphoma: results of a prospective randomized trial of the European MCL Network. Blood. 2005;105(7):2677–84.
28. Geisler CH, Kolstad A, Laurell A, Jerkeman M, Raty R, Andersen NS, et al. Nordic MCL2 trial update: six-year follow-up after intensive immunochemotherapy for untreated mantle cell lymphoma followed by BEAM or BEAC + autologous stem-cell support: still very long survival but late relapses do occur. Br J Haematol. 2012;158(3):355–62.
29. Bernstein SH, Epner E, Unger JM, Leblanc M, Cebula E, Burack R, et al. A phase II multicenter trial of hyperCVAD MTX/Ara-C and rituximab in patients with previously untreated mantle cell lymphoma; SWOG 0213. Ann Oncol Off J Eur Soc Med Oncol/ESMO. 2013;24(6):1587–93.
30. Rosenbluth BD, Yahalom J. Highly effective local control and palliation of mantle cell lymphoma with involved-field radiation therapy (IFRT). Int J Radiat Oncol Biol Phys. 2006;65(4):1185–91.
31. Haque W, Voong KR, Shihadeh F, Arzu I, Pinnix C, Mazloom A, et al. Radiation therapy is an effective modality in the treatment of mantle cell lymphoma, even in heavily pretreated patients. Clin Lymphoma Myeloma Leuk. 2014;14(6):474–9.
32. Dietrich S, Boumendil A, Finel H, Avivi I, Volin L, Cornelissen J, et al. Outcome and prognostic factors in patients with mantle-cell lymphoma relapsing after autologous stem-cell transplantation: a retrospective study of the European Group for Blood and Marrow Transplantation (EBMT). Ann Oncol Off J Eur Soc Med Oncol/ESMO. 2014;25(5):1053–8.
33. Wang ML, Rule S, Martin P, Goy A, Auer R, Kahl BS, et al. Targeting BTK with ibrutinib in relapsed or refractory mantle-cell lymphoma. N Engl J Med. 2013;369(6):507–16.
34. Rodriguez J, Gutierrez A, Palacios A, Navarrete M, Blancas I, Alarcon J, et al. Rituximab, gemcitabine and oxaliplatin: an effective regimen in patients with refractory and relapsing mantle cell lymphoma. Leuk Lymphoma. 2007;48(11):2172–8.
35. Witzig TE, Geyer SM, Kurtin PJ, Colgan JP, Inwards DJ, Micallef IN, et al. Salvage chemotherapy with rituximab DHAP for relapsed non-Hodgkin lymphoma: a phase II trial in the North Central Cancer Treatment Group. Leuk Lymphoma. 2008;49(6):1074–80.

36. Wang M, Fayad L, Cabanillas F, Hagemeister F, McLaughlin P, Rodriguez MA, et al. Phase 2 trial of rituximab plus hyper-CVAD alternating with rituximab plus methotrexate-cytarabine for relapsed or refractory aggressive mantle cell lymphoma. Cancer. 2008;113(10):2734–41.
37. Forstpointner R, Unterhalt M, Dreyling M, Bock HP, Repp R, Wandt H, et al. Maintenance therapy with rituximab leads to a significant prolongation of response duration after salvage therapy with a combination of rituximab, fludarabine, cyclophosphamide, and mitoxantrone (R-FCM) in patients with recurring and refractory follicular and mantle cell lymphomas: results of a prospective randomized study of the German Low Grade Lymphoma Study Group (GLSG). Blood. 2006;108(13):4003–8.
38. Rummel MJ, Al-Batran SE, Kim SZ, Welslau M, Hecker R, Kofahl-Krause D, et al. Bendamustine plus rituximab is effective and has a favorable toxicity profile in the treatment of mantle cell and low-grade non-Hodgkin's lymphoma. J Clin Oncol Off J Am Soc Clin Oncol. 2005;23(15):3383–9.
39. Fisher RI, Bernstein SH, Kahl BS, Djulbegovic B, Robertson MJ, de Vos S, et al. Multicenter phase II study of bortezomib in patients with relapsed or refractory mantle cell lymphoma. J Clin Oncol Off J Am Soc Clin Oncol. 2006;24(30):4867–74.
40. Belch A, Kouroukis CT, Crump M, Sehn L, Gascoyne RD, Klasa R, et al. A phase II study of bortezomib in mantle cell lymphoma: the National Cancer Institute of Canada Clinical Trials Group trial IND.150. Ann Oncol Off J Eur Soc Med Oncol/ESMO. 2007;18(1):116–21.
41. O'Connor OA, Moskowitz C, Portlock C, Hamlin P, Straus D, Dumitrescu O, et al. Patients with chemotherapy-refractory mantle cell lymphoma experience high response rates and identical progression-free survivals compared with patients with relapsed disease following treatment with single agent bortezomib: results of a multicentre Phase 2 clinical trial. Br J Haematol. 2009;145(1):34–9.
42. Habermann TM, Lossos IS, Justice G, Vose JM, Wiernik PH, McBride K, et al. Lenalidomide oral monotherapy produces a high response rate in patients with relapsed or refractory mantle cell lymphoma. Br J Haematol. 2009;145(3):344–9.
43. Wang M, Fayad L, Wagner-Bartak N, Zhang L, Hagemeister F, Neelapu SS, et al. Lenalidomide in combination with rituximab for patients with relapsed or refractory mantle-cell lymphoma: a phase 1/2 clinical trial. Lancet Oncol. 2012;13(7):716–23.
44. Russo AL, Chen YH, Martin NE, Vinjamoori A, Luthy SK, Freedman A, et al. Low-dose involved-field radiation in the treatment of non-hodgkin lymphoma: predictors of response and treatment failure. Int J Radiat Oncol Biol Phys. 2013;86(1):121–7.
45. White EC, Advani R, Hoppe RT. 2 Gy x 2 for palliative treatment of mantle cell lymphoma. Leuk Lymphoma. 2016;57(9):2219–21.

Extranodal NK/T-Cell Lymphoma, Nasal Type

11

Yexiong Li

Abstract

Extranodal natural killer (NK)/T-cell lymphoma (NKTCL), nasal type, has been defined as a distinct clinicopathologic entity since 1994 (Harris et al. Blood 84:1361–1392, 1994; Chan et al. Extranodal NK/T-cell lymphoma, nasal type. In: Jaffe ES, Harris NL, Stein H, Vardiman JW (eds) World Health Organization classification of tumours: pathology and genetics of tumours of haematopoietic and lymphoid tissues. IARC Press, Lyon. p. 204–207, 2001; Chan et al. Extranodal NK/T-cell lymphoma, nasal type. In: Jaffe ES, Harris NL, Stein H, Vardiman JW (eds). World Health Organization classification of tumours: pathology and genetics of tumours of haematopoietic and lymphoid tissues. IARC Press, Lyon. p. 285–288, 2008), with an aggressive clinical course. It is rarely diagnosed in Europe and North America, but relatively common in East Asia and South America, accounting for 10–30% of all cases of non-Hodgkin's lymphomas (NHL) in these countries (Vose et al. J Clin Oncol 26:4124–4130, 2008; Au et al. Blood 113:3931–3937, 2009; Sun et al. Am J Clin Pathol 138:429–434, 2012; Yang et al. Diagn Pathol 6:77, 2011). This disease can arise within any extranodal organ or tissue, but usually involves the upper aerodigestive tract (UADT), such as the nasal cavity and Waldeyer's ring (Aviles et al. Clin Lab Haematol 22:215–220, 2000; Li et al. Cancer 83:449–456, 1998; Li et al. J Clin Oncol 24:181–189, 2006; Li et al. Blood 112:3057–3064, 2008; Li et al. Clin Cancer Res 15:2905–2912, 2009). Clinically, it is characterized by predominance in adult males, a large proportion of early-stage diseases, good performance status, extensive primary tumor invasiveness, low-risk score by International

Y. Li, MD
Department of Radiation Oncology,
Cancer Hospital and Institute, Chinese Academy of Medical Sciences (CAMS) and Peking Union Medical College (PUMC),
Beijing 100021, People's Republic of China
e-mail: yexiong@yahoo.com; yexiong12@163.com

B.S. Dabaja, A.K. Ng (eds.), *Radiation Therapy in Hematologic Malignancies*,
DOI 10.1007/978-3-319-42615-0_11

Prognostic Index (IPI), and a propensity for extranodal spread (Au et al. Blood 113:3931–3937, 2009; Aviles et al. Clin Lab Haematol 22:215–220, 2000; Li et al. Cancer 83:449–456, 1998; Li et al. J Clin Oncol 24:181–189, 2006; Li et al. Blood 112:3057–3064, 2008; Li et al. Clin Cancer Res 15:2905–2912, 2009).

The prognosis of NKTCL varied, mainly depending on the prognostic factor and treatment (Cheung et al. Int J Radiat Oncol Biol Phys 54:182–190, 2002; Chim et al. Blood 103:216–221, 2004). The rarity and heterogeneity of NKTCL and the lack of prospective trial data have resulted in a variety of treatment options, chemotherapy regimens, and radiotherapy volumes and doses at different institutions. However, radiotherapy is the backbone of curative intent for early-stage NKTCL. New regimen chemotherapy shows promising results against refractory or advanced NKTCL.

Clinical Presentation

Case 1

A 39-year-old man presented with chronic sinusitis. A computed tomography (CT) scan was done showing an abnormality in the right nasal cavity and right maxillary area. A core biopsy of the right nasal cavity lesion was consistent with NKTCL, nasal type. Pathology showed a polymorphic proliferation of small, medium size, and large lymphocytes with high number of admixed histiocytes. Tissue necrosis was present in multifocal areas and blood vessels. Neoplastic lymphocytes were positive for CD3 and CD56, non-immunoreactive for CD4, CD8, CD5, and CD20. In situ hybridization for EBV (EBER) was strongly positive within the tumor.

The nasal cavity is the prototypic site of involvement in NKTCL [4, 6–8]. The patient in case 1 presented with disease involving the right nasal cavity as well as the medial side of the right maxillary sinus. Inflammatory enhancement was suspected to be admixed with the areas of disease including the right sinus walls as well as the part of the right nasal and left nasal cavity (Figs. 11.1 and 11.2).

In the 2008 WHO criteria [3], update of the REAL classification [2], "nasal" NKTCL was defined as a disease occurring in the UADT, whereas "extranasal" NKTCL was defined as a disease occurring outside the UADT. Based on recent data, NKTCL consists of three distinct subgroups: nasal NKTCL, extranasal UADT NKTCL, and extra-UADT NKTCL [11, 12, 18]. The various clinical presentation and prognosis between the three subgroups are summarized in Table 11.1.

UADT NKTCL is characterized by predominance in young male, good performance status, elevated lactate dehydrogenase (LDH) in a large proportion of patients, high frequency of early-stage disease, and low-risk group according to International Prognostic Index (IPI) [10]. Patients usually have local tumor invasion or adjacent structure involvement (40–60 %). For nasal NKTCL, the most frequently involved adjacent sites are the maxillary and ethmoid sinuses, followed by the nasopharynx [15, 26]. The major pathway of lymph node spread for nasal NKTCL is to the submandibular and cervical lymph nodes [9]. The primary pattern of failure is distant extranodal sites such as the skin, lung, and liver. The propensity for NKTCL spread to the extranodal organs, especially the skin, is related to the homing capacity of NK/T-cell.

Extranasal UADT NKTCL represents different clinical features and prognosis [11, 12, 18]. The most frequent presenting symptoms for Waldeyer's ring NK/T-cell lymphoma (WR NKTCL) are odynophagia, dysphagia, and cervical lymphadenopathy [11]. Patients are more likely to present with regional nodal involvement (60 %) and advanced-stage diseases (20–40 %) and have a relatively favorable prognosis [11, 12, 18]. The majority of patients with extranasal

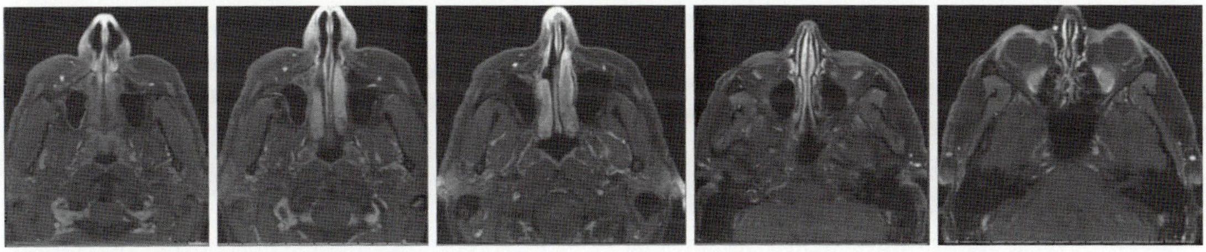

Fig. 11.1 Initial staging MRI of case 1

Table 11.1 Clinical and immunophenotypic differences between the three subgroups of extranodal nasal-type NK/T-cell lymphoma

	UADT-NKTCL		
Feature	*Nasal NKTCL*	*Extranasal UADT-NKTCL*	*Extra-UADT-NKTCL*
Primary site	Nasal cavity or paranasal sinus with or without extension into adjacent structures	Waldeyer's ring (nasopharynx, tonsil, oropharynx, base of the tongue), hypopharynx, larynx, and oral cavity	The skin and soft tissue, gastrointestinal tract, testis, et al. Accounts for 10–30 % of all cases
Phenotype	High expression of EBV (>90 %), CD3ε, CD56, and Ki-67. All cases express cytotoxic proteins.	High expression of EBV (>90 %). CD56 expression is less common than nasal variant, low proliferation index	EBV expression is relatively diverse (40–100 %). High proliferation index
Age	Usually adults, median age of 44 years	Usually adults, median age of 38–50 years	Usually adults, median age of 50 years
Sex	Male predominance, M/F = 2–4:1	Male predominance, M/F = 2.6:1	Male predominance, M/F = 1.5–2.3:1
Stage	Usually present with early-stage disease, majority with stage I (60–80 %); less common with stage III and IV (10–25 %).	Usually present with early-stage disease, stage I <20 %, stage II 50–60 %; more advanced-stage disease (20–30 %)	Usually present with disseminated and advanced-stage disease (>50 %)
Performance status	Good	Good	Poor, frequently ECOG ≥ 2
Elevated LDH	Frequency (20–50 %)	Frequency (20–50 %)	High frequency (50–70 %)
Lymph node involvement	Low frequency of lymph node involvement at diagnosis (<20 %)	Frequent involvement of the cervical lymph node (>50 %)	High frequency of regional lymph node involvement
IPI	Usually low risk, IPI 0–1 > 90 %	Usually low risk, IPI 0–1 ≥ 80 %	Usually high risk, IPI 0–1 25–58 %
Failure patterns	Extranodal organs. The skin is the most common site	Lymph nodes and extranodal organs	Extranodal organs
Clinical course	Aggressive	Less aggressive	Highly aggressive
Prognosis	Favorable outcome in stage I patients treated with appropriate radiotherapy, poor for stage II–IV patients	Relatively favorable outcome compared with nasal or extra-UADT variants	Extremely poor prognosis; median survival, 3–20 months

Modified from Liu et al. [18]

Abbreviations: *UADT* upper aerodigestive tract, *NKTCL* extranodal nasal-type NK/T-cell lymphoma, *EBV* Epstein-Barr virus, *ECOG* Eastern Cooperative Oncology Group, *LDH* lactate dehydrogenase, *IPI* International Prognostic Index

UADT NKTCL or WR NKTCL present with Ann Arbor stage II to IV disease, whereas only 10–20 % patients have stage I disease. This differed from reports in which the frequency distribution (60–80 %) of stage I disease was predominant in patients with nasal NKTCL [10, 14, 27]. Several studies have demonstrated that UADT NKTCL and extra-UADT NKTCL have different clinical features and prognoses [5, 16, 28–32, 34, 35, 41]. Extra-UADT NKTCL constitutes only 10–30 % of all NKTCL cases and is characterized by poor performance status, high frequency of elevated LDH, advanced-stage disease, high-risk IPI, and extremely poor prognosis (Table 11.1).

Pathology

Extranodal nasal-type NK/T-cell lymphoma was formerly named angiocentric lymphoma in REAL classification in 1994 [1]. Other terms such as lethal midline granuloma, malignant granuloma, midline malignant reticulosis, and angiocentric immunoproliferative lesion were used before 1994.

The typical morphology of this disease includes frequent angiocentricity with zone necrosis and polymorphism of individual cells with small or medium size of tumor cells and polymorphous inflammatory infiltrate. The histological features are similar irrespective of the anatomical sites involved [3]. Repeated biopsy is usually required for pathologic diagnosis, due to necrosis and small size of specimens.

NKTCL is derived mostly from activated NK cell, and rarely from cytotoxic T lymphocyte. The typical phenotype is CD2+, CD3s−, CD3ε+, CD56+, CD20−/CD79a−, and cytotoxic molecules (T-cell intracellular antigen-1 [TIA-1], granzyme B, perforin)+. The tumor cells are infected by Epstein-Barr virus (EBV), which is detected by in situ hybridization (ISH) for EBV-encoded RNA (EBER). Some cases also show a cytotoxic T-cell phenotype that is negative for CD56 but positive for CD3ε, cytotoxic molecules (TIA, Gram B, perforin), and EBER with TCR gene rearrangement. Patients with CD56-negative NKTCL have similar clinical features as those with CD56-positive NKTCL [15, 26]. However, NK-cell or T-cell lymphoma may have different prognosis [16]. Extranodal lymphomas that are CDε + CD56−, but negative for cytotoxic molecules and EBV should be defined as peripheral T-cell lymphoma, not otherwise specified (PTCL-NOS).

TCR rearrangement is absent for NK-cell lineage, but present for T-cell lineage. NKTCL is strongly associated with EBV infection, which is observed in more than 90 % of cases [17, 18]. Gain of 1q and 7q and loss of 6q and 7p are relatively frequent genomic aberrations [19]. Mutation of JAK3, activation of STAT3, overexpression of matrix metalloproteinase 9, and interleukin-9 have been observed in this disease [20–22]. The inactivation or mutation of p53 is common [23, 24]. High expression of Ki-67 is associated with poor survival [18, 25].

Staging Procedure

Initial Evaluation

Our patient had a careful physical (including inspection of the skin) and endoscopic examination. Imaging included an MRI, CT of the head and neck, and a PET/CT (Figs. 11.1 and 11.2). *Initial complete blood count, biochemistry, liver and renal function, and LDH were normal. Bone marrow biopsy was normal. Although it is rarely involved, bone marrow assessment is a crucial part of the staging* [36, 37].

To accurately determine local disease extent in both the soft tissue and bone, both MRI and CT scan of the head and neck are recommended in all cases [38–40]. Additionally, PET/CT can alter the original staging and affect treatment planning in 20–50 % of patients [38]. Moreover, a high tumor FDG uptake was associated with poor prognosis in patients with NKTCL [35, 41].

Although it is not done in our case, many institutions perform quantitative measurement of circulating EBV-DNA viral load for the diagnosis, monitoring, and predicting prognosis of the disease. High load of plasma EBV-DNA correlates with advanced-stage disease, elevated lactate dehydrogenase (LDH), initial response to therapy, and poor survival [42–44, 56].

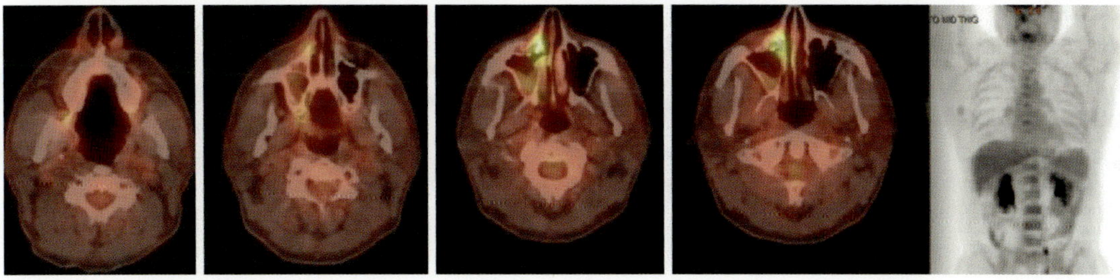

Fig. 11.2 Initial staging PET-CT of case 1

Stage and Risk Stratification

The Ann Arbor staging system is widely used for diffuse large B-cell lymphoma. However, it is not readily applicable to NKTCL. Primary tumor invasion (PTI) or local tumor invasion is an important prognostic factor for NKTCL [45–47, 105]. A modified Ann Arbor staging system is recommended, and stage I disease is subclassified into limited stage I or extended stage I disease [9, 10]. Limited stage I disease is defined as tumor confined to a single primary site without extension of adjacent organs, as in case 1, whereas extended stage I disease extends beyond the primary site into any neighboring structure or organ, without the presence of nodal or distant dissemination. Ann Arbor stage II disease is defined as involvement of supradiaphragmatic lymph node(s).

The International Prognostic Index (IPI) and Korean Prognostic Index (KPI) are commonly used for NKTCL. The IPI model includes five independent prognostic factors: age, stage, Eastern Cooperative Oncology Group (ECOG) performance status (PS), LDH, and extranodal involvement. The KPI identifies four risk factors: B symptoms, stage, LDH, and regional lymph node [30]. The Ann Arbor stage, IPI, and KPI assign patients to four risk groups with different survivals but are not consistent to segregate patients into risk groups or predict prognosis [12, 31, 45–47, 105]. Patients with NKTCL were predominantly young males with early-stage disease and good PS, which placed the majority of patients in the low-risk groups (0–1) according to the IPI or KPI. On the other hand, the value of KPI model in early-stage patients is limited because regional lymph node involvement duplicates Ann Arbor stage II disease. Based on a recent large, multi-institutional analysis of 1383 patients, a NKTCL-specific prognostic nomogram has been developed and validated as a reliable tool to individually predict overall survival (OS) and has been shown to be superior to Ann Arbor staging, IPI, or KPI [45, 47]. The nomogram model consisted of five variables from routine clinical practice: stage, PS, age, LDH, and primary tumor invasion (PTI). PTI was defined as the presence of primary disease that extended into adjacent structures or organs or the involvement of multiple, contiguous primary sites. Furthermore, patients with early-stage NKTCL can be classified as low-risk or high-risk group based on the absence or presence of risk factors including age >60 years, elevated LDH, ECOG PS ≥ 2, stage II disease, and PTI [45, 47]. Calculation of NKTCL prognostic index should be considered as part of initial work-up. In case 1, the patient belongs to the low-risk group, with normal LDH, PS < 2, age <60, and stage I disease.

Treatment Management

Our patient presented with an early-stage, low-risk disease [45, 47]. Although radiotherapy alone would have been a viable option, this patient was treated with radiation therapy followed by chemotherapy using VIPD (etoposide, ifosfamide, cisplatin, dexamethasone) for a total of three cycles, started 2 weeks after the completion of radiation.

Table 11.2 Treatment outcome of radiotherapy with or without chemotherapy compared with that of chemotherapy alone in patients with early-stage extranodal nasal-type NK/T-cell lymphoma

Authors	Time	No	Primary site	Stage	Treatment	5-year OS (%)	*P*
You et al.	2004	46	Nasal	I–II	RT: 6	83.3	0.027
					CT ± RT: 40	28.5	
Li et al.	2004	56	Sinonasal	I–II	RT: 11	50	0.01
					RT + CT: 27	59	
					CT: 18	15	
Huang et al.	2008	82	Nasal	I–II	RT ± CT: 74	62.1 (3-years)	0.000
					CT alone: 8	12.5 (3-years)	
Kim et al.	2008	280	All sites	I	RT ± CT: NA	90.3	0.022
					CT alone: NA	19.3 (median)	
Au et al.	2009	57	UADT	I–II	RT + CT: 34	57	0.045
					CT alone: 23	30	
Yang et al.	2009	177	UADT	I–II	RT ± CT: 140	53.4	<0.01
					CT alone: 37	18.3	
Nie et al.	2010	85	Nasal	I–II	RT + CT: 17	54	0.03
					CT + RT: 48 CT alone: 20	47 13	0.049
Luo et al.	2010	60	Nasal	I–II	RT + CT: 37	56.7	<0.05
					CT alone: 16	18.8	
Yang et al.	2009	177	UADT	I–II	RT ± CT: 140	53.4	<0.01
					CT alone: 37	18.3	
Vazquez et al.	2014	123	UADT	I	RT: NA	63.5	<0.05
					CT alone: NA	47.7	
		65	Extra-UADT	I	RT: NA	52.3	<0.005
			Extra-UADT		CT alone: NA	23.8	
Ahn et al.	2012	20	Skin	I	RT ± CT: 10	About 60	<0.005
					CT alone: 10	12 m (median)	
Yang et al.	2015	1273	All sites	I–II	RT ± CT: 1103	67.7	<0.001
					RT alone: 253	69.6	<0.001
					CT alone: 170	33.9	

OS overall survival, *RT* Radiotherapy, *CT* Chemotherapy, *UADT* upper aerodigestive tract, *NA* not available

Current data have indicated that radiotherapy is a critical component of curative treatment for early-stage NKTCL. Radiotherapy has been effective in achieving high complete response (CR) rates and favorable long-term survival. Except for two early studies with small-field and low-dose RT [48, 49], radiotherapy alone resulted in complete response (CR) rates of 70–90 %, 5-year locoregional control (LRC) rate of approximately 90 %, and 5-year OS of 50–90 % [10, 15, 26, 45–47, 50–52, 55, 105]. In contrast, outcome with doxorubicin-based chemotherapy alone in early-stage NKTCL has been poor, with CR rates of 10–50 % and overall response rate (ORR) of 60–80 %, 5-year OS rates of 10–35 %, and even lower progression-free survival (PFS) [5, 27, 32, 33, 50, 51]. The low initial response and poor prognosis after chemotherapy reflect the chemoresistance, which may be associated with high expression of P-glycoprotein and p53 mutation [23, 24, 54]. In 105 patients with early-stage nasal NKTCL who received primary radiotherapy, the 5-year OS and PFS rates were 71 and 59 % for all patients, with 78 and 63 % for stage I disease, and 46 and 40 % for stage II disease [10]. Tables 11.2 and 11.3 summarize series demonstrating the critical role of radiation therapy compared to chemotherapy alone for early-stage disease.

The addition of chemotherapy to radiation therapy in the treatment of early-stage disease is

Table 11.3 Treatment outcome stratified by combined modality therapy and radiotherapy alone in patients with early-stage extranodal nasal-type NK/T-cell lymphoma

Authors	Time	No	Primary site	Stage	Treatment[a]	5-year OS (%)	P
Cheung et al.	2002	79	Nasal	I–II	CT+RT: 61	40.3	0.870
					RT: 18	29.8	
				I	CT+RT: 47	36.7	0.892
					RT: 16	46.0	
Kim et al.	2001	143	UADT	I–II	CT+RT: 39	35	0.93
					RT: 104	38	
Kim et al.	2005	53	UADT	I–II	CT+RT: 20	59	0.27
					RT: 33	76	
Li et al.	2006	105	Nasal	I–II	RT+CT: 34	77	0.518
					CT+RT: 37	74	
					RT: 31	66	
Ma et al.	2008	64	Nasal	I–II	RT+CT: 41	61.5	0.469
					RT: 23	57.9	
Aikema et al.	2008	57	Nasal	I	RT+CT: 20	61.9	>0.05
					RT alone: 15	57.1	
Luo et al.	2010	60	Nasal	I–II	RT+CT: 20	56.7	>0.05
					RT alone: 7	60.2	
Li et al.	2011	214	Nasal	I–II	RT+CT: 118	74.4	0.529
					RT alone: 96	69.8	
Li et al.	2009	67	WR	II	CMT: 54	79	0.092
					RT alone: 13	57	
Li	2012	69	UADT	I–II	CMT: 33	76.6 (3-years)	0.313
					RT alone: 36	88.5 (3-years)	
Aviles	2013	427	UADT	I–II	CMT: 202	86	<0.01
					RT alone: 109	64	
					CT alone: 116	45	
Fang	2014	124	UADT	II	CMT: 84	71.2	<0.001
					CT or RT: 40	26.7	
Yang et al.	2015	276	All sites	Low-risk stages I–II	RT+CT: 54	86.9	0.896
					CT+RT: 132	86.3	0.794
					RT alone: 90	88.8	
Yang et al.	2015	827	All sites	High-risk stages I–II	RT+CT: 155	72.2	0.017
					CT+RT: 509	58.3	0.004
					RT alone: 163	59.6	

OS overall survival, *CT* chemotherapy, *RT* radiotherapy, *CMT* combined modality therapy, *UADT* upper aerodigestive tract, *WR* Waldeyer's ring

[a]Most patients received doxorubicin-based chemotherapy

controversial in Asia, with some studies showing limited benefit [10, 13, 15, 26, 46, 59, 60–63, 105], while others have demonstrated a better outcome with combined modality therapy (CMT)[11, 45, 47, 64, 65]. In the Western world, combined modality approach is generally favored.

Currently Used Combined Modality Therapy

Modern chemotherapy regimens for early-stage NKTCL (Table 11.4) including DeVIC, VIPD (etoposide, ifosfamide, cisplatin, dexamethasone), and GDP (gemcitabine, dexamethasone

Table 11.4 Treatment outcome of concurrent or sequential new regimen chemotherapy and radiotherapy in patients with stage I and II extranodal nasal-type NK/T-cell lymphoma

Authors	Time	No	Treatment	RT dose (Gy)	OS (%)	PFS (%)
Yamaguchi	2009	33	CCRT and DeVIC	Median: 50	73 (5-years)	67
Kim	2009	30	CCRT and VIPD	Median: 50	86 (3-years)	85
Tsai	2014	33	CCRT and VIPD	Median: 50.4	66 (5-years)	60
Ke	2014	32	CCRT (IMRT) and GDP	Median: 56	87.5 (3-years)	84.4
Lee	2013	27	CCRT and VIPD or SMILE	44–54	59 (3-years)	41
Kim	2014	30	CCRT and VIDL	40–44	60 (5-years)	73
Jiang	2012	26	Sandwich LVP/RT	56	88.5 (2-years)	80.6
Wang	2013	27	Sequential GELOX/RT	56	86 (2-years)	86
Wang	2014e	93	Sequential GELOX/RT: 40	56 (40–60)	78.9 (5-years)	79
			Sequential epoch/RT: 53		50.4 (5-years)	46.5
Zang	2015	64	Sequential CHOP-L, SMILE et al. and RT	Median: 56	84.2 (3-years) 57.6 (3-years)	74.3 (early RT) 55.9 (late RT)

RT radiotherapy, *OS* overall survival, *PFS* progression-free survival, *CCRT* concurrent chemoradiotherapy, *IMRT* intensity-modulated radiation oncology, *DeVIC* dexamethasone, etoposide, ifosfamide, carboplatin; *VIPD* etoposide, ifosfamide, cisplatin, dexamethasone, *GDP* (gemcitabine, dexamethasone, and cisplatin), *SMILE* dexamethasone, methotrexate, ifosfamide, L-asparaginase, etoposide; *VIDL* (etoposide, ifosfamide, dexamethasone, L-asparaginase), *LVP* L-asparaginase, vincristine, prednisone, *GELOX* (gemcitabine, oxaliplatin, L-asparaginase), *CHOP-L* cyclophosphamide, doxorubicin, vincristine, prednisone, L-asparaginase

Table 11.5 Relationship of local failure and radiation field and dose in extranodal nasal-type NK/T-cell lymphomas

		Primary	RT dose	Total	Local failure		
Author	Stage	site	(Gy)	No	No	%	P
Isobe 2006 [49]	I–II	UADT	≥50 <50	26 9	6 6	23 67	0.038
Koom 2004 [101]	I–II	UADT	≥45 <45	77 25	29 16	38 64	0.02
Shikama 2001 [103]	I–II	Nasal lymphoma	>46 ≤46	22 20	1 5	5 24	0.087
Cheung 2002 [13]	I–II	Nasal cavity	>50 ≤50	25 44	3 12	12 27.3	0.400
Wu 2008 [104]	I–II	Nasal cavity	≥50 <50	66 14	22 9	32 64	NA
Huang 2008 [27]	I–II	UADT	≥54 <54	28 46	75 % (5-year OS) 46 % (5-year OS)	60 % (5-year DFS) 33 % (5-year DFS)	$P<0.05$ for both

RT radiotherapy, *UADT* upper aerodigestive tract, *NA* not available, *OS* overall survival, *DFS* disease-free survival

and cisplatin), in combination with radiotherapy, have all been shown to be associated with improved outcome compared to historical control of radiotherapy alone [67–72]. Less common regimens used include sandwich or sequential LVP (L-asparaginase, vincristine, prednisone), GELOX (gemcitabine, oxaliplatin, L-asparaginase) or CHOP-L (cyclophosphamide, doxorubicin, vincristine, prednisone, L-asparaginase), and radiotherapy ([66, 73, 74]) with limited follow-up and experience.

Treatment Volume and Technique

Our patient received intensity-modulated radiation therapy (IMRT) to a total dose of 54 Gy in 28 treatments; IMRT is the preferred technique, as it offers more conformal target dose distribution and better normal tissue sparing [42, 56, 57, 99, 100]. Adequate radiation dose, typically >50 Gy, is critical for early-stage NKTCL based on extensively published data as shown in Table 11.5 ([9–13, 15, 26, 27, 35, 41, 42, 46, 48, 49, 52, 53, 55–57, 60, 67, 100, 101, 103–105]). Additionally, data also clearly show a linear relationship between crude or 5-year LRC and 5-year OS rates. High LRC rates of ≥90 % correlate with 5-year OS rates of 70–82 % ([10, 11, 15, 26, 52]).

Our patient was simulated using CT simulator with a mask for immobilization. The images from the MRI and PET were fused with the planning CT to help guide the contouring of the targeted area. NKTCL represents locally destructive clinical behavior and shows a tendency for extensive submucosa infiltration beyond macroscopic disease. As such, all abnormal areas seen on initial imaging were contoured as the gross tumor volume (GTV), including areas interpreted as possible inflammation by the radiologist. An additional 1 cm was added uniformly to create the clinical target volume (CTV) but edited off the eyes and optic nerves. Any area of abnormality suspicious for microscopic disease involvement was included as part of the CTV. Finally, the planning target volume (PTV) was created, by adding 3 mm uniformly [58]. In cases in which the volume is too large, it is acceptable to use two planning targets, with differential dosing of 54 Gy to the gross disease and 45–50.4 Gy to areas suspicious for harboring microscopic disease. Prophylactic lymph node radiation was not necessary in this case based on the very low incidence of cervical lymph node failure in stage I disease (<6 %) [15, 26, 61, 75, 86, 101, 102].

For NKTCL adequate coverage and control of the target volume take priority over minimizing doses to critical organs, which is a notion that quite often does not apply to other types of lymphoma. This is mainly due to the fact that radiotherapy constitutes a critical component for the treatment of the disease, in which local control is directly linked to cure. Additionally, chemotherapy, as will be discussed below, is not as effective as radiotherapy for this disease.

The treatment plan and dose volume histograms are shown in Figs. 11.3, 11.4, and 11.5. The use of IMRT has offered sparing of the eyes, optic nerves, chiasm, and most of the bilateral parotid glands. The latter had a mean dose of 3.09 Gy (right) and 4.13 (left).

In other case scenarios of early-stage disease, the CTV should include the nasopharynx when primary disease is close to the choanae (limited stage I) or extends into the nasopharynx (extended stage I). If the bilateral nasal cavity is involved, the CTV should cover bilateral maxillary sinuses. For extended stage I disease, CTV extends to encompass the involved paranasal organs or tissues with appropriate margin. If anterior ethmoid sinuses are involved, the CTV should extend the posterior ethmoid sinuses. For stage II NTKCL with involvement of the cervical lymph node, CTV also encompasses the bilateral cervical lymph nodes. The CTV of WR NKTCL should include the whole Waldeyer's ring, adjacent organs or structures with disease extension, and cervical lymph nodes [11] (Fig. 11.6).

Constraints to critical organs should follow the well-established guidelines similar to the one treated for head and neck cancers.

Posttreatment Consideration

The patient in case 1 developed grade 2 mucositis of the hard palate, grade 2 dermatitis especially in the dose entrance areas. As of the third week of treatment, he lost the hair in his nose and developed dryness in his nostril and as of week 4 had streaks of blood when blowing his nose. The symptoms were managed with saline spray. Since he was on chemotherapy, non-codeine pain medications were avoided so as not to mask a fever.

The patient has been in remission for 34 months, which is usually an indication of possibility for a long-term cure, although late relapses have been reported even the past year **five** after remission. At the last follow-up, the patient has no complaints specifically related to the area that received radiation; he does not have any indication of his salivary glands dysfunction, visual compromise, or auditory deficits, which is a reflection of how IMRT can spare normal organs even with a prescribed dose of 54 Gy. Figure 11.7 shows a complete remission but with residual sinusitis as reflected by the opacification seen in the right maxillary sinus.

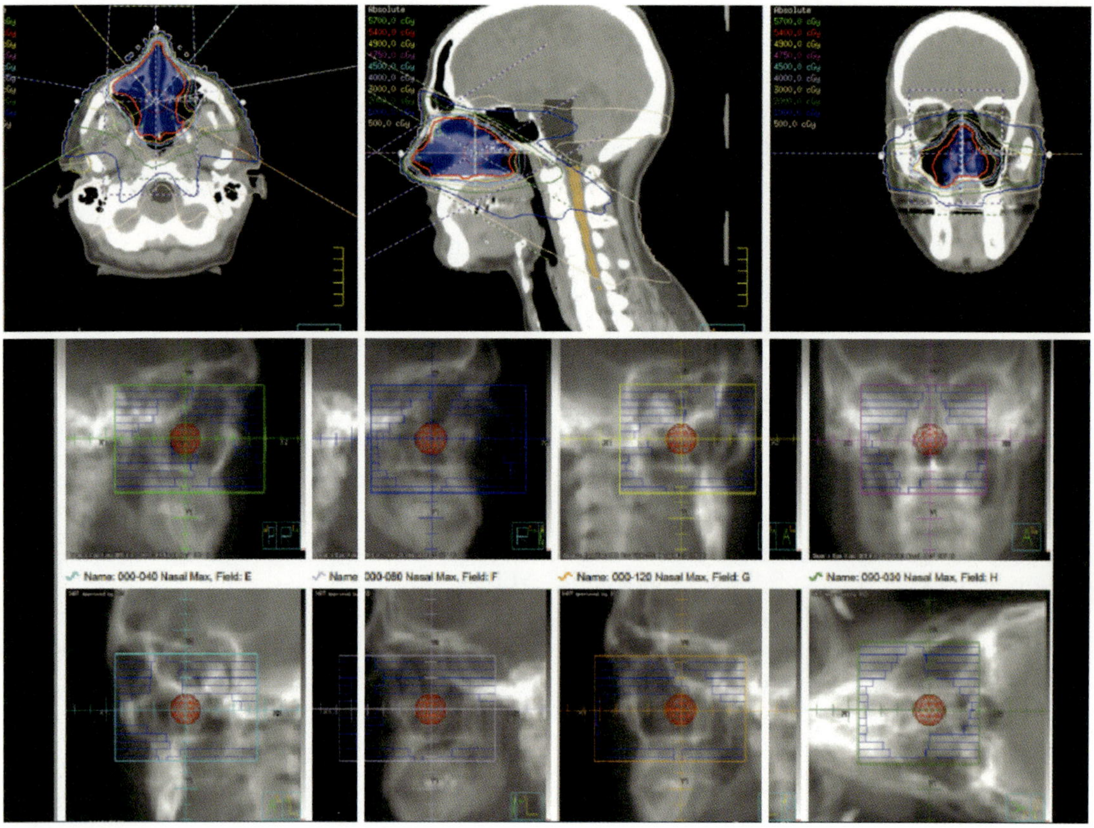

Fig. 11.3 Primary tumor localized in the left, anterior nasal cavity. Clinical target volume (CTV) included the bilateral nasal cavity, medial wall of right maxillary sinus, palate, bilateral anterior ethmoid sinuses, but not the nasopharynx

Case 2

A 43-year-old man, worked as a nurse, noted severe pain in his left cheek associated with fullness. Work-up showed a mass arising from the left maxilla infiltrating into the left orbit (Fig. 11.8). *Core biopsy was consistent with NKTCL, nasal type. The patient elected to go for alternative therapy using herbal medicine until he presented 5 months later with local progression of the disease, now infiltrating into the skin with an open ulcer in the right cheek, as well as infiltration into the soft and hard palate. MRI showed a large mass in the left naso-ethmoid and maxillary sinus extending into the left orbit, displacing the eye up and inward and causing necrosis in the lower eyelid. Additionally, multiple small lymph nodes (1–1.5 cm) were noted bilaterally at levels II, III, and IV. The patient was still able to see with his left eye* (Fig. 11.9).

Staging

This patient has a locally advanced invasive disease with regional nodal involvement. His staging work included a PET/CT scan, blood work, and a bone marrow biopsy, which showed *no evidence of distant disease or end-organ damage.*

Treatment Management

It was decided to start him on radiation therapy concurrently with chemotherapy with DeVIC regimen. Before initiating therapy, a gastric tube was inserted in preparation for treatment-related mucositis as well as in anticipation of possible development of a communicative ulcer in the right hard palate. He was also referred to head and neck surgery to prepare for an obturator, but this was deemed infeasible due to severe trismus (opening around 2 cm) caused by the disease.

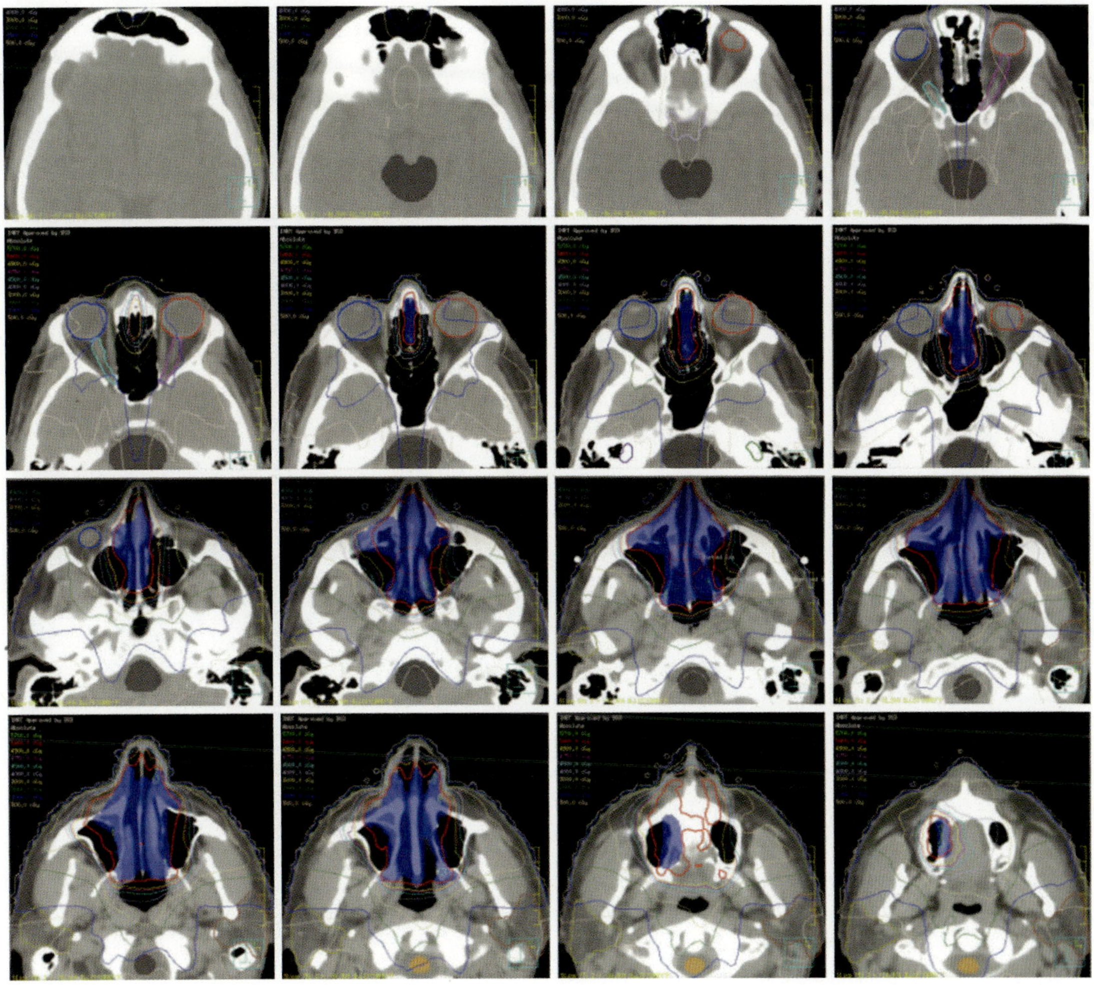

Fig. 11.4 IMRT plan of case 1

Treatment Volume and Technique

The patient was simulated with mouth open using a stent to avoid treating the tongue and bottom oral cavity while trying to target the ulcer in the palate. A facemask was used for daily reproducibility. The staging MRI and the PET scan were fused with the CT simulation scan. The patient was consented for side effects including blindness in the left eye, dryness of the mouth, brain injury, and formation of communication between the hard palate and the left maxilla that will affect his speech and swallowing. The GTV included all radiographic abnormalities, and a 1cm margin was added for the CTV but excluding the left eye, optic nerve, chiasm, and salivary glands. An additional 3 mm was added for expansion to PTV. IMRT was used, and Fig. 11.10a–d *shows isodose lines covering the GTV to full dose of 54 at 2 Gy per fraction while delivering 45 Gy at 1.8 per fraction to other areas at risk including the regional lymph nodes. After 3 weeks of treatment to a dose of 30 Gy, the patient's disease responded quite well to a point that a re-planning had to be performed to avoid doses falling into critical organs* (Fig. 11.11). *As expected, an opening through the hard palate developed mid treatment. By this time, the head and neck team was able to fit the patient with an obturator since he was then to open his mouth to over 4 cm. He*

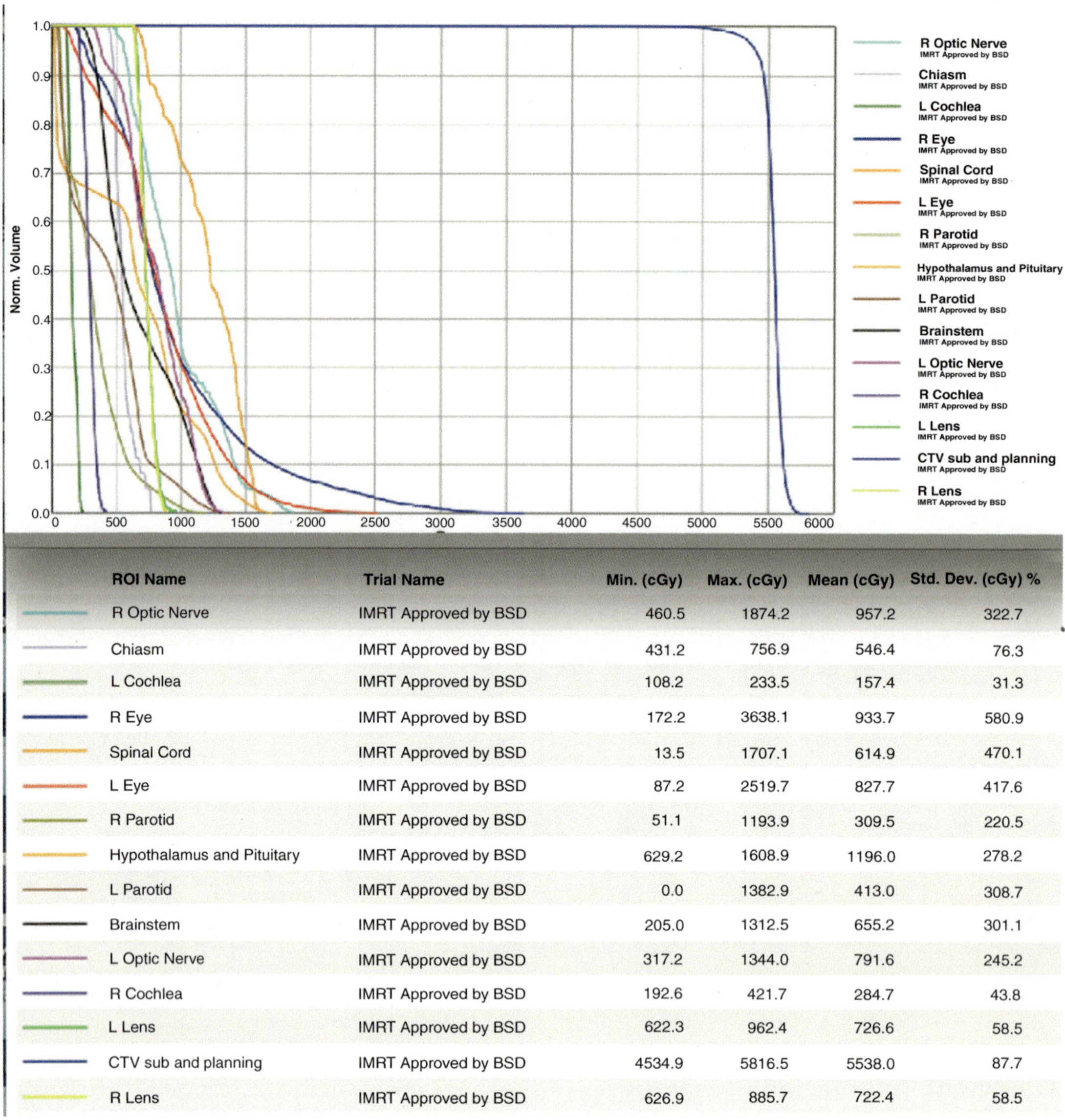

ROI Name	Trial Name	Min. (cGy)	Max. (cGy)	Mean (cGy)	Std. Dev. (cGy) %
R Optic Nerve	IMRT Approved by BSD	460.5	1874.2	957.2	322.7
Chiasm	IMRT Approved by BSD	431.2	756.9	546.4	76.3
L Cochlea	IMRT Approved by BSD	108.2	233.5	157.4	31.3
R Eye	IMRT Approved by BSD	172.2	3638.1	933.7	580.9
Spinal Cord	IMRT Approved by BSD	13.5	1707.1	614.9	470.1
L Eye	IMRT Approved by BSD	87.2	2519.7	827.7	417.6
R Parotid	IMRT Approved by BSD	51.1	1193.9	309.5	220.5
Hypothalamus and Pituitary	IMRT Approved by BSD	629.2	1608.9	1196.0	278.2
L Parotid	IMRT Approved by BSD	0.0	1382.9	413.0	308.7
Brainstem	IMRT Approved by BSD	205.0	1312.5	655.2	301.1
L Optic Nerve	IMRT Approved by BSD	317.2	1344.0	791.6	245.2
R Cochlea	IMRT Approved by BSD	192.6	421.7	284.7	43.8
L Lens	IMRT Approved by BSD	622.3	962.4	726.6	58.5
CTV sub and planning	IMRT Approved by BSD	4534.9	5816.5	5538.0	87.7
R Lens	IMRT Approved by BSD	626.9	885.7	722.4	58.5

Fig. 11.5 Dose-volume histogram for case 1

completed the remainder of his treatment, during which he developed grade 3 mucositis, epistaxis, xerostomia, grade 2 dermatitis, and hair loss.

Posttreatment Considerations

Six weeks after completion of his treatment, the G-tube was removed, and the patient was able to start eating per mouth with the obturator in place to prevent food from entering his left maxilla. Figure 11.12 *shows the patient 4 weeks past completion of treatment with an excellent response including healing of the facial ulcer, lower left eyelid ulcer, and almost complete resolution of the left ptosis.*

Unfortunately, 3 months after completing four cycles of DeVIC and 5 months after completing his radiation treatment, he presented with extensive systemic disease (Fig. 11.13). *Treatment*

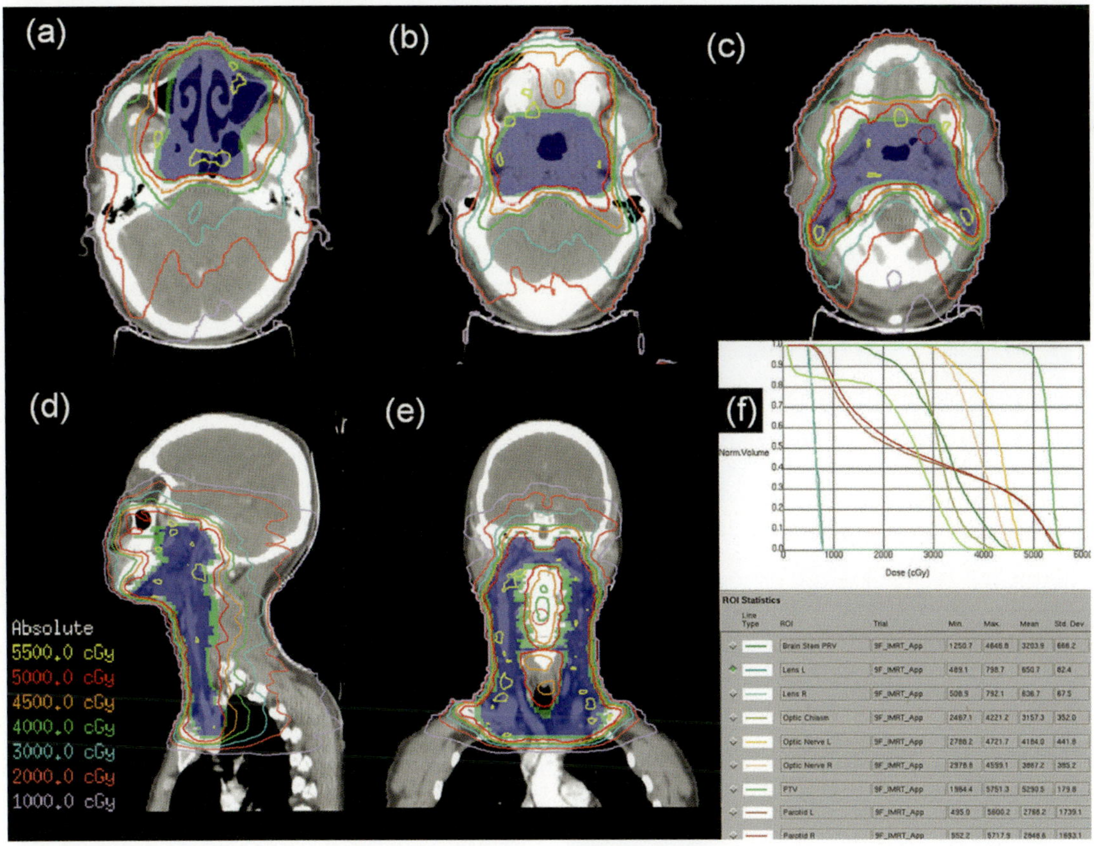

Fig. 11.6 Primary tumor involved the left nasal cavity, nasopharynx, and oropharynx with spread to cervical lymph nodes. Clinical target volume (CTV) included the nasal cavity, left maxillary sinus, bilateral anterior ethmoid sinuses, Waldeyer's ring, and bilateral cervical lymph nodes. (**a–c**) oxial. (**d**) sagittal. (**e**) coronal views of isodose distribution. (**f**) dose volume histogram

with salvage chemotherapy was attempted but failed to achieve a meaningful remission, and he passed away shortly after.

Treatment of Locally Advanced and Advanced Cases

For high-risk patients with stage II UADT NKTCL, CMT significantly improved OS and PFS compared to radiotherapy alone or chemotherapy alone (5-year OS, 71.2 % versus 26.7 %, $p < 0.001$) [64]. Additionally, patients with early-stage WR NKTCL may benefit from CMT [11, 12]. The 5-year OS and PFS rates were 79 % and 65 % for patients treated with CMT compared with 57 % ($p = 0.092$) and 41 % ($p = 0.065$) for those treated with radiotherapy alone [11]. Recently, a risk-adapted therapy has been created for early-stage NKTCL based on a large cohort analysis of 1283 patients [45, 47]. For high-risk early-stage patients with any risk factors, radiotherapy consolidated by chemotherapy proved to be the most effective treatment. Radiotherapy followed by chemotherapy significantly improved survival compared to radiotherapy alone or induction chemotherapy and radiotherapy. The 5-year OS rate was 72.2 % for radiotherapy followed by chemotherapy compared to 59.6 % for radiotherapy alone ($p = 0.017$) and 58.3 % for chemotherapy followed by radiotherapy ($p = 0.004$), with comparable OS for the latter two groups ($p = 0.913$) [45, 47]. Several studies have also demonstrated that up-front or early radiotherapy improved survival in localized NKTCL [27, 66].

Patients with advanced-stage NKTCL is traditionally treated with doxorubicin-based chemotherapy. Recently, new non-multidrug resistance (MDR)-dependent regimens such as L-asparaginase-based or gemcitabine-based regimen have shown promising activity against advanced or relapsed disease [75, 77–88, 102].

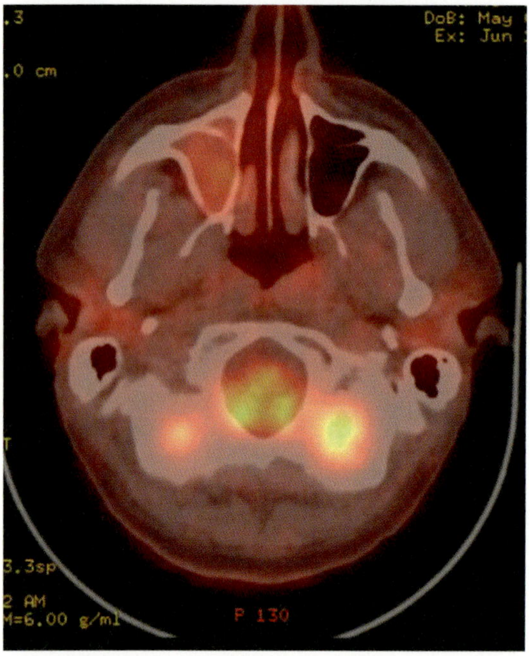

Fig. 11.7 Complete remission at 3 months after completing chemotherapy and radiation; there is secretion in the right sinus as part of the radiation side effects that might be there for months after the treatment

The ORR and CR rates were 27–66 % and 50–90 %, respectively (Table 11.4). However, prognosis in patients with advanced-stage disease is still poor [75, 86–88, 102]. Patients with locoregionally relapsed or refractory disease showed a relatively favorable prognosis. Most of these studies included newly diagnosed early-stage disease or locoregionally relapsed or refractory disease. These patients with localized disease usually received salvage or planned radiotherapy. In a phase II study of chemotherapy with SMILE for advanced-stage, refractory, or relapsed NKTCL [81], 38 patients had stage I and II disease, and 49 had stage III and IV disease. Nineteen patients received additional radiotherapy. The CR and 5-year OS rates for all patients were 56 and 50 %. Grade III–IV acute toxicities were observed in 50–95 % of patients. High level of acute toxicity induced by dose intensity or new regimen chemotherapy in these studies is a critical concern when treating advanced-stage disease or defining radiotherapy/chemotherapy sequences in early-stage disease.

Successful treatment with autologous stem cell transplantation has been reported in several small series of studies [89–92]. However, due to the limited data with inclusion of early-stage disease in these studies, further investigation is needed.

Central nerve system (CNS) chemoprophylaxis for early-stage NKTCL is not necessary, because of an apparently low incidence of CNS failure [15, 26, 93].

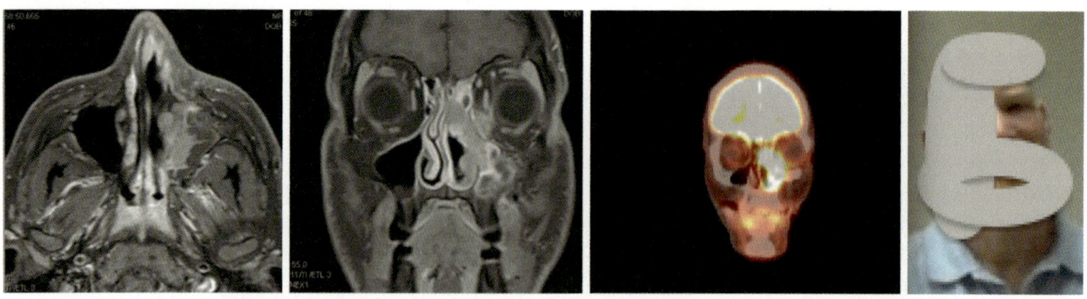

Fig. 11.8 Case 2

Salvage Radiotherapy

Salvage radiotherapy or reirradiation is a treatment option for patients with locoregional failure. Previous studies have shown that patients with locoregionally relapsed or refractory disease after initial chemotherapy can be successfully salvaged with radiotherapy [13, 76]. In 61 early-stage patients receiving initial chemotherapy [13], 31 (51 %) patients developed disease progression and 17 of them had locoregional failure. Nine of the latter patients were successfully salvaged by radiotherapy [13]. Another study has shown that salvage radiotherapy significantly improved survival compared with salvage chemotherapy alone for patients with locoregionally recurrent disease [76]. Of 29 patients with locoregional recurrence only, 19 patients received radiotherapy with or without chemotherapy, and 10 patients received chemotherapy alone. The 2-year and 5-year OS rates after recurrence were 77 % and 69 % for radiotherapy, compared with 2-year OS rate of 50 % and median OS time of 16 months for chemotherapy alone ($p=0.006$). For 24 patients who developed locoregional recurrence only after initial radiotherapy, 15 patients were reirradiated, and 9 patients were treated with chemotherapy alone. The CR rate was 100 % for reirradiation and 43 % for chemotherapy; the 2-year and 5-year OS rates after recurrence were 85 % and 74 % for reirradiation, compared with 2-year OS rate of only 30 % and median OS time of 16 months for chemotherapy alone ($p=0.004$).

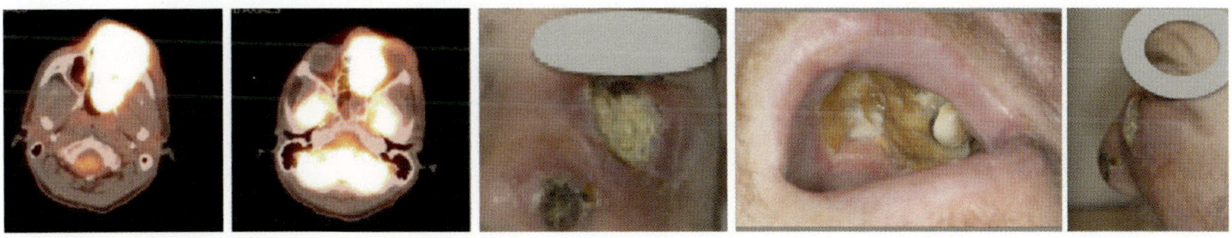

Fig. 11.9 Disease progression, case 2

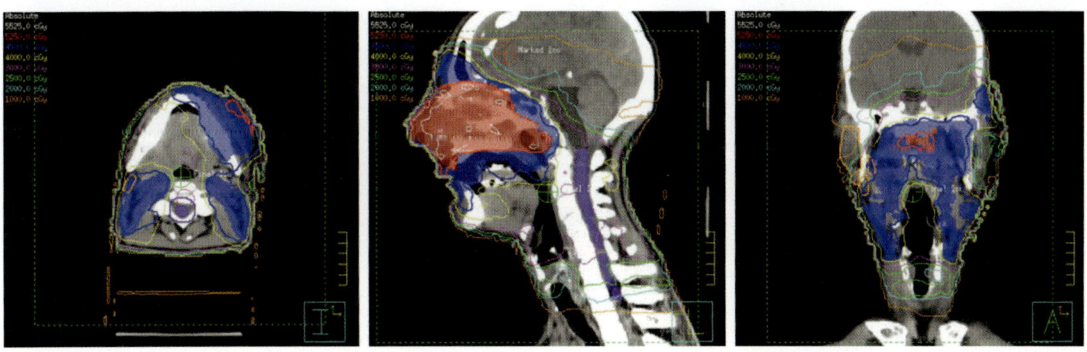

Fig. 11.10 (**a**) IMRT for case 2. *Red* represents the disease receiving 54 Gy and blue the areas receiving 45 G. (**b**) Showing the isodose lines and coverage of the tumor (*red*) to 54 Gy as well as the areas at risk including lymph node regions at risk to 45 Gy (*blue*). (**c**) Showing the isodose lines and coverage of the tumor (*red*) to 54 Gy as well as the areas at risk including lymph node regions at risk to 45 Gy (*blue*). (**d**) DVH for case 2

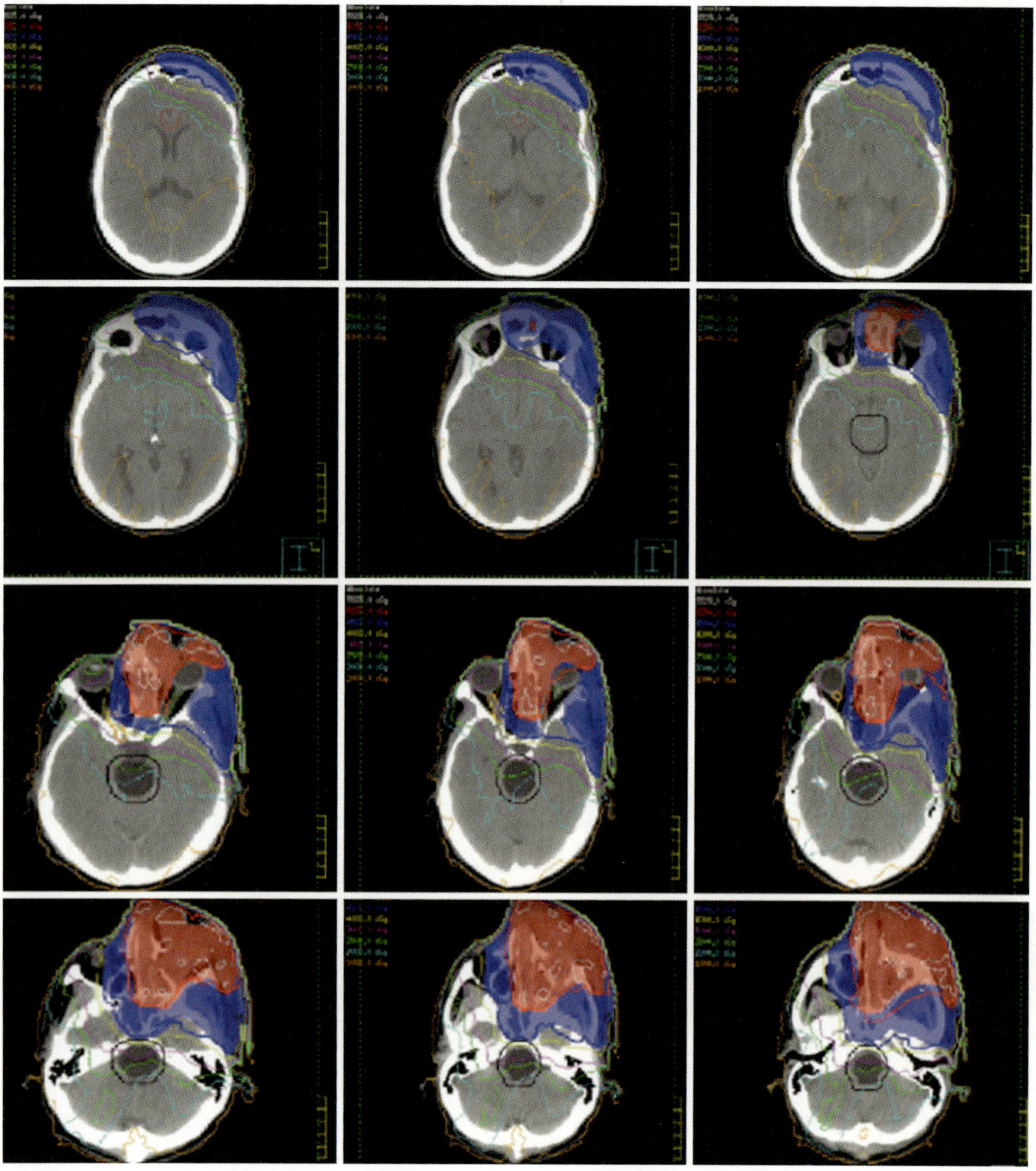

Fig. 11.10 (continues)

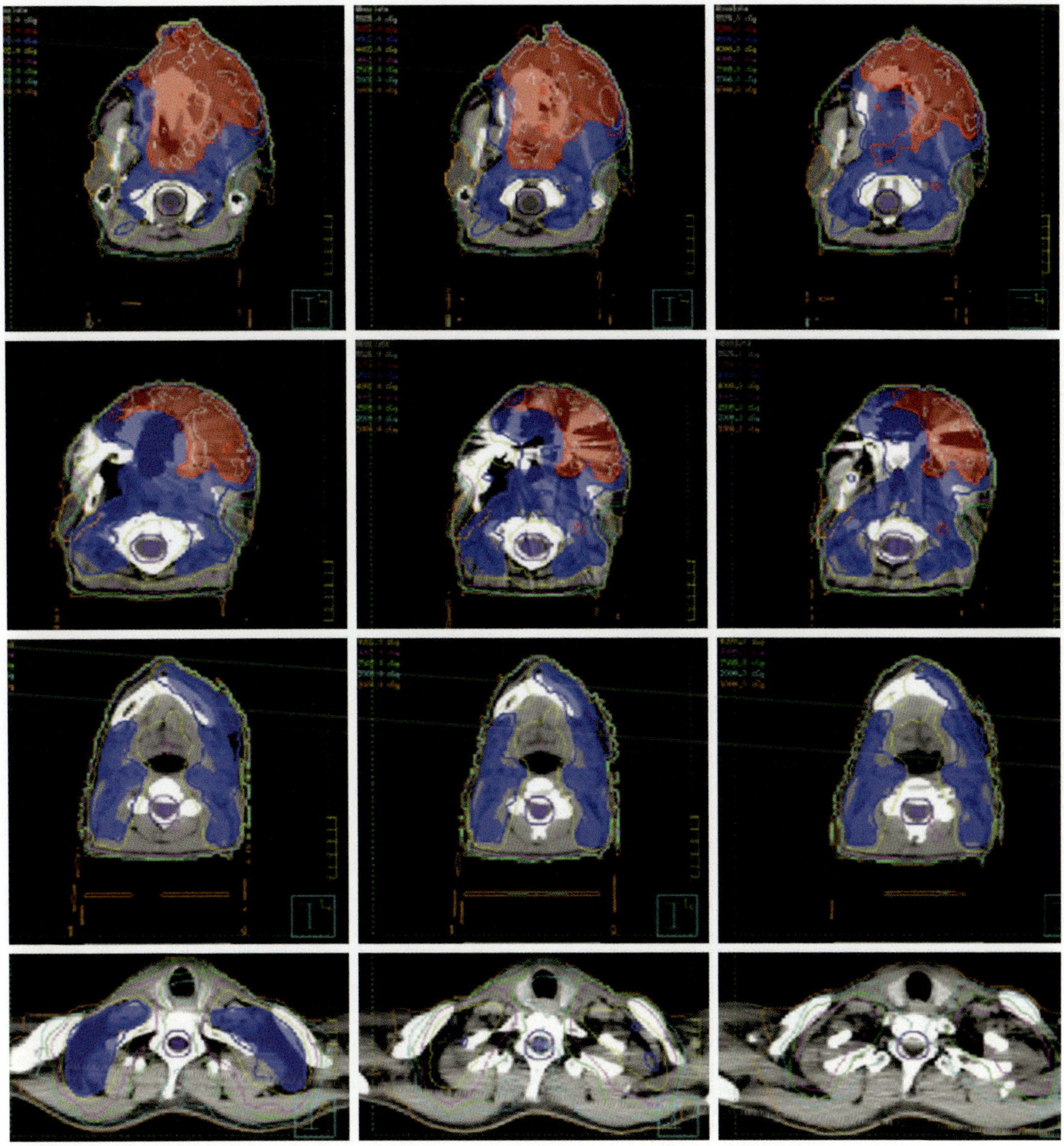

Fig. 11.10 (continues)

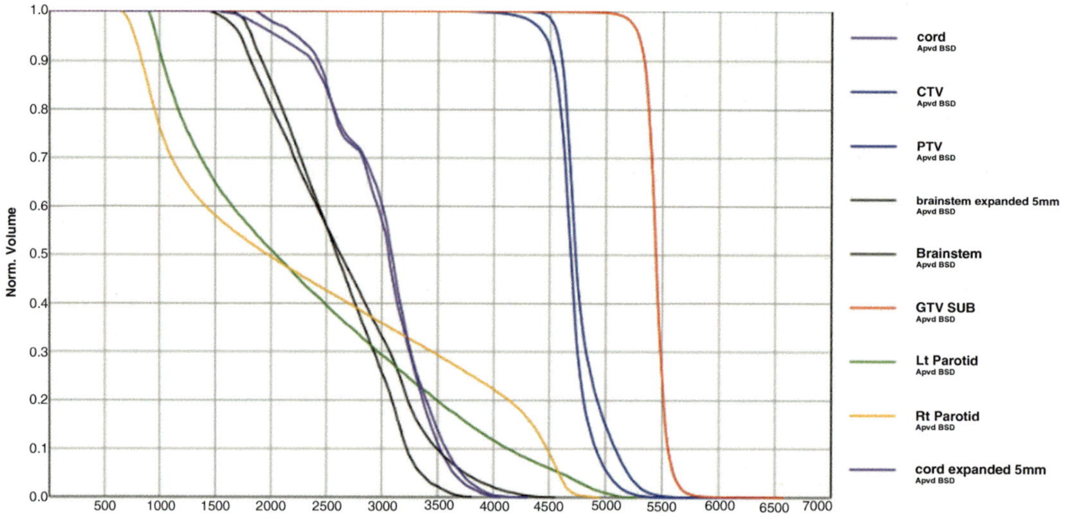

ROI Name	Trial Name	Min. (cGy)	Max. (cGy)	Mean (cGy)	Std. Dev. (cGy)
cord	Aprvd BSD	1831.4	4066.9	2994.8	436.7
CTV	Aprvd BSD	1245.0	6406.4	4786.5	200.1
PTV	Aprvd BSD	1245.0	5737.8	4698.5	180.7
brainstem expanded 5mm	Aprvd BSD	1333.2	4558.2	2651.0	644.9
Brainstem	Aprvd BSD	1592.8	3811.1	2591.2	493.3
GTV	Aprvd BSD	0.0	6583.9	5440.1	173.9
Lt Parotid	Aprvd BSD	541.3	5276.7	2321.2	1179.9
Rt Parotid	Aprvd BSD	628.2	4953.0	2370.1	1412.1
cord expanded 5mm	Aprvd BSD	1473.4	4311.0	3002.7	488.2

Fig. 11.10 (continues)

Recommendation

Based on current findings, risk-adapted therapy involving radiotherapy alone in carefully selected cases of very low-risk patients and radiotherapy and consolidation chemotherapy for intermediate to high-risk patients should be considered the optimal strategy for early-stage NKTCL. Although radiation therapy alone can be advocated based on the large database presented in this chapter, most practices still use combined modality approach for all cases, sequential for early favorable and concurrent for advanced disease. This approach could be inspired by the standard of care with chemotherapy followed by optional radiotherapy for early-stage diffuse large B-cell lymphoma (DLBCL). But the reality is that NKTCL, as opposed to DLBCL, is generally resistant to chemotherapy but sensitive to radiotherapy. Radiotherapy alone achieved similar 5-year OS in early-stage NKTCL as chemotherapy alone in early-stage DLBCL (50–90 %) [10, 45, 47, 94–96]; however, chemotherapy alone achieved a similarly low OS in early-stage NKTCL as radiotherapy alone in early-stage DLBCL (30–50 %) [96, 97, 98]. Henceforth, it is reasonable to accept radiotherapy followed by optional chemotherapy as initial therapy for early-stage NKTCL.

It should be emphasized that treatment strategy for NKTCL is different from that for DLBCL because of different chemosensitivity. Chemotherapy is primary treatment for

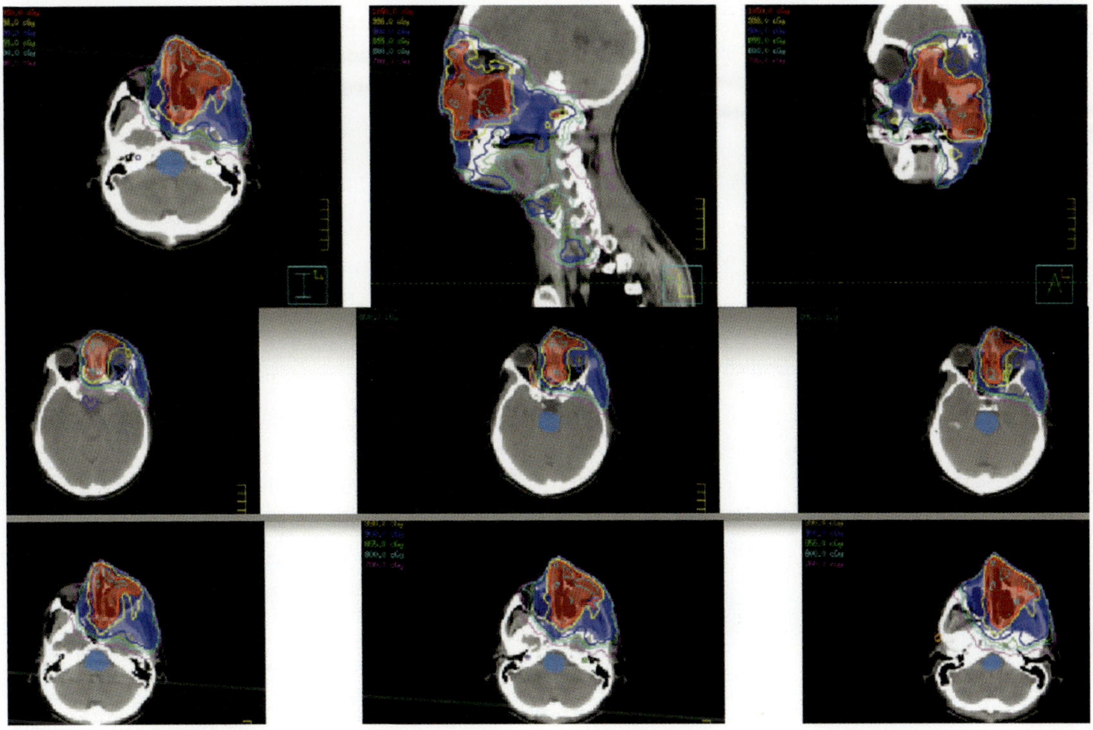

Fig. 11.11 Representative slices of re-planning

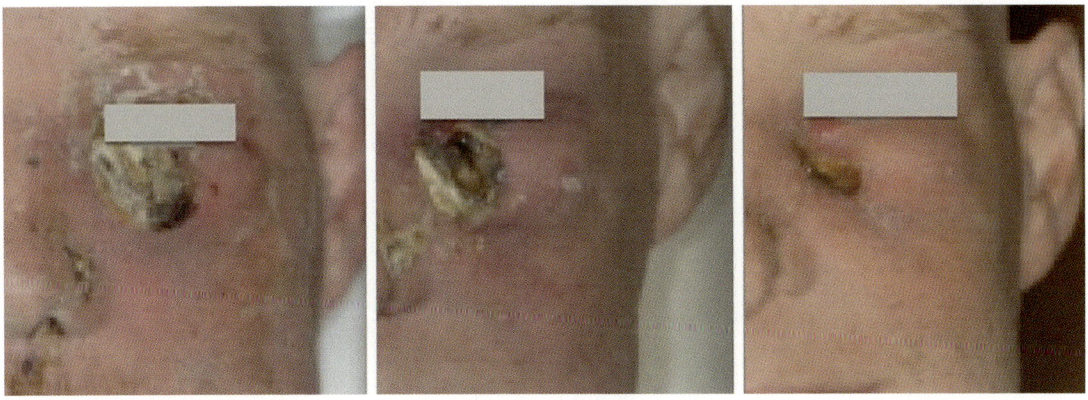

Fig. 11.12 Showing on the left, the response at the end of the treatment with radiation, 4 weeks later (*middle*) and 8 weeks later (*right*)

all stage DLBCL, whereas radiotherapy is primary therapy for early-stage NKTCL, but not for advanced-stage disease, and chemotherapy is primary treatment for advanced-stage NKTCL. Patients with localized NKTCL should be managed differently from advanced-stage diseases. Considering effective initial or salvage radiotherapy for localized NKTCL, evaluation of the efficacy and safety with new regimen-based chemotherapy should be limited to patients with advanced-stage disease. The value of these new regimens in early-stage disease needs to be refined when combined with effective radiotherapy.

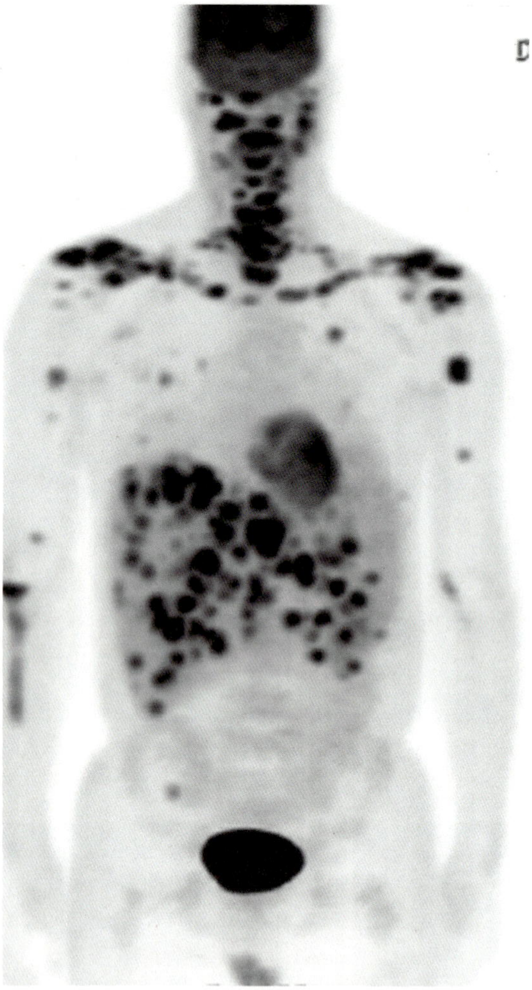

Fig. 11.13 Showing progression in case 2

Future Direction

Several important progresses have been made in the last decade: better understanding of clinicopathologic characteristics, accurate staging with modern diagnostic imaging, establishment of new dedicated prognostic model and risk stratification, risk-adapted therapy with introducing primary radiotherapy for early-stage disease, and L-asparaginase-based combination chemotherapy for advanced-stage disease. Identification of additional clinical, pathological, or molecular predictors and incorporation of more effective diagnostic and therapeutic strategies into risk-adapted therapy warrants further investigation.

References

1. Harris NL, Jaffe ES, Stein H, et al. A revised European-American classification of lymphoid neoplasms: a proposal from the International Lymphoma Study Group. Blood. 1994;84:1361–92.
2. Chan JKC, Jaffe ES, Ralfkiaer E. Extranodal NK/T--cell lymphoma, nasal type. In: Jaffe ES, Harris NL, Stein H, Vardiman JW, editors. World Health Organization classification of tumours: pathology and genetics of tumours of haematopoietic and lymphoid tissues. Lyon: IARC Press; 2001. p. 204–7.
3. Chan JKC, Quintanilla-Martinez L, Ferry JA, Peh SC. Extranodal NK/T-cell lymphoma, nasal type. In: Jaffe ES, Harris NL, Stein H, Vardiman JW, editors. World Health Organization classification of tumours: pathology and genetics of tumours of haematopoietic and lymphoid tissues. Lyon: IARC Press; 2008. p. 285–8.
4. Vose J, Armitage J, Weisenburger D, et al. International peripheral T-Cell and natural killer/T-cell lymphoma study: pathology findings and clinical outcomes. J Clin Oncol. 2008;26:4124–30.
5. Au WY, Weisenburger DD, Intragumtornchai T, et al. Clinical differences between nasal and extranasal natural killer/T-cell lymphoma: a study of 136 cases from the International Peripheral T-Cell Lymphoma Project. Blood. 2009;113:3931–7.
6. Sun J, Yang Q, Lu Z, et al. Distribution of lymphoid neoplasms in China: analysis of 4,638 cases according to the World Health Organization classification. Am J Clin Pathol. 2012;138:429–34.
7. Yang QP, Zhang WY, Yu JB, et al. Subtype distribution of lymphomas in Southwest China: analysis of 6,382 cases using WHO classification in a single institution. Diagn Pathol. 2011;6:77.
8. Aviles A, Diaz NR, Neri N, et al. Angiocentric nasal T/natural killer cell lymphoma: a single center study of prognostic factors in 108 patients. Clin Lab Haematol. 2000;22:215–20.
9. Li YX, Coucke PA, Li JY, et al. Primary non-Hodgkin's lymphoma of the nasal cavity: prognostic significance of paranasal extension and the role of radiotherapy and chemotherapy. Cancer. 1998;83:449–56.
10. Li YX, Yao B, Jin J, et al. Radiotherapy as primary treatment for stage IE and IIE nasal natural killer/T-cell lymphoma. J Clin Oncol. 2006;24:181–9.
11. Li YX, Fang H, Liu QF, et al. Clinical features and treatment outcome of nasal-type NK/T cell lymphoma of Waldeyer ring. Blood. 2008;112:3057–64.

12. Li YX, Liu QF, Fang H, et al. Variable clinical presentations of nasal and Waldeyer ring natural killer/T-cell lymphoma. Clin Cancer Res. 2009;15:2905–12.
13. Cheung MMC, Chan JK, Lau WH, et al. Early stage nasal T/NK-cell lymphoma: clinical outcome, prognostic factors, and the effect of treatment modality. Int J Radiat Oncol Biol Phys. 2002;54:182–90.
14. Chim CS, Ma SY, Au WY, et al. Primary nasal natural killer cell lymphoma: long-term treatment outcome and relationship with the international prognostic index. Blood. 2004;103:216–21.
15. Li YX, Wang H, Feng XL, et al. Immunophenotypic characteristics and clinical relevance of CD56+ and CD56- extranodal nasal-type NK/T-cell lymphoma. Leuk Lymphoma. 2011;52:417–24.
16. Jhuang JY, Chang ST, Weng SF, et al. Extranodal natural killer/T-cell lymphoma, nasal type in Taiwan: a relatively higher frequency of T-cell lineage and poor survival for extranasal tumors. Hum Pathol. 2015;46:313–21.
17. Ko YH, Cho EY, Kim JE, et al. NK and NK-like T-cell lymphoma in extranasal sites: a comparative clinicopathological study according to site and EBV status. Histopathology. 2004;44:480–9.
18. Liu QF, Wang WH, Wang SL, et al. Immunophenotypic and clinical differences between the nasal and extranasal subtypes of upper aerodigestive tract natural killer/T-cell lymphoma. Int J Radiat Oncol Biol Phys. 2014;88:806–13.
19. Karube K, Nakagawa M, Tsuzuki S, et al. Identification of FOXO3 and PRDM1 as tumor-suppressor gene candidates in NK-cell neoplasms by genomic and functional analyses. Blood. 2011;118:3195–204.
20. Siu LL, Wong KF, Chan JK, Kwong YL. Comparative genomic hybridization analysis of natural killer cell lymphoma/leukaemia. Recognition of consistent patterns of genetic alterations. Am J Pathol. 1999;155:1419–25.
21. Koo GC, Tan SY, Tang T, et al. Janus Kinase 3–activating mutations identified in natural killer/T-cell lymphoma. Cancer Dis. 2012;2:591–7.
22. Huang Y, de Rynies A, de Leval A, et al. Gene expression profiling identifies emerging oncolgenic pathways operating in extranodal NK/T-cell lymphoma, nasal type. Blood. 2010;115:1226–37.
23. Takahara M, Kishibe K, Bandoh N, et al. P53, N- and K-Ras, and -Catenin gene mutations and prognostic factors in nasal NK/T-cell lymphoma from Hokkaido. Jpn Hum Pathol. 2004;35:86–95.
24. Quintanilla-Martinez L, Kremer M, Keller G, et al. p53 mutations in nasal natural killer/T-cell lymphoma from Mexico: association with large cell morphology and advanced disease. Am J Pathol. 2001;159:2095–105.
25. Kim SJ, Kim BS, Choi CW, et al. Ki-67 expression is predictive of prognosis in patients with stage I/II extranodal NK/T-cell lymphoma, nasal type. Ann Oncol. 2007;18:1382–7.
26. Li YX, Liu QF, Wang WH, et al. Failure patterns and clinical implications in patients with early stage nasal NK/T-cell lymphoma treated with primary radiotherapy. Cancer. 2011;117:5203–11.
27. Huang MJ, Jiang Y, Liu WP, et al. Early or up-front radiotherapy improved survival of localized extranodal NK/T-cell lymphoma, nasal-type in the upper aerodigestive tract. Int J Radiat Oncol Biol Phys. 2008;70:166–74.
28. Lee J, Kim WS, Park YH, et al. Nasal-type NK/T cell lymphoma: clinical features and treatment outcome. Br J Cancer. 2005;92:1226–30.
29. Lee J, Park YH, Kim WS, et al. Extranodal nasal type NK/T-cell lymphoma: elucidating clinical prognostic factors for risk-based stratification of therapy. Eur J Cancer. 2005;41:1402–8.
30. Lee J, Suh C, Park YH, et al. Extranodal natural killer/T-cell lymphoma, nasal-type: a prognostic model from a retrospective multicenter study. J Clin Oncol. 2006;24:612–8.
31. Jo JC, Yoon DH, Kim S, et al. Clinical features and prognostic model for extranasal NK/T-cell lymphoma. Eur J Haematol. 2012;89:103–10.
32. Kim TM, Lee SY, Jeon YK, et al. Clinical heterogeneity of extranodal NK/T cell lymphoma, nasal type: a national survey of the Korea Cancer Study Group. Ann Oncol. 2008;19:1477–84.
33. Pongpruttipan T, Sukpanichnant S, Assanasen T, et al. Extranodal NK/T-cell lymphoma, nasal type, includes case of natural killer cell and αβ, γδ, and αβ/γδ T cell origin: a comprehensive clinicopathologic and phenotypic study. Am J Surg Pathol. 2012;36:481–99.
34. Ai WZ, Chang ET, Fish K, et al. Racial patterns of extranodal natural killer/T-cell lymphoma, nasal type, in California: a population-based study. Br J Haematol. 2012;156:626–32.
35. Li S, Feng X, Li T, et al. Extranodal NK/T-cell lymphoma, nasal type: a report of 73 cases at MD Anderson Cancer Center. Am J Surg Pathol. 2013;37:14–23.
36. Lee J, Suh C, Huh J, et al. Effect of positive bone marrow EBV in situ hybridization in staging and survival of localized extranodal natural killer/T-cell lymphoma, nasal-type. Clin Cancer Res. 2007;13:3250–4.
37. Suzuki R, Suzumiya J, Yamaguchi M, et al. Prognostic factors for mature natural killer (NK) cell neoplasms: aggressive NK cell leukemia and extranodal NK cell lymphoma, nasal type. Ann Oncol. 2010;21:1032–40.
38. Moon SH, Cho SK, Kim WS, et al. The role of ^{18}F-FDG PET/CT for initial staging of nasal type natural killer/T-cell lymphoma: a comparison with conventional staging methods. J Nucl Med. 2013;54:1039–44.
39. Kako S, Izutsu K, Ota Y, et al. FDG-PET in T-cell and NK-cell neoplasms. Ann Oncol. 2007;18:1685–90.

40. Tsukamoto N, Kojima M, Hasegawa M, et al. The usefulness of ^{18}F-fluorodeoxyglucose positron emission tomography (^{18}F-FDG-PET) and a comparison of ^{18}F-FDG-pet with ^{67}gallium scintigraphy in the evaluation of lymphoma. Cancer. 2007;110:652–9.
41. Li YJ, Li ZM, Xia XY, et al. Prognostic value of interim and posttherapy ^{18}F-FDG PET/CT in patients with mature T-cell and natural killer cell lymphomas. J Nucl Med. 2013;54:1–9.
42. Wang ZY, Liu QF, Wang H, et al. Clinical implications of plasma Epstein-Barr virus DNA in early-stage extranodal nasal-type NK/T-cell lymphoma patients receiving primary radiotherapy. Blood. 2012;120:2003–10.
43. Ito Y, Kimura H, Maeda Y, et al. Pretreatment EBV-DNA copy number is predictive of response and toxicities to SMILE chemotherapy for extranodal NK/T-cell lymphoma, nasal type. Clin Cancer Res. 2012;18:4183–90.
44. Kwong YL, Pang AWK, Leung AYH, Chim CS, Tse E. Quantification of circulating Epstein-Barr virus DNA in NK/T-cell lymphoma treated with the SMILE protocol: diagnostic and prognostic significance. Leukemia. 2014;28:265–870.
45. Yang Y, Zhang YJ, Zhu Y, et al. Prognostic nomogram for overall survival in previously untreated patients with extranodal NK/T-cell lymphoma, nasal-type: a multicenter study. Leukemia. 2015;29:1571–7.
46. Kim TM, Park YH, Lee SY, et al. Local tumor invasiveness is more predictive of survival than International Prognostic Index in stage IE/IIE extranodal NK/T cell lymphoma, nasal type. Blood. 2005;106:3785–90.
47. Yang Y, Zhu Y, Cao JZ, et al. Risk-adapted therapy improves outcome in early-stage extranodal nasal-type NK/T-cell lymphoma: a comprehensive analysis from a multicenter study. Published on line in 24 June 2015. http://dx.doi.org/10.1182/blood-2015-04-639336.
48. Kim GE, Cho JH, Yang WI, et al. Angiocentric lymphoma of the head and neck: patterns of systemic failure after radiation treatment. J Clin Oncol. 2000;18:54–63.
49. Isobe K, Uno T, Tamaru JI, et al. Extranodal natural killer/T-cell lymphoma, nasal type: the significance of radiotherapeutic parameters. Cancer. 2006;106:609–15.
50. Li CC, Tien HF, Tang JL, et al. Treatment outcome and pattern of failure in 77 patients with sinonasal natural killer/T-cell or T-cell lymphoma. Cancer. 2004;100:366–75.
51. You JY, Chi KH, Yang MH, et al. Radiation therapy versus chemotherapy as initial treatment for localized nasal natural killer (NK)/T-cell lymphoma: a single institute survey in Taiwan. Ann Oncol. 2004;15: 618–25.
52. Ma HH, Qian LT, Pan HF, et al. Treatment outcome of radiotherapy alone versus radiochemotherapy in early stage nasal natural killer/T-cell lymphoma. Med Oncol. 2010;27:798–806.
53. Yang Y, Zhang YJ, Lin XB, et al. Role of radiotherapy in the combined treatment of patients with early stage extranodal nasal type NK/T-cell lymphoma and analysis of prognostic factors. Chin J Radiat Oncol. 2009;18:285–9.
54. Yamaguchi M, Kita K, Miwa H, et al. Frequent expression of P-glycoprotein/MDR1 by nasal T-cell lymphoma cells. Cancer. 1995;76:2351–6.
55. Li YX, Wang H, Jin J, et al. Radiotherapy alone with curative intent in patients with stage I extranodal nasal-type NK/T-cell lymphoma. Int J Radiat Oncol Biol Phys. 2012;82:1809–15.
56. Wang H, Li YX, Wang WH, et al. Mild toxicity and favorable prognosis of high-dose and extended involved-field intensity-modulated radiotherapy for patients with early-stage nasal NK/T-cell lymphoma. Int J Radiat Oncol Biol Phys. 2012;82:1115–21.
57. Bi XW, Li YX, Fang H, et al. High-dose and extended-field intensity modulated radiotherapy for early stage NK/T-cell lymphoma of Waldeyer's ring: dosimetric analysis and clinical outcome. Int J Radiat Oncol Biol Phys. 2013;87:1086–93.
58. Yahalom J, Illidge T, Specht L, et al. Modern radiation therapy for extranodal lymphomas: field and dose guidelines from the International Lymphoma Radiation Oncology Group. Int J Radiat Oncol Biol Phys. 2015;92:11–31.
59. Luo YK, Yang T, Fu BY, et al. Prognostic factors and curative efficacy of nasal NK/T-cell lymphoma. China Mod Doct. 2010;48:7–9.
60. Kim GE, Lee SW, Chang SK, et al. Combined chemotherapy and radiation versus radiation alone in the management of localized angiocentric lymphoma of the head and neck. Radiother Oncol. 2001;61:261–9.
61. Aikemu W, Wang RZ, Li PD. A clinical study of 57 patients with extranodal natural killer/T-cell lymphoma, nasal-type. J Xinjiang Med Univ. 2008;31:1507–9.
62. Deng T, Zhang C, Zhang X, et al. Treatment outcome of radiotherapy alone versus radiochemotherapy in IE/IIE extranodal nasal-type natural killer/T cell lymphoma: a meta-analysis. PLoS One. 2014;9:e106577.
63. Jiang L, Li SJ, Jiang YM, et al. The significance of combining radiotherapy with chemotherapy for early stage extranodal natural killer/T-cell lymphoma, nasal type: a systematic review and meta-analysis. Leuk Lymphoma. 2014;55:1038–48.
64. Fang H, Jin J, Wang WH, et al. Prognostic factors and treatment outcomes for patients with stage II extranodal nasal-type natural killer/T-cell lymphoma of the upper aerodigestive tract. Leuk Lymphoma. 2014;55:1832–7.
65. Avilés A, Neri N, Fernández R, et al. Combined therapy in untreated patients improves outcome in nasal NK/T lymphoma: results of a clinical trial. Med Oncol. 2013;30(3):637.
66. Zang J, Li C, Luo SQ, et al. Early radiotherapy has an essential role for improving survival in patients with stage I-II nasal-type of NK/T cell lymphoma treated

with l-asparaginase-containing chemotherapy – a single institution experience. Ann Hematol. 2015;94:583–91.
67. Yamaguchi M, Tobinai K, Oguchi M, et al. Phase I/II study of concurrent chemoradiotherapy for localized nasal natural killer/T-cell lymphoma: Japan Clinical Oncology Group Study JCOG0211. J Clin Oncol. 2009;27:5594–600.
68. Kim SJ, Kim K, Kim BS, et al. Phase II trial of concurrent radiation and weekly cisplatin followed by VIPD chemotherapy in newly diagnosed, stage IE to IIE, nasal, extranodal NK/T-cell lymphoma: consortium for improving survival of lymphoma study. J Clin Oncol. 2009;27:6027–32.
69. Tsai HJ, Lin SF, Chen CC, et al. Long-term results of a phase II trial with frontline concurrent chemoradiotherapy followed by consolidation chemotherapy for localized nasal natural killer/T-cell lymphoma. Eur J Haematol. 2015;94:130–7.
70. Kim SJ, Yang DH, Kim JS, et al. Concurrent chemoradiotherapy followed by L-asparaginase-containing chemotherapy, VIDL, for localized nasal extranodal NK/T cell lymphoma: CISL08-01 phase II study. Ann Hematol. 2014;93:1895–901.
71. Ke QH, Zhou SQ, Du W, et al. Concurrent IMRT and weekly cisplatin followed by GDP chemotherapy in newly diagnosed, stage IE to IIE, nasal, extranodal NK/T-Cell lymphoma. Blood Cancer J. 2014;4:e267.
72. Lee J, Kim CY, Park YJ, et al. Sequential chemotherapy followed by radiotherapy versus concurrent chemoradiotherapy in patients with stage I/II extranodal natural killer/T-cell lymphoma, nasal type. Blood Res. 2013;48:274–81.
73. Jiang M, Zhang H, Jiang Y, et al. Phase 2 trial of "sandwich" L-asparaginase, vincristine, and prednisone chemotherapy with radiotherapy in newly diagnosed, stage IE to IIE, nasal type, extranodal natural killer/T-cell lymphoma. Cancer. 2012;118: 3294–301.
74. Wang L, Wang ZH, Chen XQ, et al. First-line combination of gemcitabine, oxaliplatin, and L-asparaginase (GELOX) followed by involved-field radiation therapy for patients with stage IE/IIE extranodal natural killer/T-cell lymphoma. Cancer. 2013;119:348–55.
75. Wang H, Wuxiao ZJ, Zhu J, et al. Comparison of gemcitabine, oxaliplatin and L-asparaginase and etoposide, vincristine, doxorubicin, cyclophosphamide and prednisone as first-line chemotherapy in patients with stage IE to IIE extranodal natural killer/T-cell lymphoma: a multicenter retrospective study. Leuk Lymphoma. 2015;56:971–7.
76. Zhao T, Li YX, Wang SL, et al. Survival benefit with salvage radiotherapy for patients with locoregionally recurrent extranodal nasal-type NK/T-cell lymphoma. Ann Hematol. 2013;92:325–32.
77. Yong W, Zheng W, Zhu J, et al. L-asparaginase in the treatment of refractory and relapsed extranodal NK/T-cell lymphoma, nasal type. Ann Hematol. 2009;88:647–52.
78. Jaccard A, Petit B, Girault S, et al. L-Asparaginase-based treatment of 15 western patients with extranodal NK/T-cell lymphoma and leukemia and a review of the literature. Ann Oncol. 2009;20:110–6.
79. Yamaguchi M, Kwong YL, Kim WS, et al. Phase II study of SMILE chemotherapy for newly diagnosed stage IV, relapsed, or refractory extranodal natural killer (NK)/T-cell lymphoma, nasal type: the NK-cell Tumor Study Group study. J Clin Oncol. 2011;29:4410–6.
80. Jaccard A, Nathalie Gachard N, Marin B, et al. Efficacy of L-asparaginase with methotrexate and dexamethasone (AspaMetDex regimen) in patients with refractory or relapsing extranodal NK/T-cell lymphoma, a phase 2 study. Blood. 2011;117:1834–9.
81. Kwong YL, Kim WS, Lim ST, et al. SMILE for natural killer/T-cell lymphoma: analysis of safety and efficacy from the Asia Lymphoma Study Group. Blood. 2012;120:2973–80.
82. Lin NJ, Song YQ, Tu MF, et al. A prospective phase II study of L-asparaginase-CHOP plus radiation in newly diagnosed extranodal NK/T-cell lymphoma, nasal type. J Hematol Oncol. 2013;6:44.
83. Ji J, Xiang B, Liu WP, et al. A study of gemcitabine, L-asparaginase, ifosfamide, dexamethasone and etoposide chemotherapy for newly diagnosed stage IV, relapsed or refractory extranodal NK/T-cell lymphoma, nasal type. Leuk Lymphoma. 2014;55: 2955–7.
84. Zhou Z, Li X, Chen C, et al. Effectiveness of gemcitabine, pegaspargase, cisplatin, and dexamethasone (DDGP) combination chemotherapy in the treatment of relapsed/refractory extranodal NK/T cell lymphoma: a retrospective study of 17 patients. Ann Hematol. 2014;93:1889–94.
85. Guo HQ, Liu L, Wang XF, et al. Efficacy of gemcitabine combined with oxaliplatin. L-asparaginase and dexamethasone in patients with newly-diagnosed extranodal NK/T-cell lymphoma. Mol Clin Oncol. 2014;2:1172–6.
86. Wang YQ, Yang Y, Zhuo HY, et al. Trial of LVDP regimen (L-asparaginase, etoposide, dexamethasone, and cisplatin, followed by radiotherapy) as first-line treatment for newly diagnosed, stage III/IV extranodal natural killer/T cell lymphoma. Med Oncol. 2015;32:435.
87. Kim SJ, Park S, Kang ES, et al. Induction treatment with SMILE and consolidation with autologous stem cell transplantation for newly diagnosed stage IV extranodal natural killer/T cell lymphoma patients. Ann Hematol. 2015;94:71–8.
88. Kim M, Kim TM, Kim KH, et al. Ifosfamide, methotrexate, etoposide, and prednisolone (IMEP) plus L-asparaginase as a first-line therapy improves outcomes in stage III/IV NK/T cell-lymphoma, nasal type (NTCL). Ann Hematol. 2015;94:437–44.
89. Murashige N, Kami M, Kishi Y, et al. Allogeneic haematopoietic stem cell transplantation as a promising treatment for natural killer-cell neoplasms. Br J Haematol. 2005;130:561–7.

90. Yokoyama H, Yamamoto J, Tohmiya Y, et al. Allogeneic hematopoietic stem cell transplant following chemotherapy containing l-asparaginase as a promising treatment for patients with relapsed or refractory extranodal natural killer/T cell lymphoma, nasal type. Leuk Lymphoma. 2010;51:1509–12.
91. Ennishi D, Maeda Y, Fujii N, et al. Allogeneic hematopoietic stem cell transplantation for advanced extranodal natural killer/T-cell lymphoma, nasal type. Leuk Lymphoma. 2011;52:1255–61.
92. Tse E, Chan T, Koh L, et al. Allogeneic haematopoietic SCT for natural killer/T-cell lymphoma: a multicentre analysis from the Asia Lymphoma Study Group. Bone Marrow Transplant. 2014;49:902–6.
93. Kim SJ, Oh SY, Hong JY, et al. When do we need central nervous system prophylaxis in patients with extranodal NK/T-cell lymphoma, nasal type? Ann Oncol. 2010;21:1058–63.
94. Miller TP, Dahlberg S, Cassady JR, et al. Chemotherapy alone compared with chemotherapy plus radiotherapy for localized intermediate- and high-grade non-Hodgkin's lymphoma. N Engl J Med. 1998;339:21–6.
95. Horning SH, Weller E, Kim KM, et al. Chemotherapy with or without radiotherapy in limited-stage diffuse aggressive non-Hodgkin's lymphoma: Eastern Cooperative Oncology Group Study 1484. J Clin Oncol. 2004;22:3032–8.
96. Phan J, Mazloom A, Medeiros LJ, et al. Benefit of consolidative radiation therapy in patients with diffuse large B-cell lymphoma treated with R-CHOP chemotherapy. J Clin Oncol. 2010;28:4170–6.
97. Qi SN, Li YX, Wang H, et al. Diffuse large B-cell lymphoma: clinical characterization and prognosis of Waldeyer ring versus lymph node presentation. Cancer. 2009;115:4980–9.
98. Persky DO, Miller TP, Unger JM, et al. Ibritumomab consolidation after 3 cycles of CHOP plus radiotherapy in high-risk limited-stage aggressive B-cell lymphoma: SWOG S0313. Blood. 2015;125:236–41.
99. Tomita N, Kodaira T, Tachibana H, et al. A comparison of radiation treatment plans using IMRT with helical tomotherapy and 3D conformal radiotherapy for nasal natural killer/T-cell lymphoma. Br J Radiol. 2009;82:756–63.
100. Shen Q, Ma X, Hu W, et al. Intensity-modulated radiotherapy versus three-dimensional conformal radiotherapy for stage I-II natural killer/T-cell lymphoma nasal type: dosimetric and clinical results. Radiat Oncol. 2013;8:152.
101. Koom WS, Chung EJ, Yang WI, et al. Angiocentric T-cell and NK/T-cell lymphomas: radiotherapeutic viewpoints. Int J Radiat Oncol Biol Phys. 2004;59:1127–37.
102. Wang L, Xia ZJ, Lu Y, Zhang YJ. Prophylactic cervical lymph node irradiation provides no benefit for patients of stage I extranodal natural killer/T-cell lymphoma, nasal type. Med Oncol. 2015;32:320.
103. Shikama N, Ikeda H, Nakamura S, et al. Localized aggressive non-Hodgkin's lymphoma of the nasal cavity: a survey by the Japan Lymphoma Radiation Therapy Group. Int J Radiat Oncol Biol Phys. 2001;51:1228–33.
104. Wu X, Li P, Zhao J, Yang X, et al. A clinical study of 115 patients with extranodal natural killer/T-cell lymphoma, nasal type. Clin Oncol (R Coll Radiol). 2008;20:619–25.
105. Kim K, Chie EK, Kim CW, et al. Treatment outcome of angiocentric T-cell and NK/T-cell lymphoma, nasal type: radiotherapy versus chemoradiotherapy. Jpn J Clin Oncol. 2005;35:1–5.

Radiation Therapy in the Management of Cutaneous T-Cell Lymphomas

12

Grace L. Smith

Abstract

Primary cutaneous T-cell lymphomas (CTCL) are a rare form of lymphomas, characterized by skin involvement without extracutaneous involvement at diagnosis. The most common type is mycosis fungoides (MF), which represent 72 % of cutaneous T-cell lymphomas with incidence of 6.4 cases per million or approximately 3000 cases per year in the USA. Following that are CD30+ lymphoproliferative diseases which include primary cutaneous anaplastic large-cell lymphoma (pcALCL). Both MF and pcALCL generally follow a chronic, indolent course, but with frequent skin relapses and risk of extracutaneous spread. Radiation therapy (RT) is an important palliative treatment modality in both advanced and localized cases. In this chapter, patients with advanced and early stage MF and pcALCL will be discussed. RT management in each of these cases will be addressed.

Background

Primary cutaneous T cell lymphomas (CTCL) are a rare form of lymphomas, characterized by skin involvement without extracutaneous involvement at diagnosis. The most common type is mycosis fungoides (MF), which represent 72 % of cutaneous T-cell lymphomas with incidence of 6.4 cases per million or approximately 3000 cases per year in the USA. Following that are CD30+ lymphoproliferative diseases which include primary cutaneous anaplastic large-cell lymphoma (pcALCL). Both MF and pcALCL generally follow a chronic, indolent course, but with frequent skin relapses and risk of extracutaneous spread. Radiation therapy (RT) is an important palliative treatment modality in both advanced and localized cases. In this chapter, patients with advanced and early stage MF and pcALCL will be discussed. RT management in each of these cases will be addressed.

G.L. Smith, MD, PhD, MPH
Department of Radiation Oncology,
MD Anderson Cancer Center, 1515 Holcombe Blvd,
Houston, TX 77030, USA
e-mail: glsmith@mdanderson.org

B.S. Dabaja, A.K. Ng (eds.), *Radiation Therapy in Hematologic Malignancies*,
DOI 10.1007/978-3-319-42615-0_12

Early Stage Mycosis Fungoides

Clinical Presentation: Early Stage Case 1

A healthy 59-year-old woman presented after a 7-year history of a single pruritic plaque over the chin area of the face. Low-potency topical corticosteroid cream empirically helped the pruritis and inflammation, but eventually the patient received a biopsy of the lesion (Fig. 12.1). *Results demonstrated mycosis fungoides with the majority of lymphocytes CD3+ T cells. CD30 highlighted rare, scattered cells. Dermal CD4/CD8 ratio was 8:1. This patient demonstrated some typical and atypical epidemiologic and clinical risk features of MF. MF primarily affects older adults, with incidence peaking in patients aged 70 years and older. Black race and male gender are risk factors associated with developing CTCL, with higher T stage and poorer long-term prognosis. Early lesions often start in sun-shielded areas* [1–3].

A complete head-to-toe skin examination was performed of the patient's face, hair, scalp, neck, chest, back, abdomen, buttocks, bilateral upper extremities, bilateral lower extremities, hands, feet, palms, soles, digits, and nails. Only the 5×5 cm purplish plaque on the chin area was noted, for a body surface area (BSA) assessment of 1 % plaque and modified Severity-Weighted Assessment Tool (mSWAT) score of 2, Stage IA.

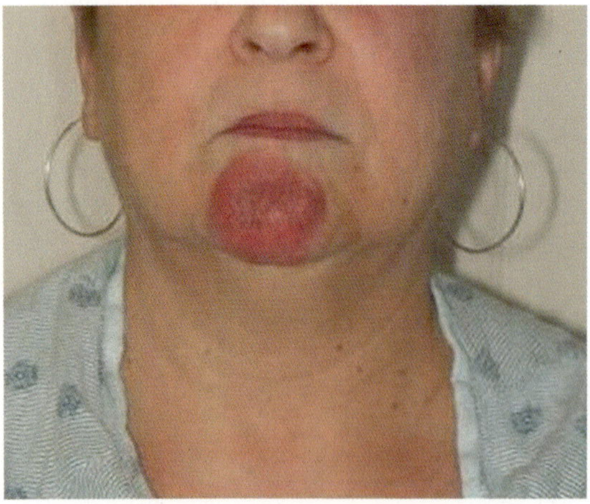

Fig. 12.1 Localized mycosis fungoides (MF) of the chin

Pathology, Staging, and Prognostic Factors

Diagnosis of MF is challenging; with the lack of a diagnostic gold standard and the many benign conditions, MF can mimic in its early stages. Diagnosis requires correlation between the clinical presentation along with histopathologic and immunophenotypic findings of the skin biopsy, including seeking to identify a clonal T-cell population clustered at the basement membrane of the epidermis. The malignant clone should bear the immunophenotype of activated, skin-homing CD4+ helper T cells that interact with antigen-presenting dendritic (Langerhans) cells in the epidermis [4]. A typical immunophenotype is CD2+, CD3+, CD4+, CD45RO+, CLA+, and CD8− (cytotoxic T cell) [5].

Early MF typically presents in patch phase, eventually progressing to plaques, tumors, and erythroderma (>80 % body surface involvement with confluent patches/plaques) (Fig. 12.2). With progression, there is loss of epidermotropism, lymphoid infiltration increasing in density and invasion into the deeper reticular dermis, and ultimately the development of tumor. The Pautrier's microabscess is considered pathognomonic but occurs in less than 20 % of early lesions. The World Health Organization-European Organization for Research and Treatment of Cancer (WHO-EORTC) established the pathologic classification scheme for CTCL including MF [6–8]. Variants include folliculotropic and granulomatous slack skin MF.

Staging and Prognostic Factors: Early Stage Case

A thorough history should demonstrate attention to duration, change, and distribution of lesion(s) and an understanding of symptoms including pruritis, pain, exfoliation, fissures, bullae, and perineal/perianal discomfort or evidence of involvement. The skin examination is critical not only for RT planning but also for staging and characterization of the percent cutaneous involvement by BSA and mSWAT scores. Skin photo-

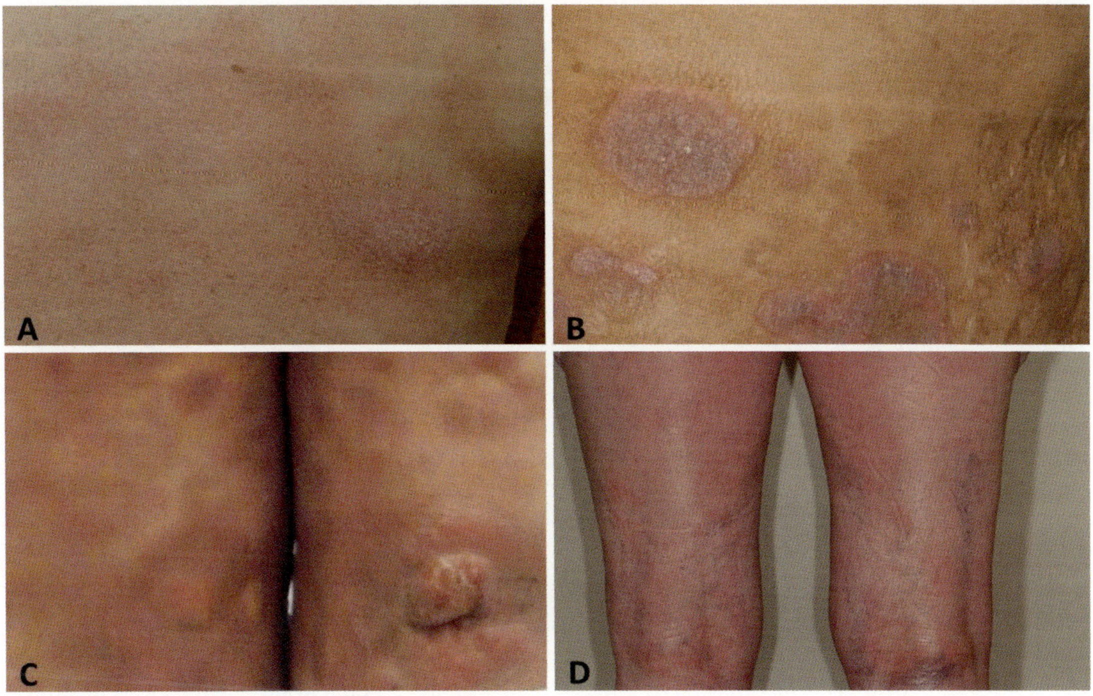

Fig. 12.2 Patch (**a**), plaque (**b**), tumor (**c**), and erythroderma (**d**) lesions

graphs are important for documentation and anticipation of the chronic waxing and waning of disease over time and treatment. Adenopathy and organomegaly should also be documented. After biopsy, complete staging evaluation for this patient included complete blood count (CBC) with differential, comprehensive metabolic panel (CMP), serum chemistries (including renal and hepatic function), and lactate dehydrogenase (LDH), all of which were normal for this patient. Concerning lymph nodes, particularly those ≥1.5 cm, may require excisional biopsy. PET/CT scan and bone marrow biopsy are not required in patients presenting with early stage, limited disease, but should be considered in patients with a higher burden of skin involvement or other concerning findings such as clinical abnormalities or large-cell transformation on pathology. Peripheral blood flow cytometry is typically performed to assess expression of CD2, CD3, CD4, CD5, CD7, CD8, CD20, and CD45RO.

Current staging is based on the TNMB system, as proposed by the European Organization for Research and Treatment of Cancer (EORTC)/International Society for Cutaneous Lymphomas (ISCL). This staging includes MF and Sézary syndrome (SS) and considers skin, nodal involvement, and clonal and tumor burden in the blood [9]. T stage consistently demonstrates strong prognostic significance. Patients with limited patch and plaque involvement (stage IA, T1 N0 M0) demonstrate 10-year survival comparable to matched controls, while a dose response in the survival curve is demonstrated in patients with extensive patches and plaques (T2), tumors (T3), and erythroderma (T4), with median 11-, 3.2-, and 4.6-year survival, respectively [10]. In contrast, the independent prognostic significance of nodal involvement on overall survival is less clear, though overall stage is still correlated with outcome [11]. Other prognostic factors previously identified in studies include older age, large-cell transformation, elevated LDH [12], increased soluble interleukin-2 receptor levels [13], lower percentage of $CD8^+$ tumor-infiltrating lymphocytes [14], or T-cell clonality within the cutaneous infiltrate, blood, and/or nodes [15–18].

Treatment and Management: Early Stage Case 1

For the patient's stage IA MF, a definitive radiation treatment approach was offered. The radiation treatment plan targeted the visible sole plaque of the skin of the chin plus a margin for penumbra and setup error (1.5 cm beyond all visible and palpable abnormality), using local appositional electrons to a total dose of 20 Gy in 10 fractions. With the consideration of decreasing toxicity to normal tissue and with the understanding that repeated courses of radiotherapy might be likely in the future, the lowest possible electron energy directed at only the involved site was chosen. Appositional 9 MeV electron treatment was adequate to cover the thickness of the lesion. Cotton rolls were placed between the lip and the gingiva to decrease the electron backscatter, avoiding excessive toxicity to the mucosa (see Fig. 12.3*). Patients will often have undergone a CT scan during their workup, and this imaging can be helpful to determine the thickness of the lesion to inform electron energy. Otherwise, for nodules or irregular skin surfaces, CT simulation may be helpful for choosing the electron energy that ensures adequate depth.*

Presentation of MF with a single cutaneous lesion is rare, with most early stage patients, though presenting with limited skin surface area involvement, still having multiple lesions. The treatment strategy for MF depends on whether it is early vs. advanced or refractory in presentation [19]. For early disease, first-line treatment strategy is based on sequential skin-directed therapies, including RT, with the goal of providing the most durable response, with the least toxicity. As the disease becomes increasingly refractory, systemic, targeted, or combined therapies are second-line considerations, though RT remains an option.

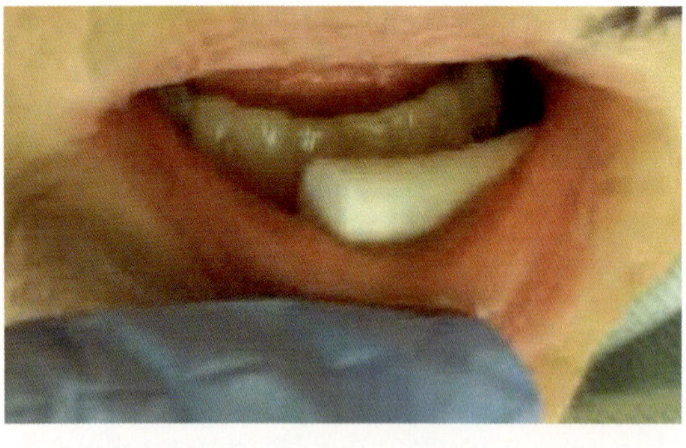

Fig. 12.3 Cotton roll between the lip and gingiva displaces the lip and decreases the electron backscatter, in order to decrease risk of treatment-associated radiation mucositis

For patients with disease limited to the skin, the skin-directed therapies including corticosteroids, mechlorethamine (nitrogen mustard), carmustine (BCNU), bexarotene gel (rexinoids), psoralen plus ultraviolet A (PUVA), ultraviolet B (UVB), and either localized or total skin electron radiotherapy all render high rates of control, particularly in patients presenting with localized uni-lesional MF or <10 % BSA involvement [20–22]. Long-term disease-free survival still ranges from 30 to 50 % in prior studies of these patients. Patients with more extensive cutaneous involvement still typically achieve initial control with these therapies, but long-term cure is unlikely [23, 24].

Radiation Field, Dose, and Technique: Early Stage Case 1

Radiation remains a highly effective treatment for MF, though determining the optimal dose is challenging [25]. The dose response with RT was well documented both for local RT and total skin electron beam therapy (TSEBT), and as a result, historically, RT doses >30 Gy were considered standard. More recently, the high rates of effective cutaneous control for lower doses has been increasingly appreciated, as high as 88 % overall response rate in a series of patients treated with 12 Gy TSEBT with mild and reversible toxicities [26, 27]. Accordingly, there is increasing consensus that the incremental local control benefit of higher RT doses may not outweigh the concomitant incremental toxicity—with a consequent shift toward low-dose RT as a standard approach. The International Lymphoma Radiation Oncology Group (ILROG) consensus field and dose guidelines consider local RT doses ranging from 6 Gy to >30 Gy as acceptable, with an emphasis on recommending lower doses for palliation and doses from 20 to 24 Gy for uni-lesional

MF. The recommended target for treatment is the lesion plus 1.0–2.0 cm margin for local palliation and the entire skin for TSEBT, using electron technique (customarily 6–9 MeV with bolus for patch, and higher energies for thicker plaques or tumors and exophytic lesions) [28].

Posttreatment Considerations: Early Stage Case 1

*The early stage MF patient developed mild erythema and dry skin with RT, completely resolved at 4-week follow-up. At the last follow-up, 20 months after treatment, the lesion remained in complete remission (*Fig. 12.4*). Unfortunately, the patient developed another similar small lesion on the left arm, which was biopsy-proven MF. This lesion is currently well controlled with topical corticosteroids only. Typical follow-up visits every 3–6 months include a history and physical examination including comprehensive skin examination, blood work (including a CBC and LDH), swab and culture of any lesions concerning for infection/colonization, and repeat imaging only as needed.*

Clinical Case 2: Patient Presenting with Stage I, Tumorous Lesion

A healthy 52-year-old female hairdresser noted an itchy lesion over the left ear. She managed it for months using topical steroids. However, the lesion kept growing, eventually forming a tumor (see Fig. 12.5*). After 18 months, biopsy confirmed MF. Careful skin examination showed another lesion in close proximity on the left ear, as well as one on the back of the neck measuring 1.5 × 2 cm. Staging workup showed no evidence of disease in the marrow, nodes, or internally. The patient was referred to receive definitive radiation therapy. The patient was simulated with an open neck position, with the area to be targeted clinically traced with radioopaque wires. The treatment was planned using a single appositional electron field with 6 MeV electrons, and in an effort to avoid the parotid gland, skin collimation was applied (see* Fig. 12.6*). To overcome the irregularity of the skin, a tissue-equivalent material was used to compensate for the gaps and form a uniform surface. A 1 cm tissue-equivalent bolus was placed over the lesion to ensure that 100% of the dose would reach the surface (see* Fig. 12.7*). A total dose of 12 Gy in six treatments was delivered. The patient was discharged with moisturizers to apply to the treated area. A picture of the lesion was taken almost on a weekly basis until complete disappearance of the lesion on week 12 (see* Fig. 12.8*).*

The patient did well for a year before she presented with another lesion over the face that was again treated with radiation. Today almost 18 months after treating her ear, the later site is still well controlled. This case is a good example of how lowering the dose can still offer a durable local control.

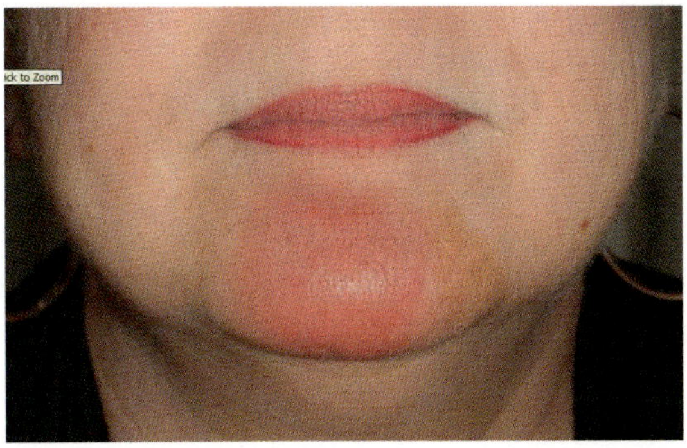

Fig. 12.4 MF lesion at 8 weeks follow-up, demonstrating an excellent clinical response

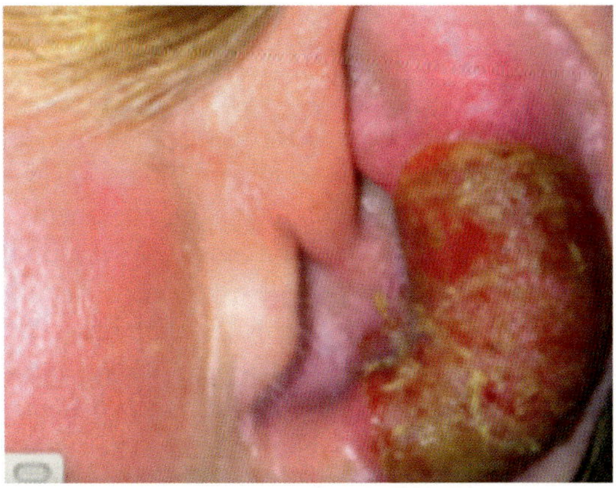

Fig. 12.5 Left ear lesion forming an ulcerative tumor. Another lesion is seen in front of the tragus

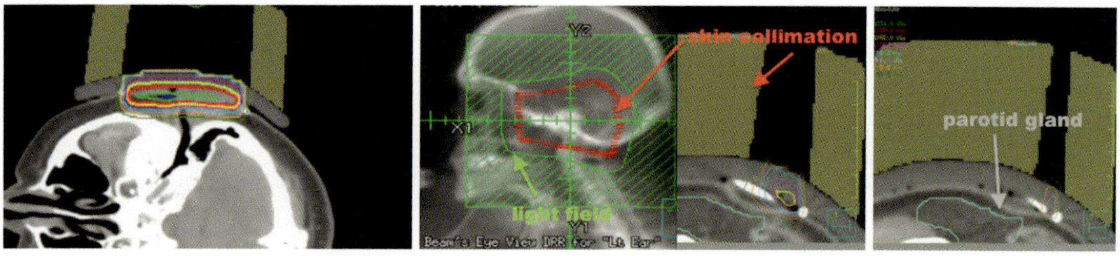

Fig. 12.6 Isodose lines encompassing the target (*left*); skin collimation placement and light field (*green*) surrounding the skin collimation (*red*) (middle photo); skin collimation blocking dose to the parotid gland (*right*)

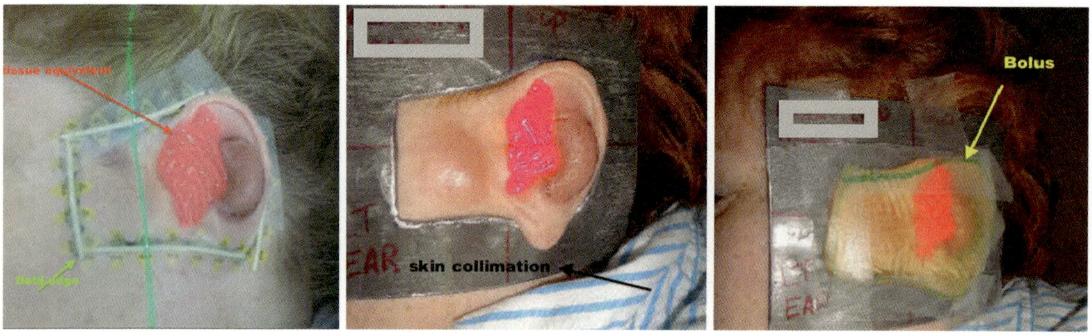

Fig. 12.7 Daily setup with bolus (*yellow*), tissue equivalent (*pink*), and the skin collimation to protect the surrounding organs including the parotid

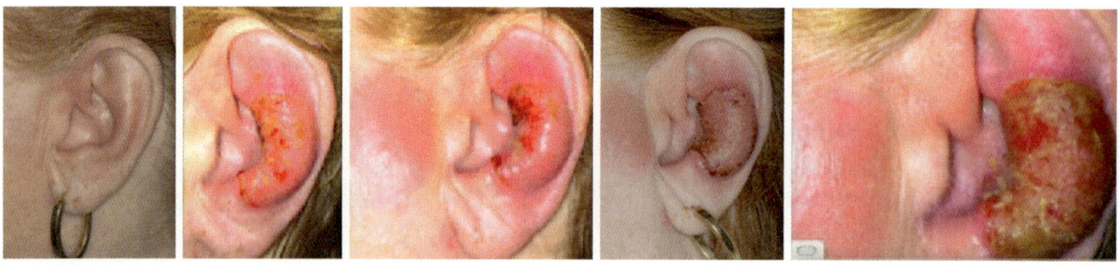

Fig. 12.8 Lesion prior to radiation (far *right*) and the progression of the response until the last one on week 12 (*left*) with complete disappearance

A key caution is to allow lesions to heal, even if healing appears slow, sometimes taking several months. As long as a continuous improvement is seen, we recommend continued observation. Patients not infrequently demonstrate a natural history consisting of local lesions only that respond very well to either topical treatment or low-dose radiation. Especially for such patients, the treatment strategy should avoid unnecessary radiation to surrounding critical organs, for instance in this case the parotid gland.

Advanced Stage MF

Clinical Presentation: Advanced Stage Case 3

A 60-year-old Caucasian woman presented with a 5-year history of progressive pruritic rash, originally thought to be psoriasis, but was eventually biopsy-proven MF. On initial presentation BSA patch was 22 %, plaque 0 %, tumor 4.5 %, and mSWAT 40. Tumors were present on the

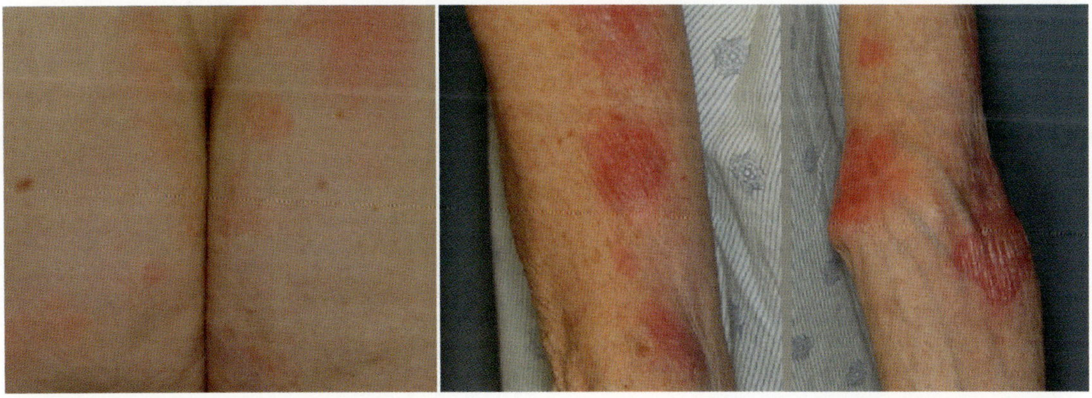

Fig. 12.9 Lesions over the arms and buttocks

arms, legs, and buttocks, with weeping, ulcerated lesions over the arms and feet; see example photos in Fig. 12.9. *The patient had a palpable right inguinal lymph node. A staging PET-CT* (Fig. 12.10) *demonstrated extensive cutaneous hypermetabolism consistent with the clinically noted skin lesions. There were several hypermetabolic right inguinal lymph nodes, the largest measuring 2.8 cm with SUV 3.9. Peripheral flow studies were negative, ruling out SS. Baseline LDH was within normal limits.*

Pathology: Advanced Stage Case

The skin biopsy demonstrated a dense dermal atypical lymphocytic infiltrate. Many of the cells were large with vesicular nuclei, irregular nuclear contours and prominent nucleoli, consistent with large-cell transformation. Immunohistochemical studies demonstrated CD3+ and CD4+ T cells with CD4/CD8 ratio >10:1. Approximately 10 % of lymphocytes expressed CD30+ in a 2+ membranous pattern. The patient also received a biopsy of the concerning inguinal lymph node, which demonstrated involvement with MF. Therefore, the patient was Stage IVA.

Large-cell transformation can occur, in up to 39 % of patients. Transformation is associated with higher stage, potentially more aggressive behavior, and CD30+ in 30 % and CD20+ in 45 % of cases [29, 30]. In advanced disease, MF can involve the lymph nodes, blood, bone marrow, and visceral organs. Sézary syndrome (SS) is characterized by erythroderma plus malignant circulating T cells (as determined by absolute Sézary cell count, flow, or polymerase chain reaction) [31].

Staging and Prognostic Factors: Advanced Stage Case

Particularly for advanced stage patients, 15 % have lymph node involvement at diagnosis, and size ≥1.5 cm is considered clinically abnormal [32, 33]. Visceral involvement, including involvement of the lungs, central nervous system, oral cavity, and oropharynx, is rarer and co-segregates with advanced skin involvement, nodal disease, and blood involvement [32, 34]. The frequency of bone marrow involvement ranges between 6 and 28 % of patients in prior studies [7, 8].

MF can progress to an erythrodermic stage and SS, or SS can arise independently. Patients can clinically present with diffuse edema and tumorous involvement of the face (leonine facies), and severe fissures of the palms and soles, accompanied by symptoms of intense pruritus and pain. In a retrospective study of 1502 patients, one of the largest cohorts assembled for MF, advanced T, N, M, and B stages were all independent predictors of worse survival, as

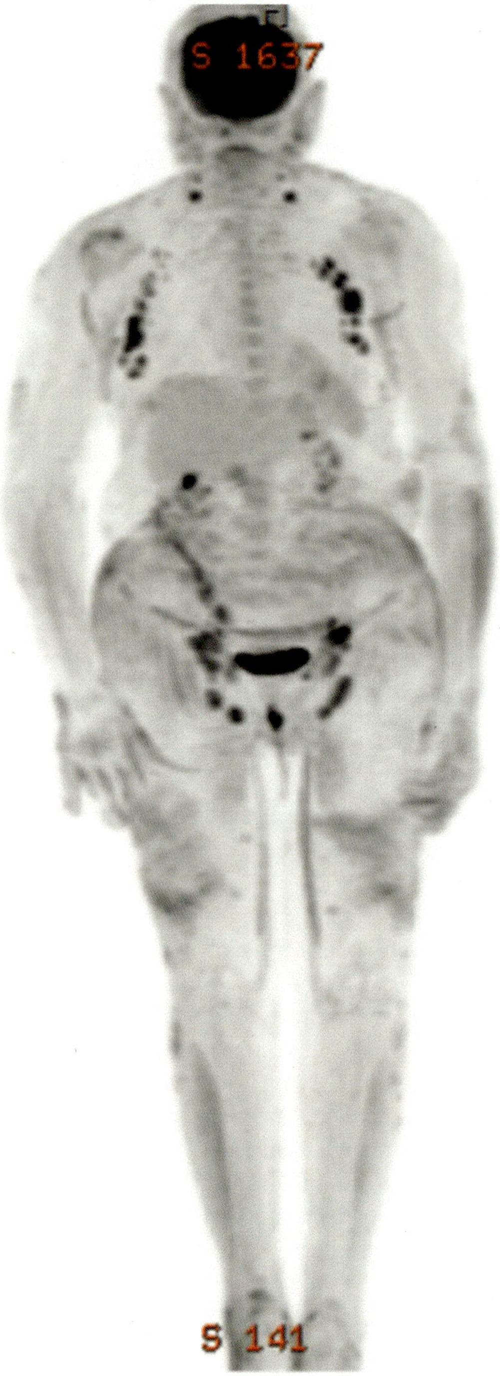

Fig. 12.10 PET/CT images of Case 1 showing lymph nodes in the neck, axillae, and groins

were older age and male sex. Large-cell transformation and tumor distribution were independent predictors of disease progression [35]. Another cohort study of 1275 patients stage IIB to IV risk stratified patients into low, intermediate, and high risk for mortality based on a prognostic index combining Stage IV, age >60 years, large-cell transformation, and increased LDH. Five-year survival for high-risk patients was 28 % in this analysis [36]. A similar prognostic index, the cutaneous lymphoma international prognostic index (CLIPi) for MF and SS demonstrated validating findings [37].

Treatment and Management: Advanced Stage Case

The patient in case 3 demonstrated a progressively refractory course. After failing topical therapies, he was started on gemcitabine, which he received for four cycles. He achieved a partial response but was unable to tolerate further therapy due to the associated nausea and fatigue. For treatment of this advanced stage case patient, oral bexarotene and topical nitrogen mustard treatment were then attempted, unfortunately with frank progression of plaques and tumors with total BSA 39.5 % and mSWAT 67.7. The patient was referred for TSEBT and concomitantly referred for workup anticipating allogeneic stem cell transplant.

Systemic chemotherapy is used in refractory disease, though with variable response rates and unfortunately less durable response for advanced and relapsed/refractory cases [38]. Gemcitabine treatment was associated with 10 % complete response and 70 % overall response rates in a prior study [39]. Other considerations include vorinostat and romidepsin, which are histone deacetylase (HDAC) inhibitors. A durable response can be achieved in a subset of patients, even lasting years in prior studies [40, 41]. Development of targeted therapies continues to be on the horizon for long-term management of MF, especially for the challenging case of advanced and refractory disease.

Radiation Field, Dose, and Technique: Advanced Stage Case 3

The ILROG guidelines accept a wide range of doses for TSEBT to be acceptable, from 8 to 36 Gy [28]. After TSEBT, patients with early stage disease can achieve as high as 90% 5-year relapse-free survival, while only 30–50% of patients with advanced disease remain without disease at 5 years. TSEBT targets the epidermis (varying from 0.05 to 0.5 mm thick, thickest in distal extremities) and dermis (varying from 2 to 4 mm, thickest in hands and feet) [26]. According to EORTC TSEBT consensus guidelines, the 80% isodose line should be ≥4 mm deep. This technique places the dose maximum at 1 mm, the 80% isodose line at 6 mm, and the 20% isodose line at 12 mm [42], thus satisfying the EORTC criteria for TSEBT [43]. Photon contamination due to bremsstrahlung scattering in the machine head, intervening air, scatterers or degraders, and patient, is acceptable at 1.2% [42]. Using six treatment positions shifts, the isodose curves toward the skin surface due to the obliquity of the incident electrons.

Overall approach At our institution, we use a modern linear accelerator using the dual-field, six treatment position technique: The machine delivers a 9 MeV beam to the patient standing 3 m from the electron source, behind a Lucite plate for x-ray attenuation. Effective energy at the skin is approximately 5 MeV. The gantry angle is set at 113 and 67° to produce dual fields (upper and lower fields). There are a total of six treatment positions, each treated with the upper and lower fields: anteroposterior (AP), posteroanterior (PA), right and left anterior oblique (RAO, LAO), and right and left posterior oblique (RPO, LPO) (Fig. 12.11). The purpose of multiple positions is to "unfold" the skin creases, to expose the "shadowed" areas as much as possible and improve *lateral* dose homogeneity. The upper and lower fields improve dose homogeneity in the *vertical*

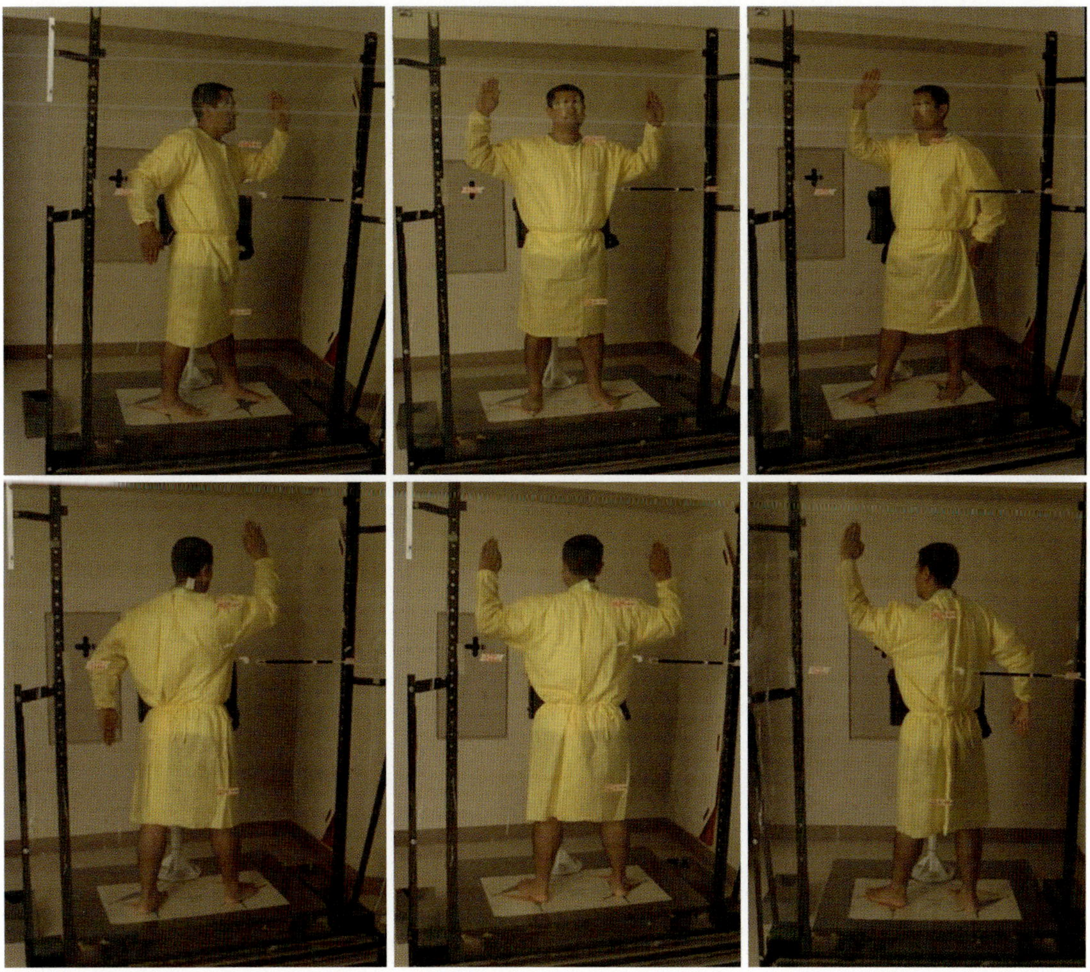

Fig. 12.11 Total skin electron beam treatment positions

dimension. At our institution, a patient typically cycles twice for each field in a single week (2 Gy × 2 fractions for a total of 4 Gy delivered to the total skin each week). Therefore, a 12 Gy treatment course is typically completed in 3 weeks, while a 32 Gy treatment course would last 8 weeks. We standardly do not exceed 2 Gy per fraction due to concern for excess toxicity [44].

To date, the conventional wisdom has preferred high-dose regimens (>30 Gy) for patients with extensive disease, higher stage, or erythroderma. Figure 12.12 shows an example of advanced cases where a dose of >30 Gy is typically used.

More recent evidence, however, including a pooled analysis from three Phase II clinical trials of a low-dose 12 Gy course in patients with stage IB to IIIA MF, underscored the effectiveness of this regimen for inducing partial to complete responses and also highlighted the benefits of shorter time on treatment, lower acute and chronic toxicities, and preservation of the option for repeat palliative skin treatment over time for an inevitably relapsing disease as well as the option for consolidative treatment doses in the setting of anticipated stem cell transplant [27]. In this study, only 11 patients had higher than stage IB disease, even after combining all data from three clinical trials, still leaving open the question of effectiveness of low-dose TSEBT in patients with worse prognostic factors or more extensive disease. Therefore, with a lack of clear comparative and guiding data, recent ILROG guidelines still supported the use of higher-dose TSEBT for such patients.

To challenge this conventional wisdom, however, we conducted a single-institution study using direct retrospective comparison of low (12 Gy) vs. conventional (≥12 Gy); the vast majority received (≥30 Gy) dose TSEBT in a heterogeneous group of 90 histologically confirmed MF patients (without Sézary). Patients with good prognostic factors achieved expected excellent partial to complete response rates assessed by mSWAT (73 % for 12 Gy vs. 83 % for ≥12 Gy TSEBT). In contrast, the direct comparison of effectiveness of low vs. conventional dose TSEBT in patients with poor prognostic factors demonstrated response rates of 30 % for 12 Gy vs. 36 % for ≥12 Gy, with no statistically significant difference in response between these two groups (unpublished data). Our direct comparative results yield several insights. First, unfortunately, the absolute response rate for patients with poor prognostic factors is low. This group with low responses may be the group of patients in whom the development and application of efficacious novel therapies may be most pressing, for example, stem cell transplant. However, secondly, the response rate in such patients is low regardless of TSEBT dose escalation. Therefore, with no perceptible benefit with dose escalation in these patients, our results suggest a new paradigm of applying low-dose

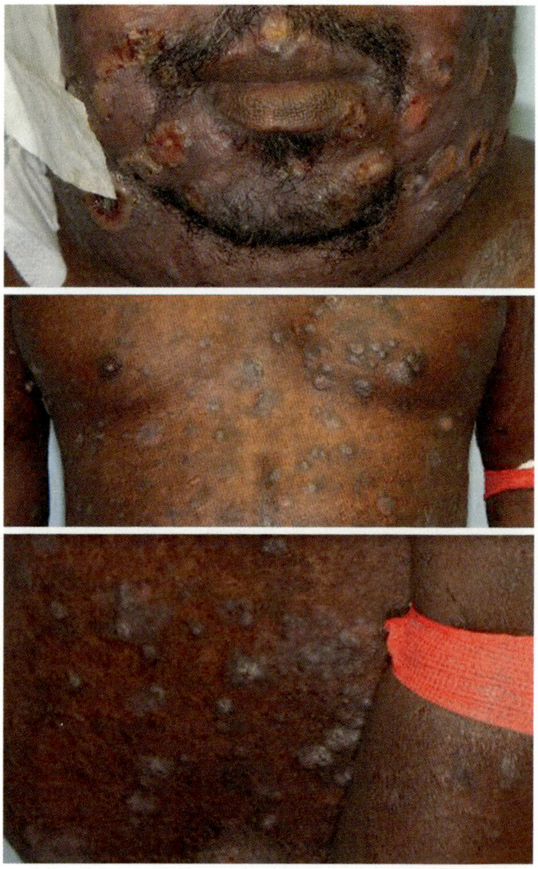

Fig. 12.12 Advanced disease where >12 Gy TSEBT is considered, either in the setting of anticipated transplant or non-transplant candidate refractory to multiple lines of therapy

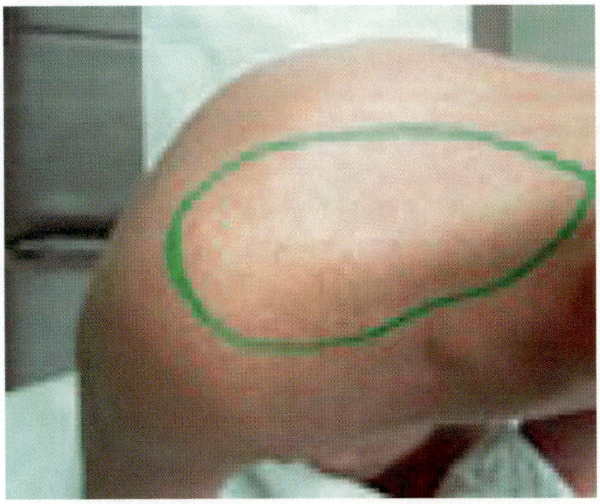

Fig. 12.13 Showing the boost drawing on the shoulder of a patient

TSEBT as the standard dose, and only high-dose TSEBT sparingly for the select circumstance of persistently refractory disease without additional nonexperimental systemic treatment options, including patients whose disease course has rendered transplant as the final available treatment option.

Boosts Electron boost fields target underdosed areas. Typically underdosed areas include the shoulders (Fig. 12.13), axillae, inframammary folds, pannus, medial thighs, perineum, and perianal area, but the patient's individual body habitus must be considered. The vertex scalp may be underdosed, but we typically deliver boosts to scalp only if there is active MF involvement, in order to decrease the risk of permanent alopecia. In vivo dosimetry is critically important, along with clinical assessment and suspicion, to determine the boost fields and ensure surfaces receive at least 50 % of the prescribed TSEBT dose [45, 46].

Shielding Hands, feet, and areas of the perineum tend to be at risk for overdosing, typically from overlap of fields or tissue heterogeneity from the anatomy of these areas [26]. These regions may require lead shielding for a part of the treatment cycles, especially for total doses beyond 24 Gy. Eyes are also customarily shielded with lead eye shields [47].

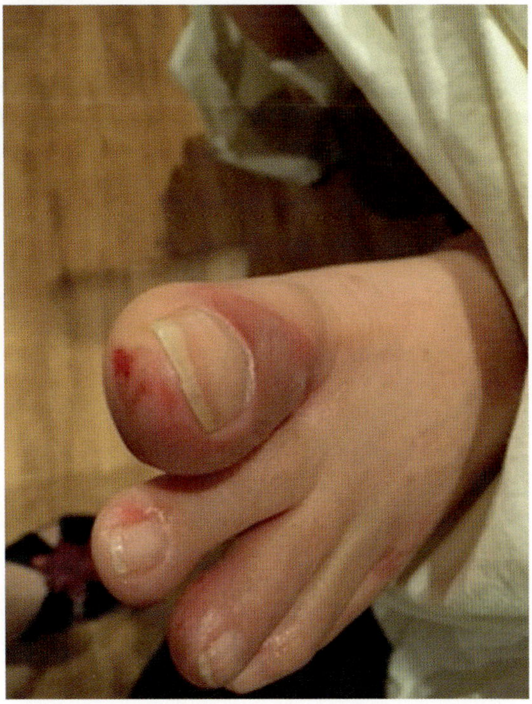

Fig. 12.14 Showing blisters that can develop in the feet when treating patients to a definitive dose of total skin electron beam, typically TSEBT >28 Gy, although the feet cannot take more than 16 Gy even if given over 6 weeks

Toxicity Skin toxicity is common, though with low-dose regimens, rarely severe. Patients will experience pruritus, dry desquamation, erythema, alopecia, xerosis, and especially with higher doses, bullae and edema of the hands and feet (Fig. 12.14), hypohidrosis (diminished perspiration) [48], and loss of fingernails and toenails [43, 49]. Side effect management should prioritize symptom relief and avoiding infection. Emollients, topical antibiotics, oral or intravenous antibiotics as needed, whirlpool, and analgesic management are critical for symptom management and helping patients complete the intended course. Treatment breaks may be required to manage these complications. Common sources of infection include *Staphylococcus aureus*, β-hemolytic streptococci, and cutaneous herpes simplex or herpes zoster [50]. *Pseudomonas aeruginosa* cellulitis can also develop, and in patients with open ulcers, bacteremia and sepsis can be a life-threatening complication with treatment. Also infections can present with lesions that mimic the disease. Therefore it is essential to treat with antibiotics when infection is at all suspected, a particularly important point to save the patient unnecessary treatment intensification of disease that appeared to be progressing. The most concerning long-term toxicity is skin fibrosis with high doses or repeated treatment courses, which can ultimately threaten function and circulation, especially in extremities and in patients with underlying comorbidities such as vasculopathy [51].

Posttreatment Considerations: Advanced Stage Case 3

The patient achieved complete clinical response, including disappearance of the lymph nodes on a follow-up PET/CT. This is commonly seen after treatment of the skin even of the lymph nodes has been proven to harbor disease. The patient's complete remission lasted only for 8 months, before she presented with new ulcerated lesions over the bilateral legs. Further treatment was initiated using brentuximab, but the ulcerated tumors continued to progress along with the appearance of new skin lesions. Targeted therapy remains a viable area of ongoing development in MF treatment. In recent studies of MF patients with variable CD30 expression levels, 50–70 % of patients treated with brentuximab demonstrated response, with peripheral neuropathy as the most common toxicity [52, 53].

The patient in case 3 was then considered for allogeneic transplant. It is our institutional practice to deliver a definitive dose of TSEB as a debulking approach just prior to allogeneic transplant. The rationale is based on the fact that allogeneic transplant is considered the only curative approach available; therefore, based on data suggesting that doses of 28–36 Gy have higher frequency of complete remission, we plan radiation treatment to this dose with the goal of optimizing debulking of gross cutaneous disease before transplant and the intent of optimizing cure rates. The patient received TSEBT to a total dose of 32 Gy delivered over 8 weeks and went on to receive allogeneic transplant using her sister as a donor. Today, 16 months later, she is still in complete remission, but with skin graft-versus-host disease (GVHD) that is being managed accordingly.

Evidence supporting the role of allogeneic stem cell transplant in treatment refractory MF continues to evolve. While autologous transplant does not appear to render durable response [54–56], allogeneic transplant with myeloablative or non-myeloablative conditioning regimens suggests improved and prolonged disease-free survival intervals, highlighting the graft-versus-lymphoma effect in producing durable remissions [57–63]. One analysis demonstrated 68 % overall response and 58 % complete response [64]. Debulking with TSEBT was the standard radiation treatment component of the regimen and therefore is now standardly adapted at our institution.

Clinical Presentation: Primary Cutaneous ALCL Case

A 67-year-old man presented with an enlarging and ulcerating tumorlike fungating lesion of the right midsole of the foot, measuring 5 × 6 cm (Fig. 12.15). *Biopsy demonstrated a CD30+ T-cell lymphoproliferative disorder, composed of small, intermediate, and large-sized lymphocytic cells with irregular nuclear contours, indistinct to distinct nucleoli, and small to abundant amounts of cytoplasm. Cells were CD3+ and CD30+* (*strong, 90 %*) *and negative for ALK-1.*

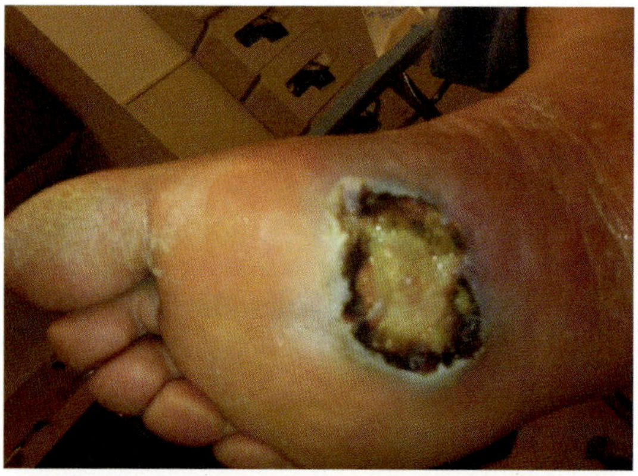

Fig. 12.15 Primary cutaneous anaplastic large-cell lymphoma (pcALCL)

The papule was not spontaneously remitting. Clinical skin examination did not demonstrate additional lesions. A staging CT scan did not demonstrate any concerning lymphadenopathy or visceral involvement.

Pathology: pcALCL Case

The diagnosis of pcALCL is challenging. The primary involvement of the disease must be restricted to the skin, though notably local nodes could be involved with extensive involvement. Concurrent systemic disease at presentation is not considered primary cutaneous. More challenging to distinguish is systemic ALCL which arises from lymph nodes and invades skin. Involvement can be superficial and deep, and in fact subcutaneous involvement can be frequent. Conversely, epidermotropism is uncommon, and cells rarely express epithelial membrane antigen (EMA). Anaplastic cytology is present, with the hallmark morphology of large, markedly pleomorphic nuclei and abundant cytoplasm. The molecular hallmark is uniform, strong CD30 expression, which is typically expressed by >75 % of large anaplastic cells. Cells demonstrate the tendency to invade lymph node sinuses. The t(2;5) chromosomal translocation and ALK expression are typically absent, unlike in systemic ALCL where approximately 70–80 % of cases are ALK positive. True pcALCL is rare, making up only 1–2 % of ALCL cases, and approximately 25 % of CTCL [65] pcALCL exists in a spectrum of overlapping primary cutaneous CD30+ lymphoproliferative diseases which also includes lymphomatoid papulosis (LyP). LyP clinically behaves distinctly, with a large portion of cases demonstrating spontaneous resolution [66].

Staging and Prognostic Factors: pcALCL Case

The ISCL/EORTC defines a unique TNM staging system for primary cutaneous lymphomas other than mycosis fungoides and Sézary syndrome, inclusive of pcALCL. T stage is based on size and distribution/involvement of lesions, N based on number and region of nodal involvement, and M based on extracutaneous involvement [67]. pcALCL is rarely found in patients under the age of 20 years and, despite the typically ALK negative status, follows a generally indolent course with a favorable prognosis. This is in contrast to systemic ALCL, where prognosis is strongly associated with ALK status [68].

Treatment and Management: pcALCL Case

For this limited disease, the patient was treated with a local electron field with a 9 MeV appositional electron beam with 1.5 cm margin to a dose of 10 Gy in 5 fractions. A 5 mm bolus applied, given the slight thickness of the nodule. Within several fractions, an immediate partial response was already noted, characterized by flattening and softening of the ulcerated area. After 3 months of continued follow-up, the ulcer underwent slow healing by second intention without further intervention, returning to near-normal skin integrity over the long term (Fig. 12.16).

Radiation Field, Dose, and Technique: pcALCL Case

ILROG consensus field and dose guidelines are still applicable, and thus local RT doses ranging

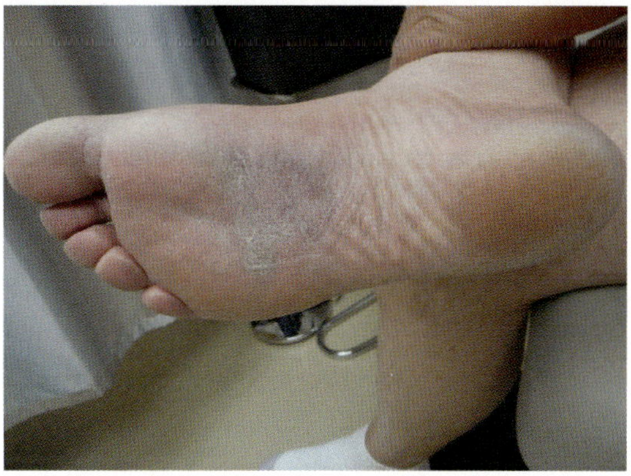

Fig. 12.16 Response to treatment after 10 Gy of radiation, 10 weeks after radiation treatment was completed

from 6 Gy to >30 Gy are largely acceptable. Unlike MF, however, the optimal treatment dose has not yet been well established. pcALCL is extremely responsive to local RT, and therefore RT is considered a treatment of choice in this disease. Though the disease is rare and reported series have small sample sizes, prior evidence suggests a response rate to local RT of 97–100 % and complete response rate greater than 80 %. Ultimately, the disease follows a relapsing course, with long-term relapse-free survival 50% or less. Nonetheless the overall disease course is still indolent, with long-term cancer-specific survival higher than 80–90 % in prior reports [66, 69–71]. In a more recent single-institution case series, RT doses still exceeded 30 Gy [72]. Little data are available on low-dose RT due to the rarity of this disease, and the question of the effectiveness of lower doses is a pressing one for patients with pcALCL. Like patients with MF, pcALCL patients can expect multiple cutaneous relapses over time and may require repeated RT courses, highlighting the need to define the minimum doses needed to achieve comparable control as historical series.

Posttreatment Considerations: pcALCL Case

The patient demonstrated durable local response at 3-year follow-up. Moreover, he was alive without evidence of any further disease. This patient's excellent response to lower-dose radiation emphasizes the possibility that low-dose RT may also be considered for this indolent CTCL, like MF. Minimizing the intensity, duration, and toxicity of RT may be an appealing treatment paradigm for this indolent, but invariably chronic disease that could require multiple RT courses over time. More data are needed to establish the optimal dose for this disease.

Conclusions

Radiation treatment is an essential component of CTCL treatment. For MF, the most commonly seen CTCL, both local electron and total skin treatments, is effective. Outcome evidence supports a shift in treatment pattern toward lower-dose RT, taking into consideration the anticipated long-term toxicity and need for repeated treatment courses over the chronic course of this disease. Along with RT, skin-directed and systemic and targeted therapies are essential components of treatment. pcALCL is a much rarer CTCL, which follows an indolent course and demonstrates very high response to RT, which can be a definitive treatment for this CTCL subtype.

References

1. Criscione VD, Weinstock MA. Incidence of cutaneous T-cell lymphoma in the United States, 1973–2002. Arch Dermatol. 2007;143(7):854–9.
2. Sun G, Berthelot C, Li Y, Glass 2nd DA, George D, Pandya A, et al. Poor prognosis in non-Caucasian patients with early-onset mycosis fungoides. J Am Acad Dermatol. 2009;60(2):231–5.
3. Cheah CY, Seymour JF, Wang ML. Mantle cell lymphoma. J Clin Oncol Off J Am Soc Clin Oncol. 2016;34:1256–69.
4. Girardi M, Heald PW, Wilson LD. The pathogenesis of mycosis fungoides. N Engl J Med. 2004;350(19):1978–88.
5. Fung MA, Murphy MJ, Hoss DM, Grant-Kels JM. Practical evaluation and management of cutaneous lymphoma. J Am Acad Dermatol. 2002;46(3):325–57.
6. Willemze R, Jaffe ES, Burg G, Cerroni L, Berti E, Swerdlow SH, et al. WHO-EORTC classification for cutaneous lymphomas. Blood. 2005;105(10):3768–85.
7. Sibaud V, Beylot-Barry M, Thiebaut R, Parrens M, Vergier B, Delaunay M, et al. Bone marrow histopathologic and molecular staging in epidermotropic T- cell lymphomas. Am J Clin Pathol. 2003;119(3):414–23.
8. Graham SJ, Sharpe RW, Steinberg SM, Cotelingam JD, Sausville EA, Foss FM. Prognostic implications of a bone marrow histopathologic classification system in mycosis fungoides and the Sezary syndrome. Cancer. 1993;72(3):726–34.
9. Olsen E, Vonderheid E, Pimpinelli N, Willemze R, Kim Y, Knobler R, et al. Revisions to the staging and classification of mycosis fungoides and Sezary syndrome: a proposal of the International Society for Cutaneous Lymphomas (ISCL) and the cutaneous lymphoma task force of the European Organization of Research and Treatment of Cancer (EORTC). Blood. 2007;110(6):1713–22.
10. Kim YH, Hoppe RT. Mycosis fungoides and the Sezary syndrome. Semin Oncol. 1999;26(3):276–89.

11. Vonderheid EC, Diamond LW, van Vloten WA, Scheffer E, Meijer CJ, Cashell AW, et al. Lymph node classification systems in cutaneous T-cell lymphoma. Evidence for the utility of the working formulation of non-Hodgkin's lymphomas for clinical usage. Cancer. 1994;73(1):207–18.
12. Diamandidou E, Colome M, Fayad L, Duvic M, Kurzrock R. Prognostic factor analysis in mycosis fungoides/Sezary syndrome. J Am Acad Dermatol. 1999;40(6 Pt 1):914–24.
13. Wasik MA, Vonderheid EC, Bigler RD, Marti R, Lessin SR, Polansky M, et al. Increased serum concentration of the soluble interleukin-2 receptor in cutaneous T-cell lymphoma. Clinical and prognostic implications. Arch Dermatol. 1996;132(1):42–7.
14. Hoppe RT, Medeiros LJ, Warnke RA, Wood GS. CD8-positive tumor-infiltrating lymphocytes influence the long-term survival of patients with mycosis fungoides. J Am Acad Dermatol. 1995;32(3):448–53.
15. Delfau-Larue MH, Dalac S, Lepage E, Petrella T, Wechsler J, Farcet JP, et al. Prognostic significance of a polymerase chain reaction-detectable dominant T-lymphocyte clone in cutaneous lesions of patients with mycosis fungoides. Blood. 1998;92(9):3376–80.
16. Guitart J, Camisa C, Ehrlich M, Bergfeld WF. Long-term implications of T-cell receptor gene rearrangement analysis by Southern blot in patients with cutaneous T-cell lymphoma. J Am Acad Dermatol. 2003;48(5):775–9.
17. Beylot-Barry M, Sibaud V, Thiebaut R, Vergier B, Beylot C, Delaunay M, et al. Evidence that an identical T cell clone in skin and peripheral blood lymphocytes is an independent prognostic factor in primary cutaneous T cell lymphomas. J Invest Dermatol. 2001;117(4):920–6.
18. Bakels V, Van Oostveen JW, Geerts ML, Gordijn RL, Walboomers JM, Scheffer E, et al. Diagnostic and prognostic significance of clonal T-cell receptor beta gene rearrangements in lymph nodes of patients with mycosis fungoides. J Pathol. 1993;170(3):249–55.
19. Smith BD, Wilson LD. Management of mycosis fungoides: part 2. Treatment. Oncology (Huntingt). 2003;17(10):1419–28; discussion 30, 33.
20. Heald PW, Glusac EJ. Unilesional cutaneous T-cell lymphoma: clinical features, therapy, and follow-up of 10 patients with a treatment-responsive mycosis fungoides variant. J Am Acad Dermatol. 2000;42(2 Pt 1):283–5.
21. Wilson LD, Kacinski BM, Jones GW. Local superficial radiotherapy in the management of minimal stage IA cutaneous T-cell lymphoma (Mycosis Fungoides). Int J Radiat Oncol Biol Phys. 1998;40(1):109–15.
22. Micaily B, Miyamoto C, Kantor G, Lessin S, Rook A, Brady L, et al. Radiotherapy for unilesional mycosis fungoides. Int J Radiat Oncol Biol Phys. 1998;42(2):361–4.
23. Quiros PA, Jones GW, Kacinski BM, Braverman IM, Heald PW, Edelson RL, et al. Total skin electron beam therapy followed by adjuvant psoralen/ultraviolet-A light in the management of patients with T1 and T2 cutaneous T-cell lymphoma (mycosis fungoides). Int J Radiat Oncol Biol Phys. 1997;38(5):1027–35.
24. Chinn DM, Chow S, Kim YH, Hoppe RT. Total skin electron beam therapy with or without adjuvant topical nitrogen mustard or nitrogen mustard alone as initial treatment of T2 and T3 mycosis fungoides. Int J Radiat Oncol Biol Phys. 1999;43(5):951–8.
25. Hoppe RT. Mycosis fungoides: radiation therapy. Dermatol Ther. 2003;16(4):347–54.
26. Jones GW, Hoppe RT, Glatstein E. Electron beam treatment for cutaneous T-cell lymphoma. Hematol Oncol Clin North Am. 1995;9(5):1057–76.
27. Hoppe RT, Harrison C, Tavallaee M, Bashey S, Sundram U, Li S, et al. Low-dose total skin electron beam therapy as an effective modality to reduce disease burden in patients with mycosis fungoides: results of a pooled analysis from 3 phase-II clinical trials. J Am Acad Dermatol. 2015;72(2):286–92.
28. Specht L, Dabaja BS, Illidge T, Wilson LD, Hoppe RT, International Lymphoma Radiation Oncology G. Modern radiation therapy for primary cutaneous lymphomas: field and dose guidelines from the International Lymphoma Radiation Oncology Group. Int J Radiat Oncol Biol Phys. 2015;92(1):32–9.
29. Diamandidou E, Colome-Grimmer M, Fayad L, Duvic M, Kurzrock R. Transformation of mycosis fungoides/Sezary syndrome: clinical characteristics and prognosis. Blood. 1998;92(4):1150–9.
30. Vergier B, de Muret A, Beylot-Barry M, Vaillant L, Ekouevi D, Chene G, et al. Transformation of mycosis fungoides: clinicopathological and prognostic features of 45 cases. French Study Group of Cutaneous Lymphomas. Blood. 2000;95(7):2212–8.
31. Vonderheid EC, Bernengo MG, Burg G, Duvic M, Heald P, Laroche L, et al. Update on erythrodermic cutaneous T-cell lymphoma: report of the International Society for Cutaneous Lymphomas. J Am Acad Dermatol. 2002;46(1):95–106.
32. de Coninck EC, Kim YH, Varghese A, Hoppe RT. Clinical characteristics and outcome of patients with extracutaneous mycosis fungoides. J Clin Oncol Off J Am Soc Clin Oncol. 2001;19(3):779–84.
33. Prince HM, Whittaker S, Hoppe RT. How I treat mycosis fungoides and Sezary syndrome. Blood. 2009;114(20):4337–53.
34. Stein M, Farrar N, Jones GW, Wilson LD, Fox L, Wong RK, et al. Central neurologic involvement in mycosis fungoides: ten cases, actuarial risk assessment, and predictive factors. Cancer J. 2006;12(1):55–62.
35. Agar NS, Wedgeworth E, Crichton S, Mitchell TJ, Cox M, Ferreira S, et al. Survival outcomes and prognostic factors in mycosis fungoides/Sezary syndrome: validation of the revised International Society for Cutaneous Lymphomas/European Organisation for Research and Treatment of Cancer staging proposal. J Clin Oncol Off J Am Soc Clin Oncol. 2010;28(31):4730–9.

36. Scarisbrick JJ, Prince HM, Vermeer MH, Quaglino P, Horwitz S, Porcu P, et al. Cutaneous lymphoma international consortium study of outcome in advanced stages of mycosis fungoides and sezary syndrome: effect of specific prognostic markers on survival and development of a prognostic model. J Clin Oncol Off J Am Soc Clin Oncol. 2015;33(32):3766–73.
37. Benton EC, Crichton S, Talpur R, Agar NS, Fields PA, Wedgeworth E, et al. A cutaneous lymphoma international prognostic index (CLIPi) for mycosis fungoides and Sezary syndrome. Eur J Cancer. 2013;49(13):2859–68.
38. Kaye FJ, Bunn Jr PA, Steinberg SM, Stocker JL, Ihde DC, Fischmann AB, et al. A randomized trial comparing combination electron-beam radiation and chemotherapy with topical therapy in the initial treatment of mycosis fungoides. N Engl J Med. 1989;321(26): 1784–90.
39. Zinzani PL, Baliva G, Magagnoli M, Bendandi M, Modugno G, Gherlinzoni F, et al. Gemcitabine treatment in pretreated cutaneous T-cell lymphoma: experience in 44 patients. J Clin Oncol Off J Am Soc Clin Oncol. 2000;18(13):2603–6.
40. Whittaker SJ, Demierre MF, Kim EJ, Rook AH, Lerner A, Duvic M, et al. Final results from a multicenter, international, pivotal study of romidepsin in refractory cutaneous T-cell lymphoma. J Clin Oncol Off J Am Soc Clin Oncol. 2010;28(29):4485–91.
41. Piekarz RL, Frye R, Turner M, Wright JJ, Allen SL, Kirschbaum MH, et al. Phase II multi-institutional trial of the histone deacetylase inhibitor romidepsin as monotherapy for patients with cutaneous T-cell lymphoma. J Clin Oncol Off J Am Soc Clin Oncol. 2009;27(32):5410–7.
42. Chen Z, Agostinelli AG, Wilson LD, Nath R. Matching the dosimetry characteristics of a dual-field Stanford technique to a customized single-field Stanford technique for total skin electron therapy. Int J Radiat Oncol Biol Phys. 2004;59(3):872–85.
43. Jones G, Wilson LD, Fox-Goguen L. Total skin electron beam radiotherapy for patients who have mycosis fungoides. Hematol Oncol Clin North Am. 2003;17(6):1421–34.
44. Rosenblatt E, Kuten A, Leviov M, Cederbaum M. Total skin electron irradiation in mycosis fungoides dose and fractionation considerations. Leuk Lymphoma. 1998;30(1–2):143–51.
45. Gamble LM, Farrell TJ, Jones GW, Hayward JE. Composite depth dose measurement for total skin electron (TSE) treatments using radiochromic film. Phys Med Biol. 2003;48(7):891–8.
46. Anacak Y, Arican Z, Bar-Deroma R, Tamir A, Kuten A. Total skin electron irradiation: evaluation of dose uniformity throughout the skin surface. Med Dosim. 2003;28(1):31–4.
47. Asbell SO, Siu J, Lightfoot DA, Brady LW. Individualized eye shields for use in electron beam therapy as well as low-energy photon irradiation. Int J Radiat Oncol Biol Phys. 1980;6(4): 519–21.
48. Price NM. Electron beam therapy. Its effect on eccrine gland function in mycosis fungoides patients. Arch Dermatol. 1979;115(9):1068–70.
49. Desai KR, Pezner RD, Lipsett JA, Vora NL, Luk KH, Wong JY, et al. Total skin electron irradiation for mycosis fungoides: relationship between acute toxicities and measured dose at different anatomic sites. Int J Radiat Oncol Biol Phys. 1988;15(3):641–5.
50. Axelrod PI, Lorber B, Vonderheid EC. Infections complicating mycosis fungoides and Sezary syndrome. JAMA. 1992;267(10):1354–8.
51. Jones GW, Kacinski BM, Wilson LD, Willemze R, Spittle M, Hohenberg G, et al. Total skin electron radiation in the management of mycosis fungoides: consensus of the European Organization for Research and Treatment of Cancer (EORTC) Cutaneous Lymphoma Project Group. J Am Acad Dermatol. 2002;47(3):364–70.
52. Kim YH, Tavallaee M, Sundram U, Salva KA, Wood GS, Li S, et al. Phase II investigator-initiated study of brentuximab vedotin in mycosis fungoides and Sezary syndrome with variable CD30 expression level: a multi-institution collaborative project. J Clin Oncol Off J Am Soc Clin Oncol. 2015;33(32): 3750–8.
53. Duvic M, Tetzlaff MT, Gangar P, Clos AL, Sui D, Talpur R. Results of a phase II trial of brentuximab vedotin for CD30+ cutaneous T-cell lymphoma and lymphomatoid papulosis. J Clin Oncol Off J Am Soc Clin Oncol. 2015;33(32):3759–65.
54. Bigler RD, Crilley P, Micaily B, Brady LW, Topolsky D, Bulova S, et al. Autologous bone marrow transplantation for advanced stage mycosis fungoides. Bone Marrow Transplant. 1991;7(2):133–7.
55. Russell-Jones R, Child F, Olavarria E, Whittaker S, Spittle M, Apperley J. Autologous peripheral blood stem cell transplantation in tumor-stage mycosis fungoides: predictors of disease-free survival. Ann N Y Acad Sci. 2001;941:147–54.
56. Sterling JC, Marcus R, Burrows NP, Roberts SO. Erythrodermic mycosis fungoides treated with total body irradiation and autologous bone marrow transplantation. Clin Exp Dermatol. 1995;20(1): 73–5.
57. Burt RK, Guitart J, Traynor A, Link C, Rosen S, Pandolfino T, et al. Allogeneic hematopoietic stem cell transplantation for advanced mycosis fungoides: evidence of a graft-versus-tumor effect. Bone Marrow Transplant. 2000;25(1):111–3.
58. Guitart J, Wickless SC, Oyama Y, Kuzel TM, Rosen ST, Traynor A, et al. Long-term remission after allogeneic hematopoietic stem cell transplantation for refractory cutaneous T-cell lymphoma. Arch Dermatol. 2002;138(10):1359–65.
59. Molina A, Zain J, Arber DA, Angelopolou M, O'Donnell M, Murata-Collins J, et al. Durable clinical, cytogenetic, and molecular remissions after allogeneic hematopoietic cell transplantation for refractory Sezary syndrome and mycosis fungoides. J Clin Oncol. 2005;23(25):6163–71.

60. Soligo D, Ibatici A, Berti E, Morandi P, Longhi E, Venegoni L, et al. Treatment of advanced mycosis fungoides by allogeneic stem-cell transplantation with a nonmyeloablative regimen. Bone Marrow Transplant. 2003;31(8):663–6.
61. Duarte RF, Canals C, Onida F, Gabriel IH, Arranz R, Arcese W, et al. Allogeneic hematopoietic cell transplantation for patients with mycosis fungoides and Sezary syndrome: a retrospective analysis of the Lymphoma Working Party of the European Group for Blood and Marrow Transplantation. J Clin Oncol Off J Am Soc Clin Oncol. 2010;28(29):4492–9.
62. Duarte RF, Schmitz N, Servitje O, Sureda A. Haematopoietic stem cell transplantation for patients with primary cutaneous T-cell lymphoma. Bone Marrow Transplant. 2008;41(7):597–604.
63. Wu PA, Kim YH, Lavori PW, Hoppe RT, Stockerl-Goldstein KE. A meta-analysis of patients receiving allogeneic or autologous hematopoietic stem cell transplant in mycosis fungoides and Sezary syndrome. Biol Blood Marrow Transplant J Am Soc Blood Marrow Transplant. 2009;15(8):982–90.
64. Duvic M, Donato M, Dabaja BS, Richmond H, Singh L, Wei W, et al. Total skin electron beam and non-myeloablative allogeneic hematopoietic stem-cell transplantation in advanced mycosis fungoides and Sezary syndrome. J Clin Oncol Off J Am Soc Clin Oncol. 2010;28(14):2365–72.
65. DeCoteau JF, Butmarc JR, Kinney MC, Kadin ME. The t(2;5) chromosomal translocation is not a common feature of primary cutaneous CD30+ lymphoproliferative disorders: comparison with anaplastic large-cell lymphoma of nodal origin. Blood. 1996;87(8):3437–41.
66. Bekkenk MW, Geelen FA, van Voorst Vader PC, Heule F, Geerts ML, van Vloten WA, et al. Primary and secondary cutaneous CD30(+) lymphoproliferative disorders: a report from the Dutch Cutaneous Lymphoma Group on the long-term follow-up data of 219 patients and guidelines for diagnosis and treatment. Blood. 2000;95(12):3653–61.
67. Kim YH, Willemze R, Pimpinelli N, Whittaker S, Olsen EA, Ranki A, et al. TNM classification system for primary cutaneous lymphomas other than mycosis fungoides and Sezary syndrome: a proposal of the International Society for Cutaneous Lymphomas (ISCL) and the Cutaneous Lymphoma Task Force of the European Organization of Research and Treatment of Cancer (EORTC). Blood. 2007;110(2):479–84.
68. Jaffe ES. Anaplastic large cell lymphoma: the shifting sands of diagnostic hematopathology. Mod Pathol Off J US Can Acad Pathol Inc. 2001;14(3):219–28.
69. Beljaards RC, Kaudewitz P, Berti E, Gianotti R, Neumann C, Rosso R, et al. Primary cutaneous CD30-positive large cell lymphoma: definition of a new type of cutaneous lymphoma with a favorable prognosis. A European Multicenter Study of 47 patients. Cancer. 1993;71(6):2097–104.
70. Liu HL, Hoppe RT, Kohler S, Harvell JD, Reddy S, Kim YH. CD30+ cutaneous lymphoproliferative disorders: the Stanford experience in lymphomatoid papulosis and primary cutaneous anaplastic large cell lymphoma. J Am Acad Dermatol. 2003;49(6):1049–58.
71. Yu JB, Blitzblau RC, Decker RH, Housman DM, Wilson LD. Analysis of primary CD30+ cutaneous lymphoproliferative disease and survival from the Surveillance, Epidemiology, and End Results database. J Clin Oncol Off J Am Soc Clin Oncol. 2008;26(9):1483–8.
72. Yu JB, McNiff JM, Lund MW, Wilson LD. Treatment of primary cutaneous CD30+ anaplastic large-cell lymphoma with radiation therapy. Int J Radiat Oncol Biol Phys. 2008;70(5):1542–5.

Index

B.S. Dabaja, A.K. Ng (eds.), *Radiation Therapy in Hematologic Malignancies*,
DOI 10.1007/978-3-319-42615-0

R

S

T

Printed by Printforce, the Netherlands